To Julie, mea alpha et omega

Take it slowly. This book is dangerous!

—Dr. Seuss

Contents

Introduction:

Doomsday Preppers

Out of such chaos, of such contradiction
We learn that we are neither devils nor divines . . .
When we come to it
We must confess that we are the possible
We are the miraculous, the true wonder of this world
That is when, and only when
We come to it.

—Maya Angelou, "A Brave and Startling Truth"
(flown into space on the NASA Orion mission)

Slowly over the past century, and now suddenly, all at once, we're suffering a collapse in Meaning. We used to find faith and comfort in organized religion, but fewer people than ever subscribe to those beliefs anymore. We can call that traditional system Meaning 1.0 and it offered salvation to the elect. Those who believed were saved. Those who didn't weren't. Harsh but fair.

For the past few hundred years, we've been trying a different experiment—one based not on salvation but inclusion. That was the promise of global liberalism—the idea that markets, democracy, and civil rights would bring us into a world where everyone, not just the elect, were entitled to a fair shot at the good life.

Except that hasn't worked out too well either. Unprecedented economic disparity, global crises, and environmental degradation have revealed that many of those promises were hollow. We can call this modern experiment Meaning 2.0 and it offered inclusion to the masses. Accept the rules, play the game, and your turn will come soon enough. Promising in theory, partial in practice.

As both Meaning 1.0 and Meaning 2.0 have collapsed, we're experiencing a global crisis. And into that vacuum have rushed a host of beliefs that threaten the fabric of civilization. Around the world, among believers and nonbelievers alike, we are finding ourselves in the grip of Rapture Ideologies.

At their heart, Rapture Ideologies share four key beliefs:

- the world as we know it is broken and unsavable.

- there is a point in the near future where everything is going to change.

- on the other side of that inflection point, everyone we value will be saved/redeemed.

- so let's get there as fast as possible, without much concern for the world we're leaving behind.

This is increasingly a problem for all of us. It's vital we regain control of the stories we're telling because they are shaping the future we're creating. To do that, we have to remember our deepest inspiration, heal our pain and apathy, and connect to each other like never before. If we don't, the Rapturists will have the last word on how this all goes down. If we do, we can remake a world that works for all of us.

* * *

For anyone who might be passingly concerned by this possibility but then thinks, "That may be the case on the extremes, but cooler heads prevail in the *Wall Street Journal, Economist,* TED Talk world we live in"—think again. Rapture philosophers are all around us. Wearing hoodies and Brooks Brothers suits as often as sackcloth and ashes. Proclaiming "The Singularity Is Near" as often as warning that "The End Is Nigh." Scrutinizing lines of computer code as often as ancient texts. You've just got to know what you're looking for.

In all the buzz predicting the Next Big Thing, few possibilities have captured our imaginations like the reboot of the space race. *The New York Times* recently reported that we're on the cusp of a watershed moment in space travel and that "trips [to Mars] could begin as soon as 2024." Beyond the livestream rocket launches and the excitement of early-bird tickets for the bravest billionaires, there's a more serious question that rarely gets asked of the would-be space colonizers: Are we *sure*?

Mars isn't where we're from. It's a long way off, and wildly hostile to human habitation. Solving for both of those problems—distance and survivability—is a *monumental* effort. Why, if we could marshal the technical expertise, capital, and drive to pull off this historic feat, wouldn't we deploy those same resources to fix the place we already live? The place we're actually from?

In two words: Rapture Ideology. It may be in a different wrapper from the religious versions we dimly remember from school. But it's the same underlying structure. Only this one isn't based on dusty scripture. It doesn't hinge on an ultimate showdown between Good and Evil. It's a Rapture Ideology nonetheless. Call it the Techno-Utopian Rapture. And it follows that same four-stage framework exactly.

- The world as we know it is doomed (not because of sin this time, but because of overconsumption).

- There's an inflection point coming soon (geopolitical/ecosystemic collapse, not the coming of the Four Horsemen).

- On the Other Side, our people will be looked after (the Singularity/Mars Colonies for the best and brightest—*Atlas Shrugged* in space).

- So let's prepare for that eventuality as fast as possible and never mind the collateral damage (build space stations and luxury bunkers rather than solve for global crises like food, water, energy, or climate).

When questioned about the obvious trade-offs and challenges of Mars, advocates, ranging from the late Stephen Hawking to Elon Musk, prove this out: "Mars colonization represents the best hope to ensure the future of our species as we exhaust the resources of our home planet," Musk has said. "Spreading out," Hawking agreed, "may be the only thing that saves us from ourselves."

When we hear comments like that, instead of sounding alarms and sparking widespread debate on our future, we go fuzzy. We're unable to grasp the severity of what we're actually talking about. We fondly remember Neil Armstrong's "one giant leap for mankind." *Star Trek*'s theme "to boldly go where no man has gone before" hums in our heads. We think back to the Jetsons and jetpacks and wonder if this is the moment when all of that science fiction finally becomes science fact. It seems so cool and familiar that we gloss over exactly how this would go down.

Let's say that Hawking and Musk are right. They're both brilliant, think deeply about subjects that most of us will never wrap our heads around, routinely solve impossible problems, and have access to the highest-quality research in the world: Neither holds much hope for our species surviving beyond the end of this century unless we come up with a radical Plan B. That conclusion alone should stop us in our tracks.

But let's go further. Within the next couple of decades we actually do establish a colony on Mars that can serve as a forward operating base for humanity's future. Then what?

One thing is certain. There won't be enough seats on the Good Ship Lollipop for all eight billion of us. And that highlights the most seductive and destructive part of all Rapture Ideologies. No matter how statistically unlikely, we secretly believe we'll personally score a ticket to ride. Against all odds, we imagine that we are one of the saved, not one of those Left Behind. Imagine how high the bar will be to nab a ticket off the Late Great Planet Earth. It will make those helicopters leaving the U.S. embassy during the fall of Saigon look like a warm-up.

*   *   *

We might not say it in mixed company, but after 9/11, the 2008 Financial Crisis, the rise of populism, and the coronavirus pandemic, we've all been thinking a lot more about the unthinkable. As far back as 2012, *National Geographic* launched a reality show called *Doomsday Preppers* about people getting ready for a time described in casually terrifying acronyms like WROL (without rule of law) WTSHTF (when the shit hits the fan) during the EOTWAWKI (End of the World as We Know It).

Its first episode racked up over four million viewers (nearly half a million *more* viewers than the top late-night comedy show pulls in). *Doomsday Preppers* has gone on to break records for the channel and become one of its top ranked shows. Baffled by their own success, *National Geographic* put out a survey to learn more about their breakout hit. It revealed that nearly *half* of Americans think that investing in bomb shelters and MREs (nonperishable military rations) is a safer bet than socking their savings away in a 401(k). The American dream of white picket fences, 2.2 happy children, and pension funds is getting eclipsed by visions of fortified bunkers, gold bullion, and bug-out bags.

We like to believe that we'll all pull together in times of crisis. We put our faith in governments, national guards, firefighters, policemen, and institutions like the Red Cross. In 2019, Brock Long, the administrator of the Federal Emergency Management Agency (FEMA) during Houston's and Puerto Rico's historic flooding, offered a reality check on disaster relief as a service: "I think FEMA faces unrealistic expectations by Congress and the American public," he said. "We've got to stop looking at FEMA as 911."

"I think, to some degree, we all collectively take it on faith that our country works," Steve Huffman, the CEO of the popular online message board Reddit, reflects. "All of these things that we hold dear work because we believe they work. While I do believe they're quite resilient, and we've been through a lot, certainly we're going to go through a lot more."

Our desire to believe it will all work out somehow lies somewhere between wishful thinking and learned helplessness. "What experience and history teach us is this," the German philosopher Georg Hegel warned, "peoples and governments have never learned anything from history."

* * *

Those same business titans investing in moon shots are covering their bases down on the ground too. And make no mistake, those with the biggest bets to place are hedging them madly.

In January 2017, Evan Osnos published "Doomsday Prep for the Super-Rich" in *The New Yorker*, detailing exactly what those with the information and resources to plan ahead are up to. The article caused an immediate sensation and spawned over half a million responses online. "Survivalism, the practice of preparing for a crackup of civilization," Osnos admits in his introduction, "tends to evoke a certain picture: the woodsman in the tinfoil hat, the hysteric with the hoard of beans, the religious doomsayer. But in recent years survivalism has expanded to more affluent quarters, taking root in Silicon Valley and New York City, among technology executives, hedge-fund managers, and others in their economic cohort." Really, it's just another Rapture Ideology in disguise. This one might not involve religious messiahs or space escapes—it just swaps out Mars colonies for converted missile silos and getaway ranches—but it shares all the telltale signs.

When Osnos interviewed LinkedIn founder Reid Hoffman about how widespread this contingency planning was among tech elites, he estimated "fifty-plus percent." "Saying you're 'buying a house in New Zealand' is kind of a wink, wink, say no more," he continued. "Once you've done the Masonic handshake, they'll be, like, 'Oh, you know, I have a broker who sells old ICBM silos, and they're nuclear-hardened, and they kind of look like they would be interesting to live in.'"

As the success of *National Geographic*'s *Doomsday Preppers* confirms, we're all interested in having a backup for when the S.H.T.F. Some of us just have more bullion and better bunkers.

A couple of summers ago, author Douglas Rushkoff (*Throwing Rocks at the Google Bus*), named one of the "world's most influential intellectuals" by MIT, wrote what amounted to an update to Evan Osnos's *New Yorker* essay. And in a couple of years, we'd moved from the hypothetical to the nearly unthinkable.

Rushkoff received an invitation to address a bunch of Wall Street financiers on the future of technology—a topic that he had spent his career tracking. And while he usually turned down those kinds of cushy speaking engagements (he was a founder of the cyberpunk movement back in the '90s, after all), he admitted that "it was by far the largest fee I had ever been offered for a talk—about half my annual professor's salary." So he swallowed his disdain and did what most reasonable people would: He took the gig.

He showed up on the appointed day in what he assumed was the greenroom (the place backstage where speakers and hosts usually congregate during conferences). Five impeccably dressed men sat down and introduced themselves. Slowly Rushkoff realized this wasn't the greenroom and there was no stage. There was no auditorium full of traders waiting to hear him talk either. These five men *were* his audience.

At first, they asked him a few easy icebreaker questions—what was the deal with blockchain and cryptocurrencies? How far off did he think quantum computing was? Can Google really upload Ray Kurzweil's mind to the cloud? Alaska or New Zealand (to escape global warming)?

But then came the real question—the one those five titans of Wall Street had paid north of $50,000 an hour to learn: "How do I maintain authority over my security force after the event?"

That sentence requires some unpacking.

Let's start at the end and work backward.

"The Event."

"That was their euphemism," Rushkoff explains, "for the environmental collapse, social unrest, nuclear explosion, unstoppable virus, or Mr. Robot hack that takes everything down." By this point, discussing, debating, or wondering about future scenarios had given way for these men to a chillingly simple placeholder. Simply, The Event. And while these men may not have been willing to bet on which particular domino would fall first, that they all would topple soon after seemed self-evident. A fixed constant in a more complex equation they were still trying to solve.

Next, the verb.

"*Maintain* authority"—carries the distinct implication that a) authority might be challenged or questioned in the near future and b) that those five men had it and intended to hold on to it.

Finally the object of that action, the noun.

"My security force." Not "my personal assistant." Not "my bodyman," "butler," or "team." My "security force." Unvarnished. Plural, even without an *s*. And judging by the urgency of their $64,000 question on how to control that group after The Event, possibly mercenary.

For the remainder of their allotted hour together, those hedge fund managers laid down a few more of their cards. How would they pay their paramilitary if the economic system collapsed and paper (and digital currency) became worthless? How would they prevent a *Lord of the Flies*–style coup once things went pear-shaped? Would secret combination locks on food supplies work? How about shock collars? Or AI robots?

"That's when it hit me," Rushkoff said. "At least as far as these gentlemen were concerned, this *was* a talk about the future of technology. Taking their cue from Elon Musk colonizing Mars, Peter Thiel reversing the aging process, or Ray Kurzweil uploading [his] mind into a supercomputer, they were preparing for a digital future that had a whole lot less to do with making the world a better place than it did with transcending the human condition altogether and insulating themselves from a very real and present danger of climate change, rising sea levels, mass migrations, global pandemics, nativist panic, and resource depletion. For them, the future of technology is really about just one thing: escape."

To his credit, Rushkoff challenged their assumptions. In response to their blunt questions he answered that the best way to maintain the loyalty of their private security forces was to start treating them really well, like family, starting now. And to not stop there. He suggested they do the same in all of their current businesses on this side of The Event. The more effectively they could do that, he suggested, the greater the odds we could all keep the wheels on civilization in the first place.

"They were amused by my optimism, but they didn't really buy it," Rushkoff admits. "They were not interested in how to avoid a calamity; they're convinced we are too far gone. For all their wealth and power, they don't believe they can affect the future. They are simply accepting the darkest of all scenarios and then bringing whatever money and technology they can employ to insulate themselves—especially if they can't get a seat on the rocket to Mars . . . the result will be less a continuation of the human diaspora than a lifeboat for the elite."

Rapturists. Every last one of them. So while it's tempting to marginalize those who embrace Rapture Ideologies, to think they only show up preaching fire and brimstone or wired up to suicide vests, the stark reality is they're all around us: wearing black mock turtlenecks and fleece vests, chatting on iPhones, tuning in to *Doomsday Preppers* on cable TV.

*   *   *

If we do nothing, and Rapturists of all stripes have their way, we'll be left to play Mad Max on an exhausted planet while a handful of tech titans upload their consciousness to computers or catch one of the last flights into space. Or maybe we'll get swept up in a Middle Eastern war en route to the Last Judgment of Revelation, or the rise of a jihadi caliphate.

None of those sound especially good.

Any one of these scenarios should provoke, at a minimum, spirited debate about our collective future, and, at a maximum, serious concern. But almost no one seems to be paying attention. We've ceded the airwaves, news cycles, and initiative to a handful of ideologues and zealots. The longer this goes unaddressed, the worse it's going to get. "A renewal of apocalyptic belief is underway that is unlikely to be confined to familiar sorts of fundamentalism," John Gray, London School of Economics philosopher, writes in *Black Mass: Apocalyptic Religion and the Death of Utopia*. "Along with evangelical revivals there is likely to be a profusion of designer religions, mixing science and science fiction, racketeering, and psychobabble, which will spread like internet viruses. Most will be harmless, but doomsday cults . . . may proliferate as ecological crisis deepens."

Here's the dangerous and seductive part: the harder and scarier the challenges we face—whether sociopolitical, economic, epidemiologic, climatic, or spiritual—the more tempting it is to believe we can leap-frog the whole train wreck.

When buying into one of those stories, we tell ourselves two lies: The first is that there's no hope for the world as we know it. The second is that, against all odds, we're one of the lucky ones who get a Golden Ticket to the other side.

* * *

In study after study, religious moderates and secular humanists around the world share a desire for stability and prosperity. Most people, across cultures, just want to live in peace and see their children get a chance for a better life. That desire unites us. Atheists, Muslims, Christians, Confucians, Buddhists, Jews, Hindus, and hipsters—all just want a shot to die in their sleep, happy and surrounded by grandchildren. It's always been this way.

But Rapturism sees the world in fundamentally different terms— it's an exponentialist approach, driven by a conviction that this world is beyond repair and that any pain and suffering in this world will be redeemed by accelerating the transition to the next. When the End is literally heaven on earth (or beyond it), the Means are always jus-tified.

Here's the problem with that logic: Even if you are a devout ji-hadi, or Christian Zionist, or have prepaid for your first-class ticket to SpaceX Mars Edition, you amount to less than 1 percent of the Earth's population. That means a fractional minority of humanity has seized the wheel of our collective future. And your "redemption" means everyone else's likely annihilation.

So what about the 99 percent—the rest of us? What about that great silent majority of people around the world who just want a decent chance to keep on keeping on?

*   *   *

While surveying the wreckage of World War I, "the war to end all wars," William Butler Yeats penned one of the classics of modern literature, his poem "The Second Coming." In fevered imagery, it overlaid biblical themes onto a traumatized Europe and reflected on what was to come. "Surely some revelation is at hand; / Surely the Second Coming is at hand," Yeats wondered. "And what rough beast, its hour come round at last, / Slouches towards Bethlehem, waiting to be born?"

It's been a fixture of popular culture ever since, giving Nigerian author Chinua Achebe the title to his seminal work *Things Fall Apart*, and Joan Didion the name of her collection of essays *Slouching Towards Bethlehem*. It even inspired an episode of the HBO series *The Sopranos* titled "The Second Coming."

A few years ago *The Wall Street Journal* reported, "Terror, Brexit and U.S. Election Have Made 2016 the Year of Yeats." A Dow Jones semantic analysis of online content revealed that there were more people around the world referencing the line "things fall apart, the centre cannot hold" in that tumultuous election year than at any time in the prior thirty years.

Since then the centrifugal forces that Yeats warned of and the number of things falling apart have only increased. "The best lack all conviction," he wrote, "while the worst are filled with a passionate intensity." And that's precisely where we find ourselves right now. A huge number of good-hearted, hardworking, live-and-let-live humans are having their fates decided by a passionately intense minority dedicated to capital "R" Rapture ideologies.

So how do the best of us, how do the rest of us rekindle an intensity passionate enough—our lowercase "r" rapture—to counterbalance the extremes, and take a stand for our lives and our future?

If we can do that, we've got a shot at solving the big problems we face. We can mend where we're broken, reconnect with each other, and live lives of passion and purpose. And if we can't? Well, the dustbin of history has swallowed civilizations far older and fancier than ours.

* * *

To get a handle on what to do next, we're going to rely on two emerging disciplines—neuroanthropology and culture architecture. Really, they're the same approach. One looks backward into the past while the other looks forward into the future. Neuroanthropology borrows from neuroscience, psychology, and history to better understand how and why humans have behaved the way we have. If you enjoyed Yuval Harari's *Sapiens* or Jared Diamond's *Guns, Germs, and Steel*, this line of inquiry will feel familiar. Culture architecture takes those insights and uses them as building blocks to design more effective solutions to social problems. If you found Richard Thaler's *Nudge* or Daniel Kahneman's *Thinking, Fast and Slow* interesting, you may be an armchair culture architect yourself.

This book is divided into three parts. **Part One: Choose Your Own Apocalypse** takes a look at our current Meaning Crisis—where we are today, why it's so hard to make sense of the world, what might be coming next, and what to do about it. It also makes a case that many of our efforts to cope, whether anxiety and denial, or tribalism and identity politics, are making things worse. It ends by outlining our pressing need to expand our awareness beyond ourselves, our tribes, and our national boundaries, and to start thinking more as members of a global species. Making that move will be hard but critical.

Part Two: The Alchemist Cookbook changes gears from cultural analysis to design thinking. In it, we'll apply the creative firm IDEO's human-centered design toolkit to the Meaning Crisis. This is where the book moves into the domains of neuroscience and optimal psychology, taking a look at the strongest evolutionary drivers that can bring about inspiration, healing, and connection. From breathing, to movement, sexuality, music, and substances—these are the everyday resources to help us harness insight, mend trauma, and work together. So whether you're a part of an existing tradition or community, or you're looking to innovate, this section offers a road map for how to gain the clarity, courage, and conviction to do what needs to be done.

Part Three: Ethical Cult Building, draws on the fields of anthropology and comparative religion to focus on the tricky nature of putting these kinds of experiences into gear and into culture. Because in the past, anytime we've figured out combinations of peak states and deep healing, we've almost always ended up with problematic communities. This section lays out a provisional road map for sparking a thousand fires without burning down the house. Think of it as an open-source tool kit for ethical culture.

It's important to note up front that any one of these three sections could be a freestanding book in itself. In fact, any one of these chapters could be. In simpler times, they probably would have. But to get to a conclusion that might be satisfying, in both a timely and a timeless sense, we'll have to move fast and cover a lot of terrain. If we can stay together on this journey, the view from the destination will be worth it. (The endnotes, which highlight amazing work being done by experts in all of these these fields, can be found online at www .recapturetherapture.com/notes. The appendix goes into detail about the research study that underpins Part Two. The glossary, which defines many of the classical and technical terms used throughout, is at the end. So even if at first, the breadth of content feels like a lot, you've got all the tools you need to make sense of it.)

In *Recapture the Rapture*, we're taking radical research out of the extremes and applying it to the mainstream—to the broader social problem of healing, believing, and belonging. It's providing answers to the questions we face: how to replace blind faith with direct experience, how to move from broken to whole, and how to cure isolation with connection. Said even more plainly, it shows us how to revitalize our bodies, boost our creativity, rekindle our relationships, and answer once and for all the questions of why we are here and what do we do now.

In a world that needs the best of us from the rest of us, this is a book that shows us how to get it done.

PART I

Choose Your Own Apocalypse

the poem at the end of the world
is the poem the little girl breathes
into her pillow the one
she cannot tell the one
there is no one to hear this poem
is a political poem is a war poem is a
universal poem but is not about
these things this poem
is about one human heart this poem
is the poem at the end of the world

—Lucille Clifton

A Cinderella Story

First, we're going to have to take stock of how we got into our current predicament. We're going to have to account for all the places we've traded courage for comfort, dedication for distraction, and inspiration for information. Put simply, as we untangle this tale, it's going to get worse before it gets better.

Which, if you think about it, shouldn't be too surprising. The whole worse-before-better roller-coaster ride is practically baked into our script. When Kurt Vonnegut, author of modern classics like *Slaughterhouse Five* and *Cat's Cradle*, studied anthropology at the University of Chicago, he found that all stories share only a handful of basic shapes.

According to Vonnegut, you can trace any narrative by the rise and fall of the main characters' fortunes. He identified certain standbys, like the well-worn "Rags to Riches" story (Down then Up), and the "Boy meets Girl" tale where a couple meets each other, then loses each other, then gets each other back (Up then Down then Up again).

But of all the possible shapes Vonnegut discovered, he noticed that the Cinderella Story (Down then Up, then *Really* Down then *Really* Up) was the most compelling. We can't get enough of her Lowly Beginnings (sweeping ashes, crummy sisters, lousy stepmother), steady Climb to the Top (fairy godmothers, fancy outfits, dancing with the prince), Precipitous Drop (stroke of midnight, pumpkin coaches, lost slipper), and a Happily Ever After that set the bar for all the rest.

And that, more or less, is the shape of our story too. Only we're joining this narrative halfway through. For almost all of history, life was nastier, more brutal, and shorter than we might have liked (Down). Then, industrial, scientific, and democratic revolutions gave us lightbulbs, indoor plumbing, voting rights, vaccines, and smartphones. We've been living longer, learning more, and lacking for little (Up).

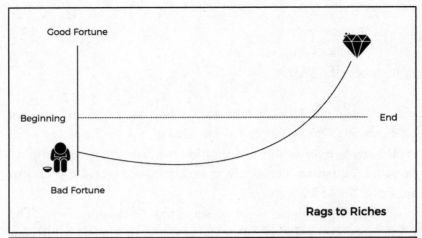

Rags to Riches

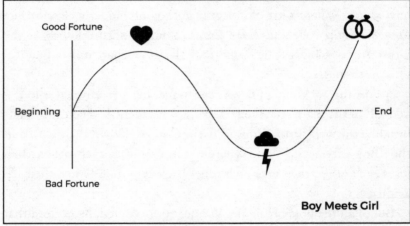

Boy Meets Girl

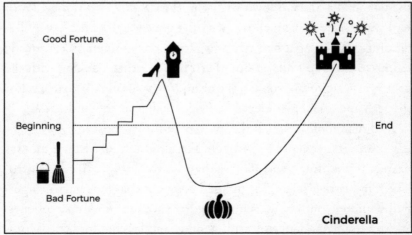

Cinderella

Until today, where we pick up the thread—at the stroke of midnight, on the verge of losing it all. As of January 2021, the *Bulletin of the Atomic Scientists'* Doomsday Clock, which tracks existential threats to humanity, reads one hundred seconds to twelve. That's the closest we've been to Armageddon since the Clock started tracking these things in 1947. The 2020 United Nations Climate Report gave us a decade to figure out the planet or face increasingly severe consequences. Geopolitics, extreme weather, famine, refugees, war, superviruses, cyberterrorism, and existential despair clog our newsfeeds and defy simple solutions (potentially *Really Really* Down).

The smartest and best informed are the most freaked out. The rest of us flip-flop between feeling anxious and pretending it's not happening. But if we can focus, there's a solid shot at redemption on the other side of that descent—a chance for the biggest Happily Ever After *ever*.

Buckminster Fuller might have said it best when he described a future that works "for 100% of humanity, in the shortest possible time, through spontaneous cooperation, without ecological offense or the disadvantage of anyone." That sounds like a pretty good Up to shoot for.

There's one important catch, though: The second half of our Cinderella story is 100 percent up for grabs. Who gets to write those final chapters is writing for all of us, and our children. And their children. So whether it's pumpkins or princes, disaster or happily ever after—all depends on what we do next.

CHAPTER 1

The Centre Cannot Hold

Exponential Everything

It wasn't until the autumn of 2018 that it finally hit me, though I should have seen it coming long before that.

I had flown into Johannesburg to give a talk at a summit dedicated to "Future Proofing Africa." As I sat in the audience listening to speakers describe the plight of that continent, its challenges and opportunities, I was alternately inspired and confused—inspired by the inventiveness of programs to bring solar and wind power to crowded townships, or ways to use nanotechnologies to make drinking water out of clouds and seawater. But also confused. Confused by the dissonance of a Californian woman excitedly describing a project to help illiterate villagers in central Africa build robots, and a ponytailed Cambridge researcher describing the promise of reversing aging so we could live forever.

What on earth did subsistence farmers need with robots? And in a world struggling to provide the basics to more people than ever, how was indefinite life extension for a fortunate few really the best move on humanity's chess board?

Surely these projects skipped a few steps on Abraham Maslow's hierarchy of needs—straight from survival to transcendence, with barely a pause in the meaty middle of the stack—where most people have always lived and died.

I scanned the program to see what else to expect. Exponential education—distributed virtual learning that could reach kids anywhere with a Wi-Fi connection. Exponential biology—gene-editing CRISPR tools to splice DNA and accelerate evolution. Exponential transportation—autonomous ride sharing apps and drone 'copter taxis to bypass the gridlock of our commutes. Exponential data— quantum computing and faster-than-light self-teaching algorithms that know what we want before we do. Exponential economics— virtual currencies to provide start-up capital to micro entrepreneurs and eliminate taxation.

But in all of that frothy, exciting future, where everything was just about to hit the hockey-stick curve of exponential acceleration, something critical was missing—and that something was exponential *meaning.* If these experts were to be believed, everything we've known about the human experience—hundreds of thousands of years of primate evolution and human culture—was about to be eclipsed by the sheer G-force of accelerating change. As Harvard biologist E. O. Wilson once put it, "We have paleolithic emotions, medieval institutions, and god-like technology." But no one was offering advice on how to make sense of it all.

Sitting in a Big Ideas conference like that one, where everyone is focused on large-scale visionary change and developments you've barely heard of are confidently identified as solutions to everything from poverty to cancer, it's almost impossible not to get swept up in the sheer audacity and optimism of it all. *Steven Pinker was right!* you think to yourself. The great Enlightenment Experiment of the last three centuries is going swimmingly, despite the Cassandras and the naysayers. Literacy and nutrition are up. War and disease are down. All signs point to an underreported but undeniable upward arc to human progress. Fully automated luxury-space communism beckons, even if we don't know precisely how we're going to get there from here.

Things, you'd be right to conclude, are undoubtedly getting exponentially better.

But then, after getting home, you scroll through your news feed and get hit with the overwhelm of a world in crisis: fires in the Arctic, the Amazon, and Malibu. Pandemics ravaging the globe. Refugees scrambling from Syria, Venezuela, or wherever is unluckiest next. Ebola. COVID. Populism. Terrorism. Sexism. Racism. All the isms. All the time.

Things, you'd be heartless to ignore, are undoubtedly getting exponentially worse.

As E. B. White, the author of the children's classic *Charlotte's Web*, once reflected, "I arise in the morning torn between a desire to improve (or save) the world and a desire to enjoy (or savor) the world. This makes it hard to plan the day."

Trying to map, plot, and plan for a world that feels like a tangled braid of conflicting and compounding exponential curves is crazy-making on the best of days. It's the kind of multivariable calculus that most of us bombed in high school. We're not any better at it now.

Two curves in particular are intersecting right now—we can call them the Coming Alive arc and the Staying Alive arc.

The Coming Alive arc starts on the bottom left and curves happily up and to the right. It's all about personal and cultural fulfillment, and the possibilities that were getting so much airtime at that exponential conference. If life were a picnic at the beach, this curve would

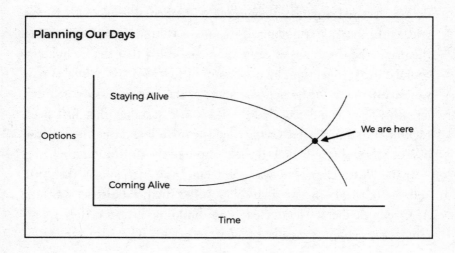

Planning Our Days

Staying Alive

Options

We are here

Coming Alive

Time

include what to pack, who to invite, and where to unfurl your blanket for the best view possible.

The Staying Alive curve starts high up on the left and plummets downward as it moves across the graph. It's not nearly so rosy. If life were a picnic at the beach, this curve would include noticing the water getting sucked out to sea, watching all the animals fleeing to higher ground, and possibly checking your blaring phone to read the tsunami warning.

Coming Alive is timeless, optimistic, and focused on maximizing choices—savoring the world. Staying Alive is time-bound, pessimistic, and focused on dwindling choices—saving the world. Right now, we seem to be caught smack-dab at their intersection. And that can make it hard to plan our days.

The Edifice Complex

It's not just that the world is changing exponentially and our ability to make sense isn't keeping up. It's that we're witnessing a collapse of meaning altogether. We experience that gap every day as uncertainty, anxiety, and confusion. Even our most familiar and trusted landmarks can't tell us which way is up anymore.

In April 2019 the famed Notre Dame Cathedral in Paris caught fire. France declared a national emergency. President Emmanuel Macron tweeted furiously and mobilized resources. Within days of containing the blaze, the think pieces came. Some reflected that the firefighters' courage and pledges from luxury brands like LVMH and Saint-Laurent were a testament to the national spirit of the French. Others felt differently. They wondered aloud if the abuse scandals that had been rocking the Church were finally catching up to it and that the collapse of Notre Dame foreshadowed the collapse of the institution itself.

If the Notre Dame fire was accidental in its symbolism, the 2001 collapse of the Twin Towers in New York's financial district was not. Al-Qaeda deliberately targeted those buildings because they represented the economic center of Western power. The vulnerability of those iconic skyscrapers sent shock waves through the world. When the towers fell, America's sense of security collapsed with them.

This broader idea of how our buildings enshrine our beliefs is helpful as we consider our current crisis in meaning. We all suffer from some version of the "Edifice Complex," where the institutions that are most prominent in a given time and place also reflect our values. They tell us at a glance exactly who's in charge and what we care about the most.

Back in the age of empires, pharaohs built pyramids and kings constructed castles, enshrining their divine right to rule. In the medieval era, monasteries and cathedrals loomed large across Europe, reflecting the power of the Church. With the emergence of the nation-state in the eighteenth century, capitols and courthouses took center stage in urban plans and skylines. By the twentieth century and the age of corporations, skyscrapers towered above everything—monuments to the barons and banks that built them. Today, silicon campuses designed by celebrity architects claim the spotlight. Power has now been harnessed in the physical world by those who invented our virtual ones.

But while the Twin Towers and Notre Dame are examples of the Edifice Complex in crisis—times where the cracks in our culture have shown up as literal cracks in our foundations—in reality, we're seeing the collapse of Benign and Divine Authority nearly everywhere we look. And it's not just in the monuments we make to power and prominence. It's in the institutions themselves.

* * *

In 2008, as storied firms like Bear Stearns and Lehman Brothers went belly-up, no one clearly understood why the market had collapsed so suddenly or so thoroughly. Politicians grabbed screen time tut-tutting greedy middle-class consumers who'd bitten off more McMansion than they could chew. By the time the postmortems like Michael Lewis's *The Big Short* came out, it was clear that at institutions like Goldman Sachs there was more self-dealing, more foreknowledge, and more disregard than most people would have thought possible.

If we believed that sort of thing, as terrible as it was, got cleared up with the passage of "never again" reform legislation like the Dodd-Frank Act, we were wrong there too—it just went underground. And overseas. In Singapore, the 1MDB scandal siphoned billions of dollars into boondoggle projects, Hollywood movie financing, and outright embezzlement, toppling a prime minister as it came undone. It, too, was overseen by the gentlemen bankers of Goldman Sachs.

The infamous Gupta brothers, in partnership with Jacob Zuma and the global consultancy firm McKinsey, bled the South African treasury of nearly $7 billion. That prompted a crash in the Rand and a crisis in power that threaten the gains of Nelson Mandela's improbably hopeful transition out of apartheid.

"The firm's willingness to work with despotic governments and corrupt business empires is the logical conclusion of seeking profit at all costs," an anonymous McKinsey staffer wrote in a widely circulated internal post. "[If you believe that capitalism's] continued practice poses an existential threat to governments, the biosphere, and poor people the world over, then the firm's role is that of a coconspirator to a crime in which we are all victims."

On its surface, these incidents of corruption between politicians and financiers aren't remarkable—they're only the latest in an uninterrupted history of well-manicured hands caught in the cookie jar. To that recent tally you can add the list of billionaire family offices, private equity–backed companies, libertarian think tanks, and megachurches that skimmed the till of the $4 trillion disaster bailouts during the COVID pandemic in 2020. And we shouldn't overlook the list of global banks implicated in over $2 trillion of money laundering for Russian oligarchs and criminal syndicates that also recently grabbed headlines. Things like this shouldn't happen, but they do. All the time.

With Goldman Sachs and McKinsey (and Deutsche Bank and Wells Fargo and many others) called out in recent scandals, the scale of impropriety threatens to undermine the promise of liberal globalism altogether.

If we've been goading the entire developing world to invest in infrastructure, take on debt, demonstrate democracy, and stamp out corruption, only to rob them blind through the very mechanism we promised was going to be their salvation, then we're going to have some pretty disenchanted neighbors.

Joseph Stiglitz, the Nobel Prize–winning economist and former chief economist at the World Bank, knows how our global system works better than most. His conclusions are stark. "The simultaneous waning of confidence in neoliberalism and in democracy is no coincidence or mere correlation. Neoliberalism has undermined democracy for 40 years. . . . The numbers are in: growth has slowed and the fruits of that growth went overwhelmingly to a very few at the top."

* * *

It's not just the bankers of Wall Street who have come under fire. That utopia of relentless optimism, Silicon Valley—where every app, start-up, and venture capitalist is earnestly committed to "Making the World a Better Place"—has lost its shine too. In the wake of the dot-com crash in 2001, the FAANG stocks (Facebook, Apple, Amazon, Netflix, Google) wired up our world in a way it had never been before.

We got drunk with the giddy wonder of what was possible in this new age of innovation. Googly Googlers pedaled colorful bikes and touted a company slogan of "Don't Be Evil" (since deleted). The Facebook, started at first as an elite digital directory for Ivy Leaguers, opened up so the rest of us (even Grandma!) could cyberstalk old crushes and Photoshop our lives.

The addictive ease of Amazon One Click shipping laid waste to small businesses and urban cores, even as sweatshop fulfillment centers across the country paid minimum-wage employees to get it to our doorstep in forty-eight hours or less (or else). It was all so good, so diverting, and so convenient, we didn't care. "Move fast and break things!" Zuck encouraged us. We believed impossibly that all that creative destruction would somehow work out for the best.

By 2016, that had all begun to change. First, the scandals of election interference in the U.K. Brexit vote and the U.S. presidential election shattered our understanding of social media platforms and their hidden downsides—how the likes of Cambridge Analytica had weaponized millions of Facebook accounts to serve up highly targeted and deliberately divisive messaging. At first it wasn't clear how negligent Facebook had been or how much of an edge case Cambridge Analytica really was. Had Facebook been pimping out our most intimate details to its third-party developers all along? What had Cambridge Analytica done in bad faith vs. with full permission?

Now it almost doesn't seem to matter. Democracy hasn't recovered from the outcomes of our last two elections or the implications of what's to come. It survived civil war, the Nazis, and the Soviets, only to be undone by AdWords and Twitter.

Suddenly the hands-off Free Speech approach of all these Silicon Valley platforms seemed woefully inadequate. When measured against deliberate efforts to game their algorithms and hack civil society, their conveniently libertarian approach seemed more negligent than principled—especially as they collected billions in advertising revenue from all sides. Facebook experienced mass walkouts in the summer of 2020 as staff protested CEO Mark Zuckerberg's seeming indifference to refereeing inaccurate and divisive political ads on their platform. Atlas, now wearing a hoodie and Allbirds sneakers, just shrugged.

In the past couple of years the cognitive dissonance has all become too much—even for those smack-dab in the middle of the hype. Dissent on the Google campus rose to a fever pitch—first sparked by a few conservative "brogrammers" declaring that they felt censured and ostracized for their right-of-center beliefs. Then women employees protested a pervasive culture of sexual impropriety and high-dollar exit packages for handsy senior executives. Finally, conscientious objectors became alarmed by the company's move to reenter China with censored search, by murky contracts to sell AI facial recognition to the Pentagon for use in drone warfare, and the unceremonious exit of one of its most prominent ethicists.

For Googlers raised on "Don't Be Evil," the lines between the good guys and the bad were getting increasingly blurred. By the summer of 2019 a *New York Times* article declared "Silicon Valley Goes to Therapy" as six-figure tech workers belatedly realized all-you-can-eat arugula and sushi weren't enough to quell the increasing queasiness they were feeling.

* * *

Even our faith in those professionals who have dedicated their lives to the Hippocratic oath—*Primum non nocere* or "first, do no harm"—hasn't come out unscathed. Starting in the 1980s and accelerating over the next two decades, doctors began freely prescribing and then grossly overprescribing synthetic opioids like OxyContin. That paved the way for a full-blown opioid epidemic that has become the largest public health crisis of the twenty-first century. One pharmacy in a small town in Appalachia prescribed nine million tablets of Oxy-Contin to a population of four hundred people. The DEA and other federal enforcement organizations bafflingly did nothing while Purdue Pharma raked in record-breaking profits.

Today, 80 percent of heroin addicts started out with a prescription for OxyContin. Add to that an equally destructive but less reported epidemic of benzodiazepines (a class of sedatives that includes Valium, Xanax, and Klonopin), and the routine over-prescription of amphetamines like Ritalin and Adderall, and it's hard not to second-guess our patient-doctor relationships. Systematic analysis by *The Lancet* reported over twenty million incidents of "iatrogenic illness" worldwide—a mouthful of a term that basically means "your doctor really screwed up and made things worse."

This collapse in faith in the medical establishment has had backlash effects too. In the midst of the 2020 COVID pandemic, formerly above-the-fray organizations like the Centers for Disease Control and World Health Organization came under intense and divisive scrutiny. Questions on their loyalty and objectivity ricocheted around social media and halls of power, massively hampering a coordinated response to a global health crisis.

* * *

Political scientists Roberto Foa and Yascha Mounk have found that nearly half of American citizens lack faith in democracy and more than one-third of young high-income earners actually favor army rule. "Young people today," Derek Thompson writes in *The Atlantic*, "commit crimes at historically low rates and have attended college at historically high rates. They have done everything right, sprinting at full speed while staying between the white lines, and their reward for historic conscientiousness is this: less ownership, more debt, and an age of existential catastrophe. . . . Why in the name of family, God, or country would such a person lust for ancient affiliations? As the kids say, #BurnItAllDown."

As things get exponentially worse and exponentially better at the same time, and our heads spin making sense of it, the collapse in Benign Authority of government, business, medicine, and academia has left us without reference points to steer by. But it's not just Benign Authority that's been collapsing. As Notre Dame's flames foreshadowed, Divine Authority has too.

The End of Faith

In the spring of 2007 in a stylish town house in Washington, D.C., the Four Horsemen gathered for what was to be their first and only meeting. The home belonged to Christopher Hitchens, journalist, pundit, and author of that year's *God Is Not Great*—a comprehensive breakdown of all the bad things done in the name of divinity. The other three attending were Richard Dawkins, the famous evolutionary biologist, author of *The Selfish Gene*, and the father of the concept of "memes"; Daniel Dennett, a preeminent cognitive neuroscientist and author of *Breaking the Spell*; and a fresh-faced youngster named Sam Harris, who'd just published the bestselling *The End of Faith*. While Hitchens pointed his dry wit and commentary toward all kinds of faith, including Buddhism and neo-paganism, Harris took particular issue with Islam and its apparent connection to the violence that had engulfed the world since 9/11. Although each thinker differed in emphasis, they could all agree on one thing: Religion, at its very roots, was a superstitious throwback, doomed to promote suffering and perpetuate ignorance.

Believing in virgin births or martyrs' paradise, or a world divided into the saved and the damned, these skeptics insisted, was incompatible with modernity, common sense, and reason. At best, they argued, it was infantilizing. At worst, it provided justification for all sorts of horror. The time for Blind Faith was up, they agreed. These Four Horsemen of the New Atheism, as they were soon called, were only too happy to celebrate the End of Faith.

Their timing was good. Demographics bore them out. From the early nineties well into this century, religiosity in America and Western Europe was waning dramatically. Attendance (and with it, revenue and impact) dropped. Churches shuttered or downsized. Dedicated lifers still attended (the blue-haired church ladies and their ilk), but the younger generations weren't showing up to take their place. The only nominal growth for Catholicism could be found in the developing world. But in the home countries of Europe and the United States, things were looking increasingly bleak for mainstream Christianity.

By 2015, the Pew Center posted a momentous survey—for the first time in history, the spiritual-but-not-religious, a.k.a. the "Nones," had surpassed all other organized denominations to become not only the largest but the fastest-growing category of belief in the United States.

The reasons this happened so suddenly are complicated. Social scientists tracked a confluence of events—ranging from the fall of the Soviet Union (and with it, the stigma associated with identifying with "godless" atheism), to the rise of the Moral Majority, which left those uncomfortable with the blurring of church and state seeking more neutral ground. And finally, there was the fire that sparked Sam Harris into action on September 11, 2001—the sudden and violent ascendance of jihadi Islam onto the world stage. Identifying as a non-believer, for the first time in history, seemed less rebellious or reactionary than simply reasonable.

Scholars of religion, meanwhile, explained sagging faith in different terms. Some focused on the growing divide between church doctrine and social issues, like women clergy, birth control, and gay marriage, that had not kept pace with changing attitudes in their congregants. Other researchers have identified the burgeoning spiritual marketplace, ranging from Oprah to Tony Robbins to *A Course in Miracles*, all offering alternate sources for solace, insight, and instruction. *Eat, Pray, Love*, after all, only cost fifteen bucks, and Elizabeth Gilbert felt guilty so you didn't have to. Church no longer had a corner on the market for inspiration and redemption.

But the New Atheists' reports of the Death of Belief were slightly exaggerated. The Four Horsemen were only half right. While the "reasonable" might have been stepping away from orthodox belief, many others were finding themselves pushed to the edges. Lacking anywhere else to center themselves, fundamentalism and nihilism were picking up the stragglers.

While mainline Protestantism and Catholicism were seeing significant drops in attendance, Evangelical megachurches have been booming. They offer a uniquely American mash-up of positive thinking and the Gospel of Wealth. These transdenominational churches encourage congregants to abandon traditional values of poverty, humility, and service in favor of dreaming their #BestLife. Stage lights, amplified "praise music," Jumbotrons, and Jesus Rock. The old Catholic standbys of penance, "smells and bells," never stood a chance.

Despite the leather-jacketed hipster pastors (a genre *GQ* skewered as "the New Hype Priests"), the doctrinal messaging has remained remarkably conservative. One of the hallmarks of the evangelical movement is literalism—that every word in the Bible is divinely inspired and nonnegotiably true. And while the most outdated mandates are overlooked (like stoning adulterous wives, or mastering slaves, or salting your enemies' fields), a large chunk of the moral code in these churches stems from word-for-word interpretation of ancient texts.

Rather than meeting in the middle and trying to adapt beliefs for a rapidly changing and modernizing world, these evangelical churches have found that doubling down on tradition (even within a self-consciously contemporary presentation) has been a surprisingly effective way to grow their reach. Awash in a sea of uncertainty, it seems that many would-be believers are happy to have a solid rock to cling to.

* * *

For seekers repelled by the tenets of fundamentalism but overwhelmed by uncertainty and complexity, the moderate middle isn't always enough to hold them. Those not drawn to the promise of the all-in-one Megachurch don't always end up where Harris and Hitchens would have imagined—in the realm of reason and rationality. They often drift to the other extreme and fall into nihilism instead.

Pew and Gallup don't survey this particular group of the unchurched and unbelieving. But public health officials do, and their findings are sobering. Diseases of despair—anxiety, depression, suicide—are rampant. One in six Americans takes psychiatric medications just to cope with the banality of modern life. To put this in harsh relief, the World Health Organization reports that more people today kill themselves than die from all wars and natural disasters *combined*. Think of all the hurricanes, floods, and fires and all the civil wars, terrorism, and military conflict that inundate our news feeds. Put together, they don't match the number of people choosing to leave this world because they cannot bear it any longer.

"We're the middle children of history, man," the ultimate nihilist character, Tyler Durden, explains in *Fight Club*. "No purpose or place. We have no Great War. No Great Depression. Our Great War is a spiritual war, our Great Depression is our lives."

Meaning 1.0—organized religion—has collapsed, the disconnected and disaffected have realized. But for them, a retreat to the fundamentalism of the faithful remains an unconvincing antidote to a hypermodern and cynical world. But Meaning 2.0—modernism—hasn't exactly panned out either. "We've all been raised on television to believe that one day we'd all be millionaires, and movie gods, and rock stars," Durden continues. "But we won't. And we're slowly learning that fact. And we're very, very pissed off." For the frustrated middle children of history, nihilism—the view that none of this matters—is their refuge of last resort.

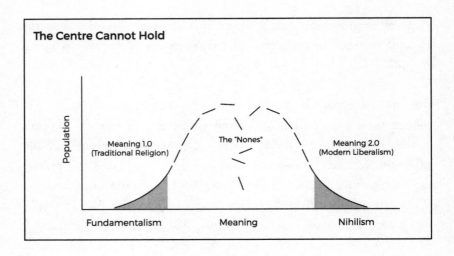

That tracks with what Nietzsche said over a century ago, when he famously pronounced God dead. Atheists interpreted that as vindication of their nonbelief. Closer readings suggest something more nuanced, and relevant for today.

For sure, Nietzsche was arguing that the reason and logic of the French Enlightenment and scientific revolution had replaced blind faith. But, he said, there are profound social consequences to lobbing the Baby Jesus out with all that backward-ass bathwater.

"When one gives up the Christian faith," Nietzsche cautioned, "one pulls the right to Christian morality out from under one's feet. This morality is by no means self-evident. . . . Christianity is a system, a whole view of things thought out together. *By breaking one main concept out of it, the faith in God, one breaks the whole*" [emphasis added].

Jonathan Haidt, New York University philosopher and author of *The Coddling of the American Mind*, agrees. "A part of being human is believing in gods and worshipping and having a sense of the sacred. And I think we have a need, we have a hole in our heart . . . it needs to be filled by something—and if you leave it empty [people] don't just feel an emptiness. A society that has no sense of the sacred is one in which you'll have a lot of anomie, normlessness, loneliness, hopelessness."

So the Four Horsemen of the New Atheism didn't get it exactly right. To be certain, the edifice of mainline religion—Meaning 1.0—has collapsed, but secularism—Meaning 2.0—hasn't been enough to hold the center in its place. As things fall apart, we've seen a migration to the extremes of fundamentalist beliefs on one hand and a drift toward nihilism on the other. And for those stuck in the moderate middle, identifying as "spiritual but not religious"? The Nones have no particular place to go.

CHAPTER 2

Stop Making Sense

A LEXICON FOR THE ESCHATON

eschaton
/'eskə,tän/

Noun: the final event in the divine plan; the end of the world.

eschatothesia
/.e-skə-tä-'thē-zhə /

Noun: a feeling of some huge event in the near future we are approaching: the end of an aeon, a marker in time after which nothing will be the same.

If we're going to talk constructively about the End of Days, we should probably define our terms. When most of us consider bigtimescarybadstuff happening in the near or distant future, we often use words like Apocalypse, Armageddon, or Rapture interchangeably.

But in reality, they're distinct. Understanding those distinctions is an essential first step in developing our eschatological literacy.

First, the Apocalypse. In the ancient Greek, *apocalypsis* means "the unveiling or revealing." As we're experiencing the collapse in both

Benign and Divine Authority, and questioning the dictates of both traditional religion and modern liberalism, there are all sorts of hidden truths that are being revealed. Not all are comforting, but they're necessary if we hope to develop an informed capacity to act.

Next, Armageddon. That's a contraction of the Hebrew *Har Megiddo* and refers to the mountain outside the Israeli town of Haifa. There, believers wait for the ultimate showdown between Good and Evil. Once this battle starts we're on the road to the final days of Judgment. There's no going back for the quick or the dead.

Lastly, Rapture. In its lowercase version, it means intense bliss or fulfillment. In its uppercase version, Rapture is a story of impending cataclysm for the many and the joyful redemption of the few. While it began as a religious belief about the End of Time, it has morphed into countless mutations since, both sacred and secular.

It's not too much of a stretch to suggest that we need very different responses to each of these three terms: We should hasten the Apocalypse—the unveiling—so that we can see and act more clearly on what is revealed. We should delay Armageddon because, after the War to End All Wars, it's literally Game Over at that point. And we should recapture both uppercase and lowercase raptures, because solutions that only work for a tiny fraction of us wreak havoc for the rest, and we're going to need to be at our absolute best to pull this off.

The first half of this chapter deliberately accelerates our apocalyptic thinking—helping us strip away distortions and misconceptions to see the future as clearly as possible. As we try to guess what the future holds, there are no singular perspectives or conclusions to assert. It's too complicated and rapidly shifting for that. But we can at least adopt the stance that a more considered position is better than a less considered position. Think of what follows as a choose-your-own-adventure Mad Libs for the Apocalypse. Mad(Max) Libs for short.

The second half of the chapter seeks to forestall Armageddon—taking a look at our increasingly volatile culture wars by exploring both the neurochemistry and psychology behind them. At a time when we all need to be rallying together, we've never felt more apart. Understanding the dynamics of unity and dissent is essential if we stand a chance of recapturing the Rapture and finding functional outcomes for everyone.

A Knee-Jerk Response

In 1847, Ignaz Semmelweis, a doctor at Vienna's General Hospital, noticed something important about the women and children he treated in the maternity ward. They died. Distressingly often. Semmelweis wondered if all of the autopsies he and his colleagues performed on cadavers were somehow contaminating the next group of children and mothers they attended. So he developed a handwashing solution of chlorine and lime for physicians to rinse with between seeing patients. It worked. Infections dropped to below 1 percent on his ward.

But, among the other doctors, the reception was less kind. His colleagues mocked him, refusing to believe on principle that a gentleman's hands could spread disease. Semmelweis himself could only offer up the vague concept of "cadaverous contamination" to justify his protocol (this was several decades before the formal articulation of germ theory). The stress drove Semmelweis to a nervous breakdown. A bitter colleague had him committed to a lunatic asylum, where he was beaten by guards, and died of an infection that his very own handwashing technique would have prevented.

But Semmelweis's legacy lives on, and not just in the grudging adoption of surgical hygiene. He's also shaped the cognitive sciences, where the Semmelweis reflex—the idea that we habitually and often violently reject new evidence or new knowledge because it runs so counter to our preexisting articles of faith—has become a standby on the list of common cognitive biases.

Our cognitive biases hamper our ability to predict with any degree of certainty what's going to happen next. That's because the Semmelweis reflex kicks us out of accepting what is staring us in the face. We can't wrap our head around it because it runs so counter to everything we hold to be self-evidently true.

Someone broke our dashboard. At this point we're flying blind.

* * *

While we are experiencing a breakdown in our ability to forecast the future, there's one thing that's almost certain—the next fifty years is going to bear little to no resemblance to the past fifty years. And that simple fact scrambles our gauges.

The soothsayers of Silicon Valley, like Peter Diamandis and Ray Kurzweil, chalk our confusion up to the exponential expansion that is rapidly coming our way—retina displays, quantum computing, gene editing, and cyborgs. We can't predict the future, they say, because it is going to be so exponentially different from the past. And while that may be true, in ways that will likely surprise even the most devout futurists, there's another even more basic explanation.

It's not just that this coming half-century will bear so little resemblance to the last one. It's that the last half-century bears so little resemblance to almost any other time and place in human history itself that's confusing us. Coming out of World War II, the past fifty-odd years were an anomaly all their own. Three generations of Americans have been living in a bubble. So if you're a baby boomer, Gen Xer, or millennial, and you're looking around for reference points and precedents to try to orient yourself around, it's crucial to recalibrate what was so unusual about the times we grew up in first.

That fluky period was so unique that historians even gave it a name—Pax Americana—or "American Peace." It began in the rubble of post–World War II Europe and Japan and witnessed the ascendance of the United States as a preeminent political, economic, and cultural force. The United States was lucky to fight all its wars overseas. Both its enemies and allies were bombed into ruin. When it came time to convert the factories churning out B-17 bombers into assembly lines turning out tail-finned Cadillacs, American industry was ready. When farms pumping out beef to feed the GIs converted to producing cheap meat for drive-in burger stands, McDonald's was born.

Publishing magnate Henry Luce called it early in the game when he claimed in a 1941 editorial in *Life* magazine that the next era was to be the American Century: "The Greeks, the Romans, the English and the French had their eras," he said, "and now it was ours."

The Cuban Missile Crisis was the closest direct conflict ever got to the United States' own backyard. With the briefest of exceptions on 9/11, Americans have always felt safe on their own soil. Six trillion dollars of military might and fifteen years of sustained operations in Afghanistan and Iraq took place entirely "over there." Wartime hardship, for most Americans today, amounts to taking off their shoes at airport security.

The entire world that baby boomers, Generation X, and millennials have grown up in (especially in the United States, but by extension in other developed countries) could be chalked up to random chance just as much as any Manifest Destiny. If you grew up in the former Soviet Union and lived through the fall of the Iron Curtain, or lived in South Africa and experienced its transition from apartheid, or called the cosmopolitan city of Kabul home, only to see it descend into decades of violence, you'd have no trouble imagining the unimaginable. That's just life, and the disorienting experience of being swept up in the broad currents of history. "The best laid schemes o' Mice and Men," the poet Robert Burns reminds us, often end badly.

Replay the American Experiment a thousand times on a computer simulation, and many of the truths we hold to be self-evident turn out to be not much more than good luck and timing. Like Shelley's optimistic King Ozymandias, we might overestimate how our past dominance will translate to future prominence. Our Magic Kingdom of Disneyfied abundance might turn out to be a castle made of sand, after all.

Mad(Max) Libs

That doesn't mean we have to give up making predictions of any kind. It just means we need to bring some basic logic to how we consider the road ahead, and what some of the more or less likely scenarios might be.

When farmers, foresters, and civil engineers are deciding when to plant, what to cut, or where to build, they estimate the likelihood of droughts, floods, and fires happening once every ten, hundred, or thousand years. A hundred-year flood or fire, for instance, has a 1 percent likelihood of occurring in any given year.

Then they figure out what to do, balanced against their willingness to tolerate a repeat disaster. Those kinds of weather events leave evidence behind them. Extreme dry spells, high-water marks, and burn deposits are traceable. They give us some sense of predictability where we might otherwise be limited by what we can guess from right here, right now. This helps counter those cognitive biases that skew us toward a present-tense focus.

Lately, once-in-a-hundred-year events have been happening several times a decade. We're needing to update our predictions. But even though our old benchmarks aren't holding like they used to, the process of updating them is essential. "Plans," said Winston Churchill, "are worthless. But planning is *priceless.*"

While we won't be able to predict exactly what is going to happen, we can make rough estimates of what type, intensity, and scale of things are most likely to occur based on our most current data. Then we can adjust our behavior accordingly. For instance, when considering the future ahead of us, do we believe it is going to bear the closest social, political, and economic resemblance to the recent past—the last decade or two? Or maybe the past century? The past millennium? Or even, the last epoch?

If we think that this coming decade is going to most closely resemble the past couple of decades, then we would reasonably expect events comparable to the Great Recession of 2008, natural disasters like hurricanes Katrina and Sandy, and conflict with state and non-state actors like ISIS and al-Qaeda. If we stretch back to include 9/11 in that accounting, we'd also expect some form of large-scale terrorist act on U.S. soil. Those are not insignificant events. We navigated them all reasonably well, but facing them again would require courage, coordination, and luck. This would mean we've taken into account the happy accident of the Pax Americana but don't believe it's going to end just yet.

If we feel that the rate of change and the amount of uncertainty we're facing now exceeds what we've just passed through, then we're in for once-in-a-century levels of disruption. Our contingency planning has to expand considerably. Two world wars and the Holocaust. Trench warfare. Gas chambers and Hiroshima. The influenza and AIDS epidemics (close to one hundred million fatalities between them). The Great Depression. The Cultural Revolution in China and Stalinism in the Soviet Union. Civil rights and the assassination of beloved political leaders. Lots of intense ground to cover.

News anchor Tom Brokaw called the cohort that lived through these upheavals the "Greatest Generation"—and it included many of our parents and grandparents. My father used to tell stories of huddling under a sturdy kitchen table during the London Blitz, before getting shipped off to a boarding school in Scotland for the rest of the war. Other families carry the memories of Normandy, Nagasaki, or Buchenwald. It may feel like ancient history, but for many of us, it's only one or two generations away.

Our ancestors' sense of how hard things can get, how resilient communities and countries must become, and how powerful ideals can be in times of crisis was directly informed by coming of age between world wars and the Depression. So while we might tease our pack rat Grandma saving rubber bands and wrapping paper in her kitchen drawer, the conditions that forged her thrift and stiffened her spine were real and present not too long ago. And if Grandma and Grandpa could pull it off, so can we.

If the once-in-a-century frame is still not spicy enough for your tastes, consider the once-in-a-millennium bracket. That includes everything we witnessed in the twentieth century, plus the U.S. Civil War, all the wars and disruptions of European colonial expansion, the Black Plague, the Inquisition, and even the empire of Genghis Khan. This frame takes us firmly out of the modern era and any sort of generational hand-me-down knowledge breaks down.

Those events unfolded in a world so foreign to our own contemporary sensibilities that it would be utterly disorienting to experience daily life back then. Things would get medieval quickly. And while that prospect might seem far-fetched and dystopian, a quick survey of narco states in the Americas and feudal warlords in Africa and Asia offers sobering evidence of how durable these forms of social organizing are. Swap out warhorses for Toyota pickups, broadswords and longbows for machetes and AK-47s, and we're pretty much there already. Coming soon to a failed state near you.

If you're profoundly bearish on our future prospects and believe that we are teetering on the brink of civilizational collapse or outright extinction—there's always the epochal time frame to consider. Extinction Rebellion is a global movement founded on this assumption, as is Dark Mountain arts collective. The recent procession of grim reports from the UN and think tanks dedicated to assessing our existential risks continually call attention to this nearly inconceivable possibility.

Depending on whom you ask, and how you date it, we're in the Anthropocene period—that chunk of time where human impact on our world has taken precedence over slower, more geological and ecological processes. If you're calibrating at this scale of future forecasting, all bets are off. You're basically saying, "It's the end of the world as we know it," and whether we go the way of the dinosaur or *Star Trek* remains to be seen. While science fiction—from *Mad Max* to the TV series *The Walking Dead*—loves to explore this scenario, we would, quite literally, be at the end of history. There would be no more precedent to lean on. In this scenario, Francis Fukuyama wasn't wrong when he wrote *The End of History and the Last Man*. He was just early.

So it's worth pausing a moment and checking in on how this actually feels to consider. Do our heads spin trying to reconcile the conflicting opinion papers, research findings, and chatter on social media? Do we find ourselves irritated or bored reading this, itching for a quick glance at our phones?

Or, do we cling to comfortable truths we take to be self-evident, like the triumphal rise of nation-states, democracy, and market capitalism? Do we cross our fingers and hold out hope for exponential technology, like fusion power, quantum computing, or geo-engineering to save us from uncertainty? Do we secretly think that some game-changing intervention, whether a new world powered by blockchain or a blossoming of human consciousness spawned by psychedelics or neural implants, will save us in the nick of time? Or how about a full-blown Rapture play—like alien disclosure or the Second Coming, to thwart all the grim predictions and deliver us, at the last minute, from evil?

BBQ Your Sacred Cows

In all this existential existentialism, there are three key drivers that affect our ability to make sense of the future: our cognitive complexity, our sacred cows, and our ability to grieve. If we are not up for tackling all three head-on, we'll get stuck.

Manage all three, and we can begin to make sense of the scope and scale of change we're facing.

First we need to make sure we have the mental complexity to map and plan for an unpredictable future. Since the recent collapse in Benign Authority, we have fewer trustable public leaders and institutions to lean on. Walter Cronkite and BBC Radio no longer define the norms of polite debate and let us know, in soothing tones, that even if all is not right with the world, that right still leads the world.

Former journals of record like *The Wall Street Journal* and *The New York Times* have courted increasingly partisan op-eds and readers. Nontraditional newsfeeds like Reddit, 4chan, and Parler gleefully bypass the gatekeepers and unite formerly fringe audiences. Even fact-checking sites, the place you're supposed to go to separate fiction from reality, have become hopelessly politicized. Extremes of opinion, whether neo-Marxist social justice revolutionaries, alt-right identitarians, or meta-conspiracists, have become increasingly mainstream.

So we have to do the heavy lifting and sort through competing and conflicting sources ourselves. That requires graduating from simple, binary, either/or thinking toward both/and/neither thinking. Not only does this require an unusually high tolerance for ambiguity, it requires cultivating what Roger Martin, the dean of the Rotman School of Management, calls an "opposable mind" that can stay above the fray. That requires practice. And time. Neither of which we feel like we've got enough of.

We need to be able to hold some of those competing and conflicting scenarios in our heads without crashing our mental browser. Then we can ask which of our a priori assumptions—those beliefs that are foundational to the way we think Life, the Universe, and Everything work—are possibly incompatible with some of the futures we're increasingly forced to reckon with.

* * *

Said another way, what sacred cows might we have to throw on the barbecue if one of those thousand-year fires comes to town?

While we discussed the collapse of faith in both sacred and secular institutions in the last chapter, our Sacred Cows live one level up from all that. They reflect our ideals, our dreams, and our cherished beliefs. Even when we experience setbacks or contradictions in real life, our Sacred Cows are what reinspire us. They are the blueprint from which we build and rebuild.

A few examples: Over the past century neoliberalism has become a popular default setting for much of our political and economic policy. Nation-states dedicated to open borders, free trade, and civil rights, the story goes, prosper. Free market capitalism and representative democracy go together like peas and carrots and provide the ultimate mechanism to raise humanity toward higher and higher levels of prosperity. Efforts to redistribute wealth, limit competition, or constrain popular dissent range from counterproductive to catastrophic.

The collapse of the Soviet Union and the rise of living standards worldwide provided powerful vindication for this paradigm. Markets work. Communism doesn't. Democracy works. Dictatorships don't. For the brief decade between the fall of the Berlin Wall in 1991 and the fall of the Twin Towers in 2001, this model appeared uncontested and ascendant.

But neoliberalism quickly fell short of explaining everything that was happening. When the second Bush administration imagined the Middle East throwing off the yoke of tyranny and embracing democracy, it backfired badly. The failure of regime change after the Arab Spring in Syria, Iraq, and Libya further destabilized the region and created the conditions that fomented ISIS.

The same rethink happened with the entry of China into the world market. Counter to the American model, it tightened rather than loosened civil liberties and prospered anyway. Democracy and capitalism, once assumed to be a package deal, had been neatly separated. "We'll take your vertically integrated supply chains, predatory lending, and profit margins," said the Chinese Communist Party. "You can keep your uppity citizenry, human rights, and elections."

Even the melting pot ideal of multicultural assimilation has melted down. Once the identities of the 9/11 bombers became widely known, it threw that theory into chaos. These men weren't desperate goatherding zealots filled with resentment, and nothing to live for. They'd spent considerable time in Europe and America, and *still* wanted to destroy it. To have people make full use of free societies and then turn that tolerance against itself posed a serious challenge to Western assumptions of universal benevolence and inclusion.

A decade later, one million refugees from Syria effectively broke the European Union, placing tremendous pressure on the tolerance of Germany and the Nordic states and sowing the seeds for Brexit and the disintegration of a once United Kingdom.

In the Western Hemisphere, a steady stream of dislocated migrants from Central America and Mexico prompted a different "sea to shining sea" vision for the United States—that of a big, beautiful wall from coast to coast, keeping out southern neighbors speaking a different language. With climate refugees slated to hit up to one billion people by 2050, those pressures are only going to increase.

*   *   *

Now let's zoom in from the global level and get down to the personal. There are some cherished assumptions we may need to let go of in our own lives as well. The "temping of America" and the gig economy have knocked the career ladder on its side. Student debt on one end and evaporating pension plans on the other have weighed down upward mobility. Job security is fading fast. Baby boomers who grew up on that promise have had to abandon it altogether as retirement at sixty-five has morphed into working hourly jobs just for the extra spending money and health insurance.

Millennials too have had to massively revise their notions of "adulting" and what it means to come of age in the aftermath of the 2008 recession and quarantine lockdowns. Home ownership, once revered as a stepping-stone to middle-class stability, has been replaced by Airbnb and couch surfing. Car ownership has been swapped for rideshares and electric scooters, marriage by dating apps, 401(k)s by Bitcoin wallets, job security by cobbling together personal brands and scrappy influencer deals. One in three millennials has a side hustle just to make ends meet.

The endless upward ascent of bigger cars and bigger houses, of higher education translating into professional opportunity, and of earning more, having more, and doing more than our parents before us and their parents before them—that whole dream, brief though it was, is unraveling right in front of our eyes.

The disruptions of the recent COVID pandemic accelerated this teetering breakdown into full-fledged collapse. Aspirational luxury brands like Rolex and Chanel are going under. Private universities, used to trading on exclusivity and mystique, are struggling to justify fifty-thousand-dollar-per-year tuition for online classes that are free just one click away. At this point, it's not just the emperor who's lacking clothes—the whole royal court has been stripped naked too. It's not a good look, but you can't unsee it either.

When twenty-six people, who could all comfortably fit on a bus together (not that they'd ever ride one), own as much wealth as the poorer *half* of the world (nearly four billion people), you know we're in a strange place. That sort of asymmetric resource accumulation has never existed in all of human history, or anywhere in nature, for that matter. And it all accrued during an era where democratic, technocratic, "rising tides lift all boats" trickle-down philosophies were the dominant story.

It's not surprising that some of us have lost the plot.

*   *   *

If we bite the bullet and shoot our sacred cows, clearing the stage for a sober look at what is going on and what we might do about it, there's one final rate-limiter, one dial that we have to tweak in order to handle what's ahead: our ability to grieve.

Because if the last few pages haven't sobered you up, if seriously considering the prospects that you might not get to show your children (or grandchildren) coral reefs teeming with Finding Nemo fish, or visit Glacier National Park and actually see any of its namesake glaciers, or continue to enjoy free and fair elections, peace in the streets, or a comfortable retirement with decent health care, if all that hasn't spurred you into clearheaded action, you're in one of two places—denial or despair—neither of which will be particularly helpful on the road ahead.

If it all seems too much, denial seems like a solid option. If we aren't able to develop the cognitive complexity to handle all this, and if we hold on to our sacred cows because shooting them feels like killing everything we hold near and dear, then we will have no choice but to reject it all. Scoff, delay, deflect. Shoot the messengers. Anything other than think the unthinkable. And with the ever present distractions of our algorithmically optimized smartphone lives, denial can take an even more banal path. "And as things fell apart," the Talking Heads sang presciently, "nobody paid much attention."

On the other hand, if we stop bargaining for the idealized future we've always imagined, despair looms large. The enormity of the problems, the natural beauty and human dignity under threat. The pissing-in-the-wind futility of any effort to change things. We will break our hearts or lose our minds. But despair isn't any more effective than outright denial.

As Supreme Court Justice Oliver Wendell Holmes once advised, "I would not give a fig for the simplicity this side of complexity; but I would give my life for the simplicity the other side of complexity." Another Wendell, MacArthur Fellow Wendell Berry, wrote that we have no choice but to "be joyful, though [we] have considered all the facts."

Put together, these two Wendells might give us a plan. We shouldn't give a fig for the joy on this side of complexity, but we should be willing to give our lives for the joy on the other side of it. And that will require facing all the facts.

Identity Politics and the Infinite Game

The first fact we need to face is that we're not really stepping up to the occasion. You'd think that if we assessed the situation and concluded we're in for a biblical flood, we'd get to work filling sandbags and setting up bucket brigades. But that's not what's happening. At all. The sheer enormity of everything—from climate, geopolitics, social unrest, and pandemics on the one hand, to the collapse in Meaning on the other—is short-circuiting both our cognition and our emotions.

It's a toxic combination that's metastasizing into rage. Right when we need to be at our best, we're at our worst. Welcome to the culture wars, circa 2021.

Culture, as conservative publisher Andrew Breitbart observed, is upstream of politics. But he neglected to mention that biology sits upstream of them both. So whatever social patterns we want to defend today, we look for in the evolution of the species and past civilizations—as positive proof that the Laws of the Jungle and the Laws of Man are built from the same natural truths. We then shape the past to justify and explain our present. That always has political ramifications.

Both the far left and the alt-right correctly intuit that controlling the narrative around both the Western legacy and evolutionary biology is strategically important for their larger goals of social change. Tell the story of the way things have always been, and you own the high ground to also frame how (and why) things are the way they are now, and what we should all do next.

The left wants to tear down the Western canon because they see it as the seedbed of historic and contemporary oppression. They want to censure biology in case contemporary findings on race or gender become weaponized.

(To be fair, the past four hundred years have a tarnished record of "scientific" arguments propping up everything from the institution of slavery to chemical castration for homosexuals to wage gaps between men and women. Social activists aren't wrong to suspect that science hasn't always been a pure pursuit of knowledge free from ideology.)

The alt-right agrees. But rather than fearing those defenses of traditionalist power, they're cheering them. Trolling the libs, melting the minds of the snowflakes. Shoring up their fever-dream Aryan patriarchy one semi-ironic Reddit post at a time. #becuzaristotle and #becuz science.

In this race to the bottom, both sides might be missing the most critical insight of all: that a careful study of biology highlights how fragile, rare, and precious the humanist experiment really is.

Evolutionary biologist Bret Weinstein, himself no stranger to the culture wars, notes that "there are really two ways in which cooperation evolves. The first one is very ancient and is based on genetic relatedness. . . . The other kind of cooperation is based on various kinds of reciprocity and *it is much newer and much more fragile* [starting 10,000 years ago]. When reciprocity-based cooperation breaks down we default to gene-based cooperation. . . . Backing people against the wall who have a genetic basis for cooperation is very dangerous because history tells us . . . they may turn into a genocidal menace."

That's what puts the power in White Power. As often as not, biology beats psychology. So when we advocate for more inclusiveness, or the righting of societal wrongs, we need to pay attention to the foundation our lives are built on.

* * *

A good place to start is the neurochemistry of connection—and what happens to it in times of crisis. While evolutionary biology looks at these dynamics playing out across hundreds of generations, neurochemistry maps the bedrock of our actual experience day to day.

When people undergo sustained chronic stress due to loss of social status, economic hardships, and general dislocation (as is increasingly happening around the world), their serotonin levels get depleted.

They're more likely to behave vengefully. "According to our experiments," Oxford researcher Molly Crockett wrote in an address to the World Economic Forum, "[when] serotonin, a neurotransmitter involved in self-regulation . . . levels are low, people become more focused on immediate rewards, and they become more impulsive and aggressive."

While most people entrenched in culture wars these days will insist that they are taking stands for justice, ethics, or some other moral principle, Crockett found that subjects with depleted neurotransmitters took revenge on others even when it cost them personally. And their vindictiveness persisted even when the other person had no idea they were being punished. It feels really good to get our licks in, even when it undermines our own interests.

When we meet in large crowds like political rallies, protests, or sporting events, something else happens—both serotonin and dopamine surge. We feel better. That's a huge part of the power of crowds. But that dopamine spike kills our "hyperaltruism"—or kindness to strangers. If you've ever had to endure someone coked up at a party, that's this effect in extremis. Doped up on dopamine, we feel better, but we behave worse.

There's a final layer of neurochemistry that drives group bonding—oxytocin. While oxytocin has been touted as the "cuddle drug," the "love hormone," and even the "moral molecule" because of its ability to prompt generosity and bond mother to child and lover to lover, it, like most explanations of the biology beneath our psychology, isn't quite that simple.

"Now these studies [showing the positive effects of oxytocin] are scientifically valid, and they've been replicated," Crockett explained at TED, "but they're not the whole story. Other studies have shown that boosting oxytocin increases envy. It increases gloating. Oxytocin can bias people to favor their own group at the expense of other groups. And in some cases, oxytocin can even decrease cooperation. So based on these studies, I could say oxytocin is an immoral molecule."

Katherine Wu, a Harvard immunologist, takes it a step further. "Oxytocin [also plays] a role in ethnocentrism, increasing our love for people in our already-established cultural groups and making those unlike us seem more foreign. Thus, like dopamine, oxytocin can be a bit of a double-edged sword."

In all of this there's a vital implication we should be sure not to miss: Tribalism is the last level of social identification and belonging we are hard-coded to support. After genes and oxytocin bond us to the ones we love, and intensify our willingness to "Other" the others, everything else we aspire to is elective and not at all guaranteed.

Left to our own devices, we regress under stress. Put simply, tribalism is destiny. Humanism is optional.

The Dark Artists

That's the peril of identity politics in general. The evolutionary instinct to bond with and protect those who look, smell, and talk like us is genetically encoded—it's quite literally foundational to our survival as tribal primates. The kind of reciprocal cooperation based on mutual interest beyond our kin groups—that's incredibly recent in historical terms, and fragile.

That fragility often gets exploited. It's an old cliché that politics make for strange bedfellows, but in the case of identity politics, it gets stranger than that. Anyone seeking to smash the System, get what's coming to them, and stick it to their enemies—no matter how righteous or seemingly justified—is, at a profoundly important and structural level, on the same team. Alt-right neo-Nazis actually have more in common with far left radicals than either would be willing to admit.

A recent study at the Queensland University of Technology proved that it's not just a tribalist philosophy they share, it's a troubling psychology as well. The researchers compared over five hundred diversely representative U.S. residents whose opinions all diverged from the mainstream. They divided them into three categories: radical left, progressive liberal, and White Identity. Then they assessed how prone each group was to favor authoritarian tendencies and what psychiatrists call the Dark Triad of personality types—narcissism, Machiavellianism, and psychopathy.

Interestingly, the centrists—those people who held pro-social values but also respected the choices of others—did not show any correlation with the Authoritarian Dark Triad. But both the radical left and alt-right did. That's the basic contrast. Omni-Considerate win-win, versus self-interested win-lose.

Even though those two groups are "thought to reflect opposing ends . . . of the political spectrum," the authors wrote in the journal *Heliyon*, they held a remarkably similar psychological orientation: "Our study indicates that an emerging set of mainstream political attitudes—most notably [radical left and alt-right], are largely being adopted by individuals high in Dark Triad traits and entitlement. Individuals high in authoritarianism—*regardless of whether [they] hold politically correct or rightwing views*—tend to score highly on Dark Triad and entitlement . . . [they're] statistically more likely than average to be higher in psychopathy, narcissism, Machiavellianism and entitlement."

This study puts in sharp relief what's at stake for all of us. It provides a twenty-first-century update to Yeats's observation that "the best lack all conviction, while the worst are filled with passionate intensity." Those with a cold Will to Power can readily infiltrate and hijack otherwise well-intentioned movements. Even the noblest philosophies can get captured by sociopaths. Robespierre is the poster boy for the Dark Triad, warping the ideals of the French Revolution into the bloody Reign of Terror.

By peddling Rapture ideologies cloaked in the language of identity and belonging, Dark Artists can capitalize on unrest to advance their own agendas. And they do it by hacking into our tribal physiology.

As cathartic as it may feel to be not just right but righteous, as justified as that rage and disillusionment may be, if we go that way, it will be our undoing. Blockchain futurists, seasteading libertarians, alt-right accelerationists, and social justice advocates often fantasize about demolishing our current system so they'll have a blank slate upon which to build their Utopia. But that's a naïve and dangerous delusion. Unleash the dogs of war and they'll almost certainly come back to bite us.

To put what's at stake into some perspective, after the Vandals sacked ancient Rome, it took until the Declaration of Independence for us to claw back to the same standard of living. It's much easier to break a few eggs than to put Humpty together again.

* * *

To get some helpful perspective on the current culture wars, we need to go back a few decades. In 1987, theologian James Carse wrote a short book called *Finite and Infinite Games: A Vision of Life as Play and Possibility*. In it, he described most of human history as consisting of finite games, i.e., discrete contests with clear winners and losers. These would include war and conquest, but also transactional business, sexual negotiations, and national politics. Anything with a one up/one down outcome.

According to Carse, there was another game, the Infinite Game— which, instead of having winners and losers, creates conditions where the purpose isn't to end the game victorious. The purpose is to tune the game so everyone can keep playing it indefinitely.

We all experienced some version of this Infinite Game as children— where a bigger brother or neighbor who was dominating a game of kickball or hide-and-seek would agree to rejigger the rules when facing mutiny by dispirited younger kids. He'd give some head starts, spot points, or award first pick of teammates so it was closer to a fair fight. The big kids still loved winning but were willing to concede just enough to the losers to entice them to keep playing rather than quit the game altogether. That's the Infinite Game in miniature.

Although Carse's book didn't come out until the last decades of the twentieth century, a deeper version of the Infinite Game he was describing had been in play for at least three hundred years. It started with the French Enlightenment and a radical commitment to the inalienable rights of Man: *liberté*, *égalité*, and *fraternité* (liberty, equality, and brotherhood) for everyone, regardless of race, color, or creed.

It gained traction in the American experiment and its lurching movement toward an open, inclusive society. This messy, contradictory legacy—the one that includes the heady idealism of the Enlightenment with the bloody and tragic realities of power, oppression, and reconciliation—is the story of our fumbling efforts to move beyond the tribal imprinting of evolution and biology.

Make no mistake: Those with a home court advantage have often pulled every trick in the book to keep their upper hand. Change comes hard fought, or not at all. Abolitionists, suffragettes, unionizers, Black Panthers, Stonewall marchers, Cesar Chávez's migrant workers, antiwar pacifists, farm protesters, Sagebrush Rebels, pro-life advocates, pro-choice defenders, Occupy Wall Street protesters, Tea Party activists, and Black Lives Matter demonstrators. All of them have had to take their grievances to the public square to be heard.

Crucially, and distinct from conservative defenses of Western Civilization, an accounting of the Infinite Game also includes Frantz Fanon's withering critiques of European colonialism. It includes Noam Chomsky's dismantling American hegemony as a tenured professor at MIT. It includes Cornel West railing against the racism embedded in American culture while teaching at Harvard, Princeton, and Yale. It includes Ta-Nehisi Coates winning the National Book Award and a MacArthur Fellowship while testifying to Congress about the need for reparations for slavery.

The Infinite Game includes all these perspectives—traditional, progressive, and radical—provided they commit to keep expanding the game to include everyone—whether their side wins or loses. If we turn our backs on that notion, we don't just tear down the Dead White Males who happened to be in the right time and place in history to first put it into words and deeds, we tear up the best road map we have for a future that works for everyone.

"Because let's be real," Pulitzer Prize–winning author and MIT professor Junot Díaz wrote in *The New Yorker*. "We always knew this shit wasn't going to be easy. Colonial power, patriarchal power, capitalist power must always and everywhere be battled, because they never, ever quit. We have to keep fighting, because otherwise there will be no future—all will be consumed. . . . This is the joyous destiny of our people—to bury the arc of the moral universe so deep in justice that it will never be undone."

* * *

Which more or less brings us back to our current moment. Cynicism is so deep on all sides that it's become incredibly tempting to conclude that the whole system needs to come down. To break this stalemate we might have to give up our search for common ground, to meet each other on higher ground.

"The dream of the 18th century was that a single, coherent set of values, rooted in rationality, could make a heaven on Earth," UC Berkeley philosopher Alison Gopnik writes. "But more-recent philosophers . . . sobered by the 20th century's failed utopias, have argued for a more modest liberal pluralism that makes room for multiple, genuinely conflicting goods. Family and work, solidarity and autonomy, tradition and innovation are really valuable, and really in tension, in both the lives of individuals and the life of a nation. One challenge for enlightenment now is to build social institutions that can bridge and balance these values."

While that kind of split-the-difference compromise is often held in contempt by revolutionaries, there is a subtle genius to M.A.D.—mutually assured dissatisfaction. At its worst, this kind of strategic stalemate leads to stagnation and frustration. At its best, this sort of agonistic liberalism leads to the kinds of hard-won compromises that delight virtually no one, frustrate nearly everyone, and perversely expand the chance to keep playing the Infinite Game with more and more players, better than any other options we've found.

What's better—supply side economics à la John Keynes, or libertarian free markets à la Milton Friedman? Safety nets or bootstraps to build a just society? Big sticks or carrots to preserve international order? Federal or states' rights to guide the governed? Investing in education or employment to empower a citizenry? Separation or integration of church and state? Multicultural melting pot or national identity? Revolution or evolution?

The only honest answer is "it depends." And we're not entirely sure.

If all of life on Earth was compressed into one twenty-four-hour day, anatomically modern man shows up at four seconds before midnight. Cave paintings at one second before the end. We've only been playing at civilization for the last fraction of a second. To put how little we know in perspective, we're still not settled on the simple fact of whether eggs, butter, and coffee are the best things ever, or are going to murder us in our sleep.

So this remains our present and most pressing challenge: Can we take Alison Gopnik's advice, and dust off the battered and bruised Enlightenment experiment—the one that stops the regression into tribalism threatening both sides of the political spectrum these days—the one that aspires to get us past win-lose gamesmanship and into the win-win Infinite Game?

Because every time we've repaid oppression with oppression, it's ended in bloodshed and more suffering. The few times our Better Angels have met oppression with compassion, we've remade the world.

*   *   *

On July 2, 1776, at the Second Continental Congress in Philadelphia, all the delegates stood frozen in fear. They had just drafted the Declaration of Independence from England, but no one wanted to be the first one to sign it.

Finally Benjamin Franklin of Pennsylvania spoke up. "Gentlemen, I understand your concerns about signing this declaration. . . . But one thing I know, we must all hang together, or most assuredly we shall hang separately."

That sentiment—of collective destruction or salvation, is just as true today. In the past thirty years, identity politics of all persuasions—the idea that your race, gender, ethnicity, or ideology constitutes a certain irreducible essence of your being and of your experience, and that the only path to justice is to seek redress from those who have denied you your due—that premise comes undone at a structural level if one other thing is also true: that the next century is going to include more instability and possible hardship for all of us than any specific group's outstanding IOUs.

If we fracture now, when we should be urgently uniting, if we dig in our heels and say, "I refuse to cooperate or acknowledge the shared humanity of those not like me until I get mine," then we increase the likelihood that we all get hurt. Badly.

If we conclude that the regression into violent win-lose tribalism as the planet strains to support eight billion humans is a catastrophically bad idea, then we must also conclude, as Muhammad advised, "The enemy of my enemy is my friend." At least for now. Maybe forever.

We will need to bury our respective hatchets and grudgingly agree to work together against the pressing threats to civilization, and even the survival of our species. This does not and should not require universal consensus, nor can it wait for it. We only need to find the broadest expanse of our shared concerns, meet there in mutuality, and get to work.

CHAPTER 3

We Are the World

THERE IS NO AWAY

In the summer of 2018 I traveled with my family to the border between the United States and British Columbia. We were heading north to visit old friends in the mountains. Part of the trip was social—our kids liked each other—but the other part was practical: We were scouting locations where we might want to move. For over a decade we'd been hunting for the Last Best Place in North America to call home. A place with wild lands to adventure in and community to raise our kids.

Except at the border we got a scratchy voice mail from our friends. "Don't bother coming up," it said. "Too much smoke in the valley. We're getting out of here until we can breathe again."

Forest fires are a fixture of the American West, and the cooler latitudes of British Columbia offer only marginal relief from dry summers, careless campers, and lightning strikes. But this was different. Our maple-leaf Shangri-la wasn't even burning this time. Sweden was. "This year, it's an incredible amount of burning," said Liz Hoy, a researcher at NASA's space flight center, "and the smoke affects air quality thousands of miles away from the Arctic region."

Our imagined refuge just wasn't going to cut it. Even the "early adopters" who'd planted gardens, raised barns, and forged community in that ideal spot were suddenly refugees from events sparked off halfway around the world.

There really is no "away."

For Doomsday Preppers rejecting Ben Franklin's advice to hang together and insisting on going it alone, the wilds of British Columbia might still seem too accessible. They'd prefer to think that their own private Idaho or New Zealand or Hawaii might provide a more pristine refuge away from our problems. But consider the most extreme and remote places on the planet, like the north and south poles.

A team of researchers has recently discovered that microplastics—those tiny little pellets that break down from all of our waste—have found their way into arctic ice cores at nearly the same rate they show up in European towns. We're all eating, breathing, and absorbing the stuff. Even Santa and his elves. Even those adorable marching penguins of Antarctica.

Conditions at the highest and lowest points on Earth—Mount Everest and the Mariana Trench—aren't much better. Trash left behind by climbing expeditions—empty oxygen bottles and abandoned gear—have been a sad fixture of Himalayan base camps for decades. But it's not just climbers leaving a black mark on that mighty mountain.

John All, of Western Washington University, reported that his team at Nepal's Everest base camp found pollution buried deep in the snowpack. The samples they processed in their makeshift mountain labs were surprisingly dark with contaminants.

"There are little pieces of pollution that the snow is forming around, so the snow is actually trapping the pollution and pulling it down," Dr. All said from Kathmandu. As alpine winds whip across the tallest summit in the world, they're bringing the smog of Mumbai and Shanghai with them. So much for "mountain air fresh."

A year after the Swedish fires prompted that evacuation from British Columbia, *National Geographic* published results from deep-sea expeditions into the Mariana Trench—the deepest spot on Earth. And there, thirty-six thousand feet below sea level, a place so remote and extreme that virtually nothing can survive, a high-tech submersible snapped a photo of a discarded plastic shopping bag.

As arresting as that image is, it wasn't a fluke. "Last February," *National Geographic* reported, "a separate study showed the Mariana Trench has higher levels of overall pollution in certain regions than some of the most polluted rivers in China . . . the chemical pollutants in the trench may have come in part from the breakdown of plastic in the water column."

We can chalk both of these examples—wildfire smoke and industrial pollution in weirdly remote places—up to two forces, the jet stream and the Gulf Stream. We're on a rotating planet and air and water circulate in strong and predictable currents. What starts in one place almost always ends up someplace else. But other elements of our hyper-connectedness are new and shrinking our world whether we like it or not.

Consider air travel and the internet. Both germs and memes spread virally.

*   *   *

As far back as the Black Death in medieval Europe, scholars have traced the same wavelike pattern of epidemic infection. A virus starts in one place and ripples out at a predictable rate, limited only by the average speed of travel. In the fourteenth century, the bubonic plague hitched along the Silk Road to the seaports of Crimea and the Black Sea. The sickness then spread across Europe at roughly the rate of horse-drawn travel—about two kilometers per day.

The advent of planes, trains, and automobiles pushed that familiar wave pattern underground. Hop on a plane in Beijing and you (and any virus you were inadvertently hosting) could be in New York fourteen hours later. Attend a conference in Boston or a political rally in London and by the time you got home and started feeling sick, thousands of participants could have carried the illness almost anywhere.

That sort of near-instantaneous teleportation confounded old models of tracking disease. But once network theorists were able to correct for these accelerated rates of transport, the algorithms began to show the familiar wave pattern of transmission again.

But there's an even more recent contagion that's virtual rather than physical. And it's all made possible by the transport of ideas through fiber-optic cables and Wi-Fi signals.

To understand how viral ideas propagate and mutate, we need to examine a horrific example of global infection that makes the others seem tame—the 2012 YouTube spread of the K-pop song "Gangnam Style." That year, a strange, atonal, numbingly repetitive song exploded in popularity, becoming the first video on YouTube to pass one billion views.

Researchers have long assumed that digital memes—whether songs, tweets, videos, or jokes—follow the same pattern of growth as biological diseases. Until recently they had no way to prove it. Trying to track that telltale viral ripple of contagion was next to impossible.

If they tried to follow the geographical trail as they had for the Black Plague, "Gangnam Style" seemed to spread randomly from ground zero in South Korea across the world. According to the old modeling, it didn't make any sense.

"Geographic distance is not the key factor in the spread of information over social networks," the researchers wrote in MIT's *Technology Review*. "That depends instead on the strength of links from one area to another—places that have lots of social ties are likely to receive information more quickly than those that have weak ties."

Once they were able to correct for social distance versus physical distance, they found that the route to the worldwide domination of "Gangnam Style" matched the old wave pattern perfectly. After first getting uploaded, it hopped from South Korea to the nearby Philippines, and from there to the United States and the rest of the English-speaking world. Google Trends and Twitter mentions of the song matched the ripple effect first noticed with the Black Death: from the speed of horseback, to the speed of airplanes, until today, when the rate of transmission is limited only by the speed of our internet routers.

"The spread of modern memes occurs in just the same way as ancient diseases," the team noted. "So the 'Gangnam Style' video pandemic spread in exactly the same way as bubonic plague. That's not really a surprise. But it does confirm the extraordinarily deep link between the physical world and the world of pure information."

The knock-on effects of a world shrunken by travel, satellites, and internet cables make it nearly impossible to escape from our challenges, even at the literal top, bottom, and ends of the Earth. Pollution, disease, and gratingly catchy dance memes are all only one click away. And, as it turns out, so are Rapture ideologies. Even at the Ends of the Earth, the End of Days will find us.

The question becomes less and less about where we might run and more and more about where we must stand.

Ground Control to Major Tom

Our loyalties must transcend our race, our tribe, our class, and our nation; and this means we must develop a world perspective. . . . We must either learn to live together as brothers or we are all going to perish together as fools.

—Martin Luther King Jr.

So we appear to be stuck with each other.

The critical challenges we face all require coordinated responses. Somehow, we need to start thinking, feeling, and acting more globally. But making that move to a perspective that includes the whole world is hard.

In fact, it's never really been done. After oxytocin-induced tribalism, everything more expansive and inclusive is up for grabs. Always has been. From time to time, in the lulls and lucky moments, small groups of idealists have entertained notions of equality and mutuality, but it has rarely lasted. And it's never been tried as a "full stack" project including everyone, everywhere, all at once.

At this point, it's not even an idealistic or romantic notion to shoot for—it's rational self-preservation. As Elon Musk said recently when challenged why he would give away all the technology behind his battery patents, "It makes no sense to be the only person sitting in the lifeboat." Even Machiavelli and Sun Tzu would have to agree.

If we're going to try to boost our collective problem-solving and decision-making to the level required, we're going to have to grow up—fast. But to do that we need to understand the research on how we grow in the first place. Because how we make our way from one level of development to the next holds a key insight we might otherwise miss.

One of the simple facts of life is the notion of "recursive development"—namely, that as we grow up we are forever going two steps forward, one step back.

One of the most familiar examples is the developmental stage every parent dreads—the Terrible Twos.

When a baby comes into the world, it has a hard time telling where Mommy ends and Me begins. It's all one embryonic fusion of food, warmth, and heartbeats. But sometime between eighteen and twenty-four months, something changes. The baby notices something profound. There's Me, and there's Not Me. And all the Not Me's (starting with Mommy) are subject to my will. Cry and they come running. Reach and I get fed. Coo and I get hugged. Look them straight in the eyes and chuck that rattle on the floor and just see what happens! And it's that specific act of the baby realizing the existence of the Other that cements their identification with themselves.

The same thing happens when we make the next move from ego-centric to ethnocentric living. In order to really bond to our family or tribe, we need to go beyond "us" to define "them." We, as a working concept, can only exist in contrast to They. The Other. The folks across the river who look, dress, and smell funny, talk funny, and worship strange gods not at all like ours. And the worse we say they are, the better We begin to sound (and feel). That's tribalism—"Us" versus "Them."

So how can we make the move from ethnocentric to global-centric perspective—where we invite all those Others into an even bigger tent—a "We" that includes everyone everywhere?

It follows that the surest way to experience a global point of view is to go one whole step beyond it to a universal perspective. We, just like the Terrible-Two-year-old, would have to peer beyond our current position. In this case, we'd have to go beyond the terrestrial world to the universe in which it sits.

In the past, that was an incredibly rare move. The saints and sages of the Axial Age—Jesus, Plato, Zoroaster, Buddha, Lao-tzu—all had some universal insight that transcended tribe and allegiance. But virtually no one truly picked up what they were laying down, and many of their profound insights got co-opted. "In truth," Nietzsche wryly observed, "there was only one Christian and he died on the cross."

* * *

These days, the best contemporary examples of the global-centric perspective we're talking about come from those who have literally left the world behind—astronauts. It wasn't until the Apollo space missions of the late 1960s that anyone had ever actually departed our home planet and come back to tell about it.

On July 20, 2019, *The Washington Post* released a report in honor of the fiftieth anniversary of the Apollo 11 moon landing. They interviewed 50 astronauts of the 570 who have ever been to space. NASA shuttle pilots. Russian cosmonauts. Afghanis, Malaysians, and cash-on-the-barrel-head civilians.

Even the famously tight-lipped Neil Armstrong couldn't help himself from marveling as he looked back on his experience. "It suddenly struck me that that tiny pea, pretty and blue, was the Earth," he said. "I put up my thumb and shut one eye, and my thumb blotted out the planet Earth. I didn't feel like a giant. I felt very, very small."

In 1988, as the Soviet-Afghan war was grinding along, Abdul Ahad Mohmand, Afghanistan's first and only cosmonaut, flew to the Mir space station with two Russians. When he reached orbit and took in the entire scene, he spoke to the Afghan president by phone. "I said that the war should end, that we should all unite. That people, particularly Afghans, didn't need this war." Cosmic perspective had yielded a strategic insight.

In 2013, Canadian astronaut Chris Hadfield had some time to kill on the International Space Station. So he picked up the guitar that was floating around, hit record on a video camera, and began singing an old David Bowie tune. Fifty million downloads later, his cover of Bowie's "Space Oddity," with its iconic "ground control to Major Tom" verse, had thoroughly captured people's imagination. Alone in space, singing a song we all knew the words to, Hadfield brought the world a little closer together.

As inspired and inspiring as these testimonies are, there's one problem: Becoming an astronaut in order to glimpse global unity is a small-batch solution to a large-scale problem. Hardly anyone makes it through NASA's grueling selection and training, and virtually no one else has a spare quarter of a million dollars (the going rate on Virgin Galactic's presale) to shoot the moon.

Meanwhile, the rest of us need whatever it was those astronauts were having. Soon.

*   *   *

Sometimes all it takes is a hint of Cosmic Otherness to bring us together. In a recent study on racial bias, researchers interviewed white householders, testing for their responses to people of color ringing their doorbell. In conservative areas, there was a noticeable increase in neutral to negative word choice by white homeowners when engaging visitors of color compared to white canvassers. They also shortened the time that they engaged the newcomers before ending the conversation and closing the door. Sad to read about, but not that surprising.

But then the team tweaked the setup: They informed the homeowners that there had been a recent discovery of alien life. Nothing especially complex about the narrative—no deep dives into Area 51 or *Independence Day* scenarios—just the simple fact that We Are Not Alone after all.

That nudge—to consider ourselves as humans together in the face of something weirder and even more Other, was enough to meaningfully boost openness and receptivity to strangers. White folks greeted

Black and Brown folks more warmly. Racism appears to be a weaker bond than species-ism. If it's humans against little green men, the color of *our* skin seems to be less important.

*   *   *

But hoping that alien contact will inspire global unity isn't a viable strategy for a simple reason—sheer probability. Sure, if it happened it would be the Black Swan to end all Black Swans. But waiting around for it, despite all the curious hints from places like the Pentagon and the Vatican, still seems like longer odds than the more certain unraveling of things we're facing. Until we have our very own Close Encounter we're going to have to explore other ways to expand our cosmic perspective.

To do that, we have to crack Fermi's paradox, named for famous physicist Enrico Fermi, who asked: If there's a nearly infinite number of planets and galaxies, how come we seem to be the only ones here? There are dozens of competing theories to explain that unavoidable fact—from the Great Filter thesis suggesting that either we're the only ones to have got this far, or every more advanced civilization has already snuffed it, to the Dark Forest theory, which suggests the best thing to do in a universe teeming with intelligent and likely hostile life is HIDE!

But in an interview with Singularity University, the futurist John Smart suggests something else again—the idea that advanced extraterrestrial life probably wouldn't still be banging about in three-dimensional space-time in the first place.

According to Smart, the reason that projects like Search for Extraterrestrial Intelligence (SETI) that ping radio- and microwaves into deep space have failed is that they are naïve and reductionist in their thinking. It's a bit like the old *Far Side* cartoon where the scientists are trying with no success to speak to dolphins and one says, "Matthews, we're getting another one of those strange 'ah-blah-es-panyol' sounds." We might not be having any luck talking to our galactic brethren because we're insisting they conform to our limited modes of communication.

"Advanced species don't colonize outer space—an idea they'd find archaic," Smart suggests, "but instead colonize inner space. . . . Evolutionary processes in our universe might lead all advanced civilizations towards the same ultimate destination; one in which we transcend out of our current space-time dimension into virtual worlds of our own design."

That idea of advanced civilizations creating immersive virtual worlds was popularized by Oxford philosopher Nick Bostrum's simulation hypothesis. It proposes that all of humanity is living in a simulation created by more intelligent beings. Smart, though, doesn't think that simulation theory takes things far enough. It's not that we're trapped inside a video game, it's that all of our cosmic brethren slipped outside 3D reality a long time ago. And they are running wild in the multiverse. According to Smart, we've been looking in the wrong place for the galactic party.

*   *   *

At first glance, a wild and speculative theory like the transcension hypothesis seems impossible to validate. But researchers are wading in anyway. Scientists at both Imperial College in London and Johns Hopkins University are beginning to map "hyperspace"—the realm users of the potent psychedelic DMT (dimethyltryptamine) report entering. It's one of the most likely stomping grounds of all those Transcended Civilizations. In one early study in the 1990s at the University of New Mexico, researcher Rick Strassman and his team found that over 50 percent of subjects under the influence of intravenous DMT contacted alien beings and had otherworldly experiences that felt "as or more real than everyday waking reality."

The same research team at Hopkins that only a few years ago was cautiously reporting that 3 grams of psilocybin mushrooms was helping patients with mundane issues like smoking cessation and anxiety, is now plainly asking study subjects if they contact entities while hurtling through hyperspace. And if so, *which kinds*? Angelic beings? Machine Elves? Grays? Or perhaps those Giant Praying Mantises?

Which brings to mind Hunter Thompson's drug-fueled hallucinations in *Fear and Loathing in Las Vegas.* "No point in mentioning these bats," he concluded. "The poor bastard[s] will see them soon enough." The fourth wall between objective materialist science and multidimensional possibility has been thoroughly kicked down. Mapping the Mysto has begun.

If that Hopkins study seems far-fetched, the Imperial College team is standing up a project that beggars the imagination. A "conventional" DMT experience usually ranges from five to fifteen minutes but often leaves users with a sense of departing that otherworldly domain almost as soon as they've arrived. Mapping that terrain is a bit like trying to paint a portrait while bouncing on a trampoline. The Imperial team has refined a process by which intravenous DMT can be delivered continuously to a subject, keeping them in hyperspace for hours at a time. With these extended sessions, Imperial hopes to begin exploring this territory in a more systematic way.

In a page eerily out of the MK-ULTRA playbook (a notorious CIA psyops project that focused on all things Weird and Weaponizable), they are hoping to test precognition and remote viewing between subjects. As these psychonauts step out of conventional time and consciousness, the researchers hypothesize that they might access information that is non-local and non-ordinary. In other words, otherworldly.

Ever since Albert Einstein first conducted his famous thought experiments scrambling past, present, and future together, we've at least known intellectually that what happened before and what comes after are more subjective than we'd like to admit. The Imperial College team is hoping that their study will take this inquiry out of the realm of thought experiment and into the world of physical experiment.

But even stranger than that, they are trying to establish contact with the entities of hyperspace and *to begin a dialogue.* Which brings to mind the cautionary tale of Dr. Faustus selling his soul for knowledge, and the setup of countless sci-fi horror movies that start out in the basement of a medical school somewhere.

Might a definitive contact with the Other be enough to knock ourselves out of our tribal fixations? That Terrible-Two-year-old needs to realize there's Mommy in order to become fully aware of Me. The tribe has to define the Other across the river to affirm the Us that lives in our village. Could we actually live into a shared humanity by spying the Great Unknown that lies beyond us?

Despite tantalizing hints and suggestions, our search for E.T. in 3D has consistently come up short. Since we can't all become astronauts adventuring outward into the universe, maybe we can become psychonauts venturing inward toward the multiverse. Or as Smart would call us, we could become "Engineers of inner space."

If we could become more skillful in the exploration of our minds, and of reality itself, we would inevitably reframe our sense of our own significance in the Big Scheme of Things. For a species that seems to forever trip over our own sense of importance, a healthy dose of awe, wonder, and humility could be good for what ails us.

Hamlet was right. There are more things on heaven and earth than we dreamt of in our philosophies after all.

The Intertwingularity

Unfortunately, it's those philosophies that are causing half the trouble.

As we approach what many people are imagining to be the End of History, it's increasingly unlikely we're heading toward a slickly choreographed Singularity. Ray Kurzweil won't be there to usher us across the silicon Pearly Gates. We're going to have to navigate this one ourselves.

Instead, it's looking more and more like an *Intertwingularity*. As we search for some kind of coherent explanation for a world in turmoil, everyone's favorite mythologies are smashing, crashing, and blending into each other. It's getting near impossible to separate signal from noise.

To be sure, there are social media algorithms amplifying our worst instincts, geopolitical players weaponizing content, and fringe theorists confusing things almightily—but these seeds are landing in especially fertile soil in our minds right now—and here's why.

Our little amygdalas, oxytocin, and dopamine.

Given that the last few years have contained decades' worth of shocks and destabilizing developments, it's fair to say that our amygdalas—our threat detection systems—have been on super high alert. Whether it's been surprise election results, natural disasters, or global pandemics, it really has mattered what's going on in other countries, other states, even right next door. Our impulse to stay on top of every breaking news item, every hot take, and every "expert opinion" has skyrocketed.

In the olden days we would've been listening to jungle drums, smoke signals, or village gossip. Now it's morphed into Facebook and Instagram posts, YouTube binge watches, and WhatsApp groups. We're all desperate to get a handle on what might save us or kill us.

Each time we listen to that amygdala alarm clock and find something that Stanford's Robert Sapolsky calls "salient"—meaning it might make us or break us—we get a strong squirt of dopamine. Even if the news is shitty, it feels perversely good to have found it. Plug that "like," click, or comment into Big Tech optimization algorithms, and we're off on a self-reinforcing ride of our lives.

But a funny thing happens when we get too much dopamine in our systems. We succumb to apophenia. It's the tendency to perceive patterns and meaning between otherwise unconnected events and facts. It shows up in early onset schizophrenia and in conspiracy theorists.

That's not all. Especially when we're all cooped up, separated from each other, unable to hug, kiss, and hang out with our friends and family, our oxytocin levels plummet. This leaves us less trusting, more suspicious, and prone to paranoia.

In the paper "Oxytocin, Dopamine, and the Amygdala: A Neurofunctional Model of Social Cognitive Deficits in Schizophrenia," Andrew Rosenfeld, a psychiatrist at the University of Vermont, and his colleagues lay it out: "Aberrant interactions between dopaminergic reward systems, a dysfunctional amygdala, and the neurohormone oxytocin engender a neural milieu that improperly assigns emotional salience to environmental stimuli. This deficit in turn results in aberrant social cognition that may ultimately lead to misguided social responses, from withdrawal and isolation to suspicion and paranoia."

Put more simply: We're overcooked, overclocked, and losing our minds. Even familiar and comforting narratives are breaking down. Into this vacuum, all sorts of wild stories are rising up to fill their place.

* * *

When we're considering End of Days Rapture Ideologies, there's less difference between what's written on ancient papyrus, celluloid, and comic books than we might think. All our mythologies, both contemporary and historic, are products of human imagination expressed in language and image—it's only the format that has changed over the years.

Take two of the most popular epic tales of recent times—*Star Wars* and *The Matrix*—and we can see how once heroic and unifying stories are splintering under the tensions of the Intertwingularity.

When *Star Wars* debuted in 1977, it told the rousing tale of Luke Skywalker, Princess Leia, Han Solo, and the rest of the Rebel Alliance battling the Evil Empire. At the eleventh hour, Luke shot an improbably lucky torpedo down the exhaust tubes of the Death Star and delivered victory to Team Good Guy. For millions of fans, the whole thing felt profoundly resonant. It was the *Odyssey* and the *Wizard of Oz* retooled for the space age.

But fast-forward forty years to the eighth installment of the franchise, *Star Wars: The Last Jedi*, and things weren't quite so simple anymore. The familiar plotline of good vs. bad was fracturing. A story that had once united audiences was now dividing them.

With the young girl Rey replacing Luke as the central character, a black Stormtrooper as her best friend, a Latino pilot (standing in for the wisecracking Han Solo), and an Asian woman all getting major screen time, traditional Hollywood casting had been turned upside down.

Many die-hard fans, often Middle American males, found themselves written out of leading roles. They weren't happy. On the review aggregator site Rotten Tomatoes, the gap between critics and fans clocked in at 90 to 42 percent in the opening weeks—the widest of any film in the history of the franchise.

"Good and evil doesn't seem quite so clear," the film critic Dave

Schilling writes about *Star Wars: The Last Jedi*. "Everyone's hands are dirty in one way or another. Greed, lust for power, and self-interested cynicism won out. Whatever New Hope *Star Wars* represented in 1977 is in retreat. How can one make a cathartic action romp about space Nazis in a time when actual Nazis are reasserting themselves in the national political conversation? Simple: you make a movie about how hope dies."

The once unifying narrative that inspired Ronald Reagan to christen his antinuclear missile defense system "Star Wars" and call the Soviet Union "the Evil Empire" has flipped. Former White House adviser Steve Bannon argues, "Darkness is good . . . Dick Cheney. Darth Vader. Satan. That's power." Meanwhile, Republican strategists celebrate the construction of an electoral "Death Star" to hijack social media and bend elections.

It's fair to say that things have taken a turn since that Long Time Ago in a Galaxy Far, Far Away when we all sat entranced, bonded by the story unfolding in front of us.

*   *   *

It's not just *Star Wars* that's gone off the rails lately. *The Matrix*—a parable about seeing behind the illusion of the conventional world into a darker but more heroic battle underneath—has also been hijacked by competing interpretations of What It All Means.

The film famously expressed the chasm between initiates and the ignorant. Neo, the main character, finds himself pulled out of his numbing cubicle job as a software programmer into an alternate reality filled with danger and purpose.

The character of Morpheus (a nod to Ovid's god of sleep) offers Neo a choice between two pills—the Red Pill and the Blue Pill. "This is your last chance," he tells Neo. "After this, there is no turning back. You take the blue pill—the story ends, you wake up in your bed and believe whatever you want to believe. You take the red pill—you stay in Wonderland, and I show you how deep the rabbit hole goes. Remember, all I'm offering is the truth—nothing more."

That was the line that launched a thousand memes. Since the film's premiere in 1999, Red Pills have come to stand in for meditation, men's work, psychedelics, leadership advice, cybersecurity, and pretty much any product or service where someone believes someone else needs to be radically disillusioned about what they hold to be true.

For the better part of twenty years, that held up. Sheeple, Muggles, Basics—those were the sort of boring or cowardly folks who opted for the simple comfort of taking the Blue Pill. But the brave, heroic, and courageous, convinced there has to be something more to life? The "Crazy Ones" who shared Apple's Think Different ad campaign with all their friends? Red Pillers, every last one of them.

That was the Big Tent Matrix, roomy enough to hold free thinkers and rebels of every stripe. Until 2016, when a growing online men's movement on Reddit and 4chan message boards shrank the tent considerably. It redefined being "Red Pilled" as the experience of white men finally waking up to a world where the deck is firmly stacked against them. According to this community, they had to band together to defeat the forces of globalism, feminism, and reverse racism directed their way.

In 2019, *Wired* magazine editor Emma Ellis wrote, "This reading of Neo's choice is so widespread that it's made its way to some very unlikely places—like Kanye West's Twitter account." Her co-author, Emily Dreyfuss, wrote, "Its meaning has been totally corrupted. . . . It's hard to talk about the Aristotelian ideal of the blue or red pill as it was meant to be. Now it's something else."

Darth Vader—unsung hero of the White House. Rebel Alliance as totalitarian thought police. Black stormtroopers, white masks. Red Pillers as freedom fighters against the machine. Red Pillers as "deluded misogynist trolls." These days it's better to never leave home than try to find our way to a happy ending.

A Lion in Zion

Given the stakes and the increasing likelihood of Intertwingular crossed wires these days, it's only going to get more intense. After all, the worst that happens when movie fans differ are flame wars on Rotten Tomatoes and Reddit. But for other, older, even more sacred stories? Some people are willing to die for them.

When it comes to holy scripture—there's text, there's subtext, and then there's context. "Both read the bible day and night," William Blake once wrote, "but where you see black, I see white!"

* * *

On May 14, 2018, something momentous but also kind of strange happened in Israel. After years of talking about it, the United States moved its embassy from Tel Aviv to the historical capital of Jerusalem.

That's the momentous part. The strange part will take a bit of explaining.

For decades, campaigning U.S. presidential candidates had promised to make that switch official, but once in office none had ever followed through. Bill Clinton made it a part of his 1992 run against George H. W. Bush, calling out the elder Bush for "repeatedly challenging Israel's sovereignty over a united Jerusalem." On the 2008 trail, Barack Obama went further: "Jerusalem will remain the capital of Israel, and it must remain undivided." On this much, at least, Republicans and Democrats seemed to agree.

But once in office, they balked. It was too tricky to navigate. Too much at stake. Move the embassy from Tel Aviv and you'd send a clear signal to Israel, one of the United States' strongest and longest-serving allies, that you were committed to both its past and its future. But take away Palestinian claim to at least part of that holy city, and you'd lose the United States' role as a good-faith meditator of Arab-Israeli peace. It was a lot for anyone to navigate.

So when a U.S. delegation showed up at the Jerusalem consulate in the middle of that May it really was momentous. Decades of positioning, posturing, and equivocating had finally been resolved. The move was happening.

But those years of hesitation proved well founded too. In the twenty-four hours leading up to the ceremony, riots broke out involving tens of thousands of protesters and military along the Gaza-Israel border.

Twenty-seven hundred people were injured. Fifty-six died. Israeli prime minister Netanyahu and Palestinian Authority president Abbas weighed in, as did the secretary-general of the United Nations.

This is where things got strange. As tear gas and tires burned in Gaza, an unassuming sixty-something Baptist minister from Dallas, Texas, took the stage in Old Jerusalem. He positioned himself behind the embassy podium, adjusted the microphone, and led the assembled dignitaries in prayer.

"We come before you, the God of Abraham, Isaac, and Jacob, thanking you for bringing us to this momentous occasion in the life of your people and in the history of our world." He praised the leadership of both governments, adding that the embassy move "boldly stands on the right side of history but more importantly stands on the right side of you, O God, when it comes to Israel."

From a typical minister, those words might have seemed innocuous. But Robert Jeffress is not your typical minister. Pastor of First Baptist Church in Dallas, Texas, he oversees a multimillion-dollar radio, media, education, and worship ministry (including a $130 million megachurch built in 2013). Jeffress has emerged as one of the more culturally and politically influential evangelical preachers of the past decade. And he's drawn as much controversy as praise.

In the week leading up to the embassy ceremony, former Republican governor, presidential nominee, and senator Mitt Romney flatly challenged Jeffress's attendance, tweeting, "Such a religious bigot should not be giving the prayer that opens the United States embassy in Jerusalem. . . . Jeffress says 'you can't be saved by being a Jew,' and 'Mormonism is a heresy from the pit of hell.'"

Those weren't awkward sound bites taken out of context, either. Jeffress doubled down on his position, tweeting back to Romney, "Historic Christianity has taught for 2,000 years that salvation is through faith in Christ alone. The fact that I, along with tens of millions of evangelical Christians around the world, continue to espouse that belief, is neither bigoted nor newsworthy."

But that day in Jerusalem it was newsworthy. If Jeffress believes that Jews, Mormons, and Muslims too are all going to hell, why was he the one offering the opening prayers at the embassy? What part could all those nonbelievers gathered in Jerusalem play in Jeffress's larger ambitions?

In two words, Christian Zionism: the idea that Jesus Christ will return to earth once Israel is a sovereign state again. That's why Jeffress was so fired up to mark the occasion. Moving the embassy was bringing us all one step closer to the fulfillment of scripture and the End of Days.

Christian Zionism has roots that stretch back centuries, with supporters ranging from U.S. presidents to Martin Luther King Jr. But it reached a tipping point in the last half-century, due in large part to Tim LaHaye's *Left Behind* Christian novels. This blockbuster series describes the aftermath of the Rapture—where all faithful Christians are brought straight up to heaven and the Leftovers have to figure out what to do next. With well over one hundred million combined copies in print, televangelist Jerry Falwell acknowledged that *Left Behind*, "in terms of its impact on Christianity, is probably greater than that of any other book in modern times, outside the Bible."

According to Christian Zionism, God restored the nation of Israel to the Jews in 1948 (not coincidentally, seventy years to the day of the recent embassy ceremony). This reestablished the kingdom of Israel and set up a clear path to the End Times foretold in the books of Revelation, Daniel, Isaiah, and Ezekiel. According to those accounts, after a cataclysmic battle with the Antichrist, Jesus will return and usher in a thousand-year reign of peace. And the Jews? They will realize what Jeffress has been talking about and all convert to Christianity.

But before that essential fulfillment of Christian theology, Israel has to rule an undivided Jerusalem and the entire Middle East has to descend into the "war to end all wars." Which, when you think back to the tinderbox of tensions surrounding the embassy announcement in May 2018, makes it a deeply puzzling diplomatic decision to put a Christian Zionist preacher onstage at all. Almost everyone else gathered there was invested in avoiding a regional meltdown. But for Jeffress that unraveling can't come soon enough.

Jeffress is in no way alone in his thinking. According to the Pew Research Foundation, 58 percent of American evangelicals believe that the Second Coming is going to occur before 2050. Consider that for a minute. Saving for retirement? No point. Transitioning off fossil fuels? Why bother? Saving endangered species or solving world hunger? That would just be playing God when He's coming again, soon enough.

To be clear, United States citizens have always enjoyed remarkable freedom to worship who, what, when, and how they wanted. That long and principled tradition separating church and state has always been one of this country's greatest strengths.

But when church and state come under the sway of powerful religious beliefs based upon outlier interpretations of texts written thousands of years ago, in times and places that bear little resemblance to our current world, we should pay attention. In the great conversations of our time, we're not only not on the same page, we're not even in the same books.

And Christian Zionists aren't the only ones betting on a final showdown in Jerusalem. As it turns out, the historic city is double-booked for the End of Days.

*   *   *

The Islamic State in Iraq and Syria (ISIS), the most recent and grisly face of Islamic extremism, has an End Times tale too, based on one of the hadiths, or holy sayings attributed to the Prophet Muhammad. According to their reading, ISIS is expecting a series of major battles against the "Armies of Rome" (loosely interpreted to mean Turkey, Israel, or the United States) where they will get massacred down to their last five thousand fighters. "On this theory, even setbacks dealt to the Islamic State mean nothing," the *Atlantic*'s Graeme Wood writes, "since God has preordained the near-destruction of his people anyway. The Islamic State has its best and worst days ahead of it."

Which is kind of weird to wrap your head around. Our usual military reference points rest on twentieth-century notions like realpolitik, détente, and mutually assured destruction. But that logic of incentives and deterrents breaks down when your adversaries think in such topsy-turvy ways.

Kill ISIS's soldiers and they're energized, because you're bringing them closer to their predicted decimation (and ultimate victory). Target their leaders with drone strikes and they inch one step closer to celebrating the arrival of the Mahdi—the twelfth (final and triumphant) caliph. No matter how nerve-racking the Cold War might have been, at least it operated on a game-theory rationale of self-preservation shared by the major players.

And the final part of ISIS's end game? You couldn't make it up. According to their script, their own near annihilation will usher in two saviors: the Mahdi—that divinely anointed caliph who will reunite the nations of Islam—and a second prophet, who will defeat the Antichrist.

But it's not the Prophet Muhammad as you might think—it's Jumping Jesus himself, praised in the Koran as the Messiah and the living "word of God." At morning prayer on the appointed day, Jesus will kill the Anti-Messiah with a spear. He will then "break the cross," a symbolic action that lets Christians know that the death and resurrection taught in their faith is mistaken, and that in reality He never actually died. In a perfect mirror of the Christian Zionists predicting that all Jews would convert at the last minute, ISIS believes that all Christians will then see the error of their faith and convert to Islam on the spot.

Which leaves us in as much of a bind as the other version. Because as polar opposite as the game plans for Christian Zionists and ISIS are, as strangely overlapping as their Jerusalem setting and cast of characters may be, they both share an underlying structure or rapture ideology. And it's this overlapping format that is proving so troubling to anyone interested in happy days on the road ahead, regardless of where you live or what you believe.

*   *   *

The Intertwingularity has become a giant muddy Meme Soup, unmoored from any kind of narrative continuity whatsoever. We might even look at the same things, agree that what we're looking at is both real and important, but come to completely opposite conclusions about what it means and what we should all do next.

Whether it's billionaire philanthropists saving the world or secretly scheming to take it over, or Deep State conspiracies plotting to hijack democracy or preserve it, or Antichrists masquerading as messiahs— it's getting nearly impossible to sort through it all and come to trustworthy conclusions.

As the Intertwingularity sucks us down the drainpipe of time and space, it's not likely to play out exactly like anyone's stories predict. It's entirely possible that the Great Sorting Hat at the End of Time won't give a damn which side we thought we were on—Rebel or Stormtrooper, Red Pill or Blue—but only on our intentions. Which flag we flew, which uniform we wore will yield to something much simpler. Were we coming from fear or love? Were we standing for all of us or only some of us? Were we playing for Team Finite, or Team Infinite?

Chapter 4

Designing Meaning 3.0

So this is where we find ourselves: in the midst of a Meaning Crisis, at the End of Time. The collapse in Meaning 1.0—organized religion—has left us with a vacuum in the center of civic life. This happened just as the rate of exponential change in everything else was going through the roof.

But Meaning 2.0, what we might term the religion of classical liberalism—the belief that free markets and democracy will usher us all forward to an era of equality and prosperity—has come up short as well. When Nobel Prize–winning economists like Joseph Stiglitz are calling foul on the entire shell game, it's fair to say that late-stage capitalism has lost its shine. The current fragmentation of identity politics suggests that if people's needs aren't met via "trickle-down globalism," they are more than willing to smash the system and grab what they feel they've got coming to them.

If Meaning 1.0 was all about salvation for the faithful, Meaning 2.0 has been about inclusion of the masses. Religion has always promised inspiration, healing, and connection, but it did so at the cost of identifying an elect who deserved such perks, and nonbelievers who didn't.

Meaning 2.0—with its extension of inalienable rights to everyone regardless of belief or background, offered inclusion—but at the price of salvation. That was what Nietzsche was talking about when he observed that "God is dead." We got the vote, the fridge, and the smartphone, but we forgot what it was all for. That has played a large part in the rise of diseases of despair.

Fundamentalism on one hand and nihilism on the other. Neither is especially helpful. *to you* .

So the question for us is what Meaning 3.0 might look like. Can we architect culture that balances the salvation of traditional religion with the inclusion of liberalism? Can we do it not by top-down fiat but rather by bottom-up mobilization?

And is truly inclusive salvation even a thing we can hope for?

Wonder Bread and Magic Pencils

September 1989, NASA Johnson Space Center, Texas. A member of a visiting Soviet delegation wanted to see a little of the "real America." So he asked his handlers to arrange a visit to a Houston grocery store.

According to a piece in the *Houston Chronicle* at the time, the Russian "roamed the aisles of Randall's grocery store nodding his head in amazement." He seemed especially taken with the open freezer bays packed with TV dinners and pudding pops. He told his delegation that if Muscovites who had to queue in long lines for daily essentials saw the conditions of U.S. supermarkets, "there would be a revolution."

"Even the Politburo doesn't have this choice. Not even Mr. Gorbachev," he said.

Afterward, it wasn't the mockup of the space station, or NASA's mission control that obsessed him. It was that grocery store. "When I saw those shelves crammed with hundreds, thousands of cans, cartons and goods of every possible sort," he later wrote in his biography, "for the first time I felt quite frankly sick with despair for the Soviet people."

Two years later, that curious delegate, Boris Yeltsin, played a major role in unwinding the Soviet Union. He'd go on to serve as Russia's first post-communist president. And what boggled his mind in Houston is something we should all pay more attention to, because it has direct implications for our road ahead.

Beyond the simple abundance he witnessed, Yeltsin couldn't wrap his head around how it all got done. Thousands of products and vendors and somehow all of it arrived fresh, on time, and in overwhelming quantity.

To which Adam Smith would have replied—the Invisible Man got it all done. Or at least, his Invisible *Hand*—the miracle of the free market. A thousand small decisions, each made in a frictionless environment by a thousand independent actors, all resulting in a sublime concert of grocery greatness (and pudding pops).

In 1958, the conservative economist Leonard Read wrote a short story called "I, Pencil." In it he described, from the point of view of a lowly pencil, how many people and decisions had to come together to make himself possible.

"I, Pencil, am a complex combination of miracles," Read wrote, "a tree, zinc, copper, graphite, and so on. But to these miracles which manifest themselves in Nature an even more extraordinary miracle has been added: the configuration of creative human energies—millions of tiny know-hows configurating naturally and spontaneously in response to human necessity and desire and in the absence of any human masterminding!"

Read's libertarian parable might sound a bit dated these days. But it does include a vital truth: All of us, unencumbered in our choices, make richer, more varied, and more adaptive decisions than even the smartest bureaucrats. In our search for collective solutions we'd do well to remember the lesson of the Little Pencil That Could.

Because the Soviet state that Yeltsin helped dismantle isn't the only top-down centralization we should be wary of. Ironically, capitalism has created its own mutation. We're in the age of philanthrocapitalism— where Bill Gates, Eric Schmidt, Mark Zuckerberg, Jeff Bezos, and others, after ruthlessly crushing competitors and exploiting offshore tax havens, are now redirecting their historic fortunes toward solving many of the problems they helped create (and to be fair, a few they had no part of).

As much as it's tempting to sit back, secretly relieved that our Iron Man Super Geniuses are going to swoop in to save us, the strategy is flawed.

There are several reasons philanthrocapitalism doesn't work as well as we need it to.

First, it absolves us of reviving dysfunctional democratic responses. Our systems for addressing social needs are broken, but the solution is to fix them at the local level, not bypass them altogether.

Second, it's a massively inefficient redistribution of capital. There's an enormous amount of humanitarian and civil engineering that is not sexy at all, and may never catch the eye of a major donor. Waiting for earmarked handouts from the digital Robber Barons is a lopsided way to address a broad portfolio of civic needs.

Third, and worth unpacking in detail, is the lesson of Yeltsin's grocery store and Mr. Pencil. Centralized decision-making is no match for a thousand micro-decisions made on the ground. No one, not even Gates or Bezos, is that smart. "Winning" in one domain, such as technology, is no guarantee of success in alternate domains. Move one step away from what made you rich and famous, Bain and Company's Chris Zook writes in *Profit from the Core*, and you have a 33 percent chance of succeeding. Move four steps away and that number has plummeted to 6 percent.

So a tech nerd like Bill Gates, who was in the right time and place in the '80s and '90s to realize his vision of "a computer on every desk running Microsoft software"—now reaching out to coordinate global health responses for the Bottom Billion people on the planet? It's not to say he can't help, but it is to say it's longer odds than the puff pieces in *Forbes* and *Bloomberg* might suggest.

The public feels increasingly uneasy about this too. The year 2020 saw a spike in conspiratorial concern over Gates's advocacy for vaccines in response to the coronavirus pandemic. It prompted deep questions about giving a nonelected individual such an outsize influence in a global health response.

But there's an even simpler test case of the unintended consequences of philanthrocapitalism—Gates's efforts to rid the world of malaria. Clever people at his foundation crunched large numbers and concluded that if you were trying to save as many lives as possible in the developing world, you'd eradicate malaria. And the best bang for your buck would be to distribute as many mosquito nets as possible.

Simple. Elegant. Efficient.

But the on-the-ground realities turned out to be different. "The narrative has always been, 'Spend $10 on a net and save a life,'" Amy Lehman, founder of the Lake Tanganyika Floating Health Clinic, told *The New York Times*. "But what if that net is distributed in a waterside, food-insecure area where maybe you won't be affecting the malaria rate at all and you might actually be hurting the environment?" Analysts found that 87.2 percent of villagers surrounding Lake Tanganyika in Africa ended up using their mosquito nets to fish. "That," Lehman added, "is not a very neat story to tell."

MacArthur fellow Paul Farmer, founder of Partners in Health, agrees. "It doesn't surprise me that as someone who has made his fortune on developing a novel technology, Bill Gates would look for 'magic bullets' in vaccines and medicines. But if we don't have a solid delivery system, this work will be thwarted. That's something that's going to be hard for the big foundations . . . they treat tuberculosis. They don't treat poverty."

It's not that the malaria net initiative was especially ill-conceived or poorly executed. It's just that solving for complex "wicked" problems is incredibly difficult. And it's exponentially harder the further you drift from grassroots response. We need to foster more localized solutions to global challenges. We need to update I, Pencil, with its emphasis on the invisible hand of the market, into We, Humans, and our collective wisdom and resourcefulness.

It might be time to put down our mosquito nets and go be fishers of men.

Riding the Lightning

While the New Atheists like Christopher Hitchens and Richard Dawkins initially celebrated that collapse in religion, we've lost many of
the pro-social elements that Faith used to convey. We're suffering in
their absence. After all, religion, as a cultural meme, would not have
persisted for tens of thousands of years if it didn't convey an adaptive
advantage.

And it does. Far beyond religion's function as an "opiate of the
masses," believers are generally wealthier, healthier, and happier than
nonbelievers. In their 2019 report *Religion's Relationship to Happiness,
Civic Engagement and Health Around the World*, the Pew Research
Foundation found that "people who are active in religious congrega-
tions tend to be happier and more civically engaged than either reli-
giously unaffiliated adults or inactive members of religious groups."
It's not about Vishnu, or Jesus, or Buddha, either. What you believe
appears to be far less important than *that you believe*.

That "God-shaped hole in our hearts" that Blaise Pascal grieved
for is real. If we don't fill it, nihilism will. But for secular progressives,
talking about belief, about faith, about meaning is the third rail of
polite conversation.

That's what threw me for a loop at that exponential ideas conference in Johannesburg. We were happily talking about tinkering with
the human genome, cheating the Reaper with life extension projects,
and uploading our consciousness to microchips—in other words,
happily *playing* God. But no one—at least, in those circles—was going to electrocute themselves on the live wire of Meaning, of talking
about God, let alone figuring out how to talk to God.

On its surface, that restraint is noble. We're all aware of the violent
and bloody potential of holy war. Protestant versus Catholic. Shia
versus Sunni. Buddhist versus Muslim. Religion was one of the first
tools to mobilize tribal energies beyond a few hundred or thousand
people into the millions. The results have been grim. That's a large
part of what prompted the rise of Enlightenment rationalism in the
first place.

But scratch the surface of this hands-off stance, and there's something of the arrogance of the New Atheists in the mix too. "Let the locals have their superstitious customs," the conversation might go at Davos. "Once they have electric lights, shopping malls, and air-conditioning, they'll grow out of their quaint beliefs and join us at the banquet of Modernity."

Except that's not what's happening. Everyone isn't marching happily along the conveyor belt of Progress. Some are running in the opposite direction back to the certainty of tribal belonging. Others are throwing sand in the gears and looking to trash the whole Enlightenment project.

"If God did not exist," Voltaire observed, "it would be necessary to invent him."

Now, perhaps more than ever, we should listen.

It might be time to grab that third rail of Meaning and ride the lightning for all we're worth. We need to reinvent religion.

WWID? (What Would IDEO Do?)

In 1991, in Palo Alto, California, a Stanford University professor named David Kelley teamed up with some colleagues and started the design firm IDEO. Originally focused on consumer products like Apple's first computer mouse and Steelcase office furniture, Kelley, and subsequent CEOs Tim Brown and Sandy Speicher, continued to push the firm into broader and broader applications of its creative process.

In 2011, they created IDEO.org to extend their impact to poor and vulnerable populations. So they developed a Guide to Human-Centered Design. The Human-Centered Design tool kit is "all about building a deep empathy with the people you're designing for," the company explains, "generating tons of ideas; building a bunch of prototypes; sharing what you've made with the people you're designing for; and eventually putting your innovative new solution out in the world." They have hundreds of successful case studies, ranging from indoor toilets for Ghana's poor to digital finance apps for urban immigrants. All developed by and for the people who needed the solutions.

IDEO's method is based on three principles: Inspiration, Ideation, and Implementation. In the first phase, Inspiration, you "learn directly from the people you're designing for as you come to deeply understand their needs." In the second phase, Ideation, "you'll prototype possible solutions." And in the final phase, Implementation, "you'll bring your solution to life and eventually, to market."

So that's what this book is about—bringing a Human-Centered Design process to the challenge of Meaning.

on page 76?

If Part One has been about deeply understanding our need for Exponential Meaning, Part Two is all about prototyping possible solutions. Part Three will take those insights and explore ways to implement these ideas in the larger world.

Finding a solution to a problem as large as a global collapse in meaning means we have to think systemically as well as locally. Bespoke answers to pressing questions—from education to addiction to sustainability—exist in droves. But they are often too expensive, too particular, or too personality-driven to grow beyond the microclimates that birthed them. The Wright brothers discovered flight at Kitty Hawk, after all, but it took the likes of KLM and Qantas to connect the world through air travel.

If Meaning 3.0 stands a chance of helping our current crises, it needs to be broadly relevant and locally adaptive. To do that, it should borrow three design criteria from scientific modernism (Meaning 2.0) to make it as inclusive as possible—Open Source, Scalability, and Anti-Fragility.

Open Source. That means that rather than insisting on a one-size-fits-all approach, it should respect the vast diversity of values and beliefs across cultures and communities and be adaptable to regional conditions. It should be *content neutral*, i.e., nondogmatic and nondoctrinal—so everyone can fill in the blanks themselves.

Rather than Microsoft Windows—a proprietary platform that cannot be modified by users, we would want to build something closer to Linux software. It's freely available to anyone who'd like to use it, and infinitely modifiable by anyone who has a specific problem they'd like to solve. Useful solutions are shared and picked up by others, who in turn add layers of functionality. The overall code base grows from grassroots efforts, not top-down release schedules.

Scalable. We've already ruled out sending everyone into orbit to experience the flyover effect. That would be too slow and too costly to ever prompt global unity. The same goes for cutting-edge solutions of most stripes. What gets proven in mice, or in labs, or with high-touch attention is largely reserved for the top 1 percent, never mind the Bottom Billion. For something to be truly scalable, it needs to be cheap or outright free, and as low-tech and user-friendly as possible.

Anti-fragile. That's NYU professor and author of *The Black Swan* Nassim Taleb's term for a solution that gets better as things get worse. As we face solid odds of increasing instability in the coming century, we need to design cultural solutions that are robust enough to cope. The complexity we're facing, the loss of comforting narratives, and the nearly overwhelming grief we face as the enormity of our situation looms, all threaten to undermine our best efforts. "We are perhaps entering an era," Harvard-trained theorist Zak Stein recently wrote, "where billions may watch while millions die." That's going to take more resilience than we've ever had.

Beyond our actual existential predicament, there's another level of anti-fragility that's essential to solve for: namely, that any cultural movement that threatens to upset the existing status quo is typically squashed by those looking to maintain business as usual.

History is littered with the stories of joyful ecstatic experiments violently suppressed by the powers that be. Think of it as the never-ending battle between the Priests and the Prometheans. Law and Order against the Freedom Fighters. Someone discovers a direct route to liberation that threatens to cut out the established middlemen, and they're rarely welcomed with open arms. Try to storm heaven and there's almost always hell to pay.

The Spanish Inquisition eradicated the Cathars, a mystical sect that thrived in medieval France and Italy. The whirling dervishes of Sufism have been persecuted for centuries in Turkey, Iran, and Pakistan for their refusal to bow to external authority. Tantric Shaivist sects in India regularly ran afoul of conservative leaders of more mainline denominations. Shakers, Quakers, and Mormons all had to flee their homelands to pursue their more direct and experiential faiths.

It's not just spiritual communities who've experienced this repression. In the late 1960s and early 1970s Richard Nixon's administration deliberately suppressed that era's move toward social justice by criminalizing drugs the activists favored.

Near the end of his life, John Ehrlichman, the Watergate coconspirator, admitted to a journalist at *Harper's*: "We knew we couldn't make it illegal to be either against the war or black, but by getting the public to associate the hippies with marijuana [and psychedelics] and blacks with heroin, and then criminalizing both heavily, we could disrupt those communities. We could arrest their leaders, raid their homes, break up their meetings. . . . Did we know we were lying about the drugs? Of course we did."

The counter to this predictable suppression of transformational movements is simple. Widely share recipes that enhance individual and communal sovereignty, using ingredients that are easily accessible. Distribute the human-centered design tool kit far and wide, so it cannot be censored or suppressed. In other words, make it open source and scalable. Make these tools a perpetual part of the commons. Share the cheat codes to the Infinite Game. Democratize transcendence. *Seed* a revolution, don't lead a revolution.

* * *

Once we have design criteria for Meaning 3.0 in place—Open Source, Scalable, and Anti-fragile that support inclusion—we should decide what functionality we need to include from traditional religion (Meaning 1.0) that prompt salvation.

There are a lot of ways to map the functions of faith, but the Sacred Design Lab at Harvard Divinity School has distilled them down to three core elements: Beyond, Becoming, and Belonging. Three essential nutrients vital to human flourishing. Or put another way, inspiration, healing, and connection. The ancient Greeks called those

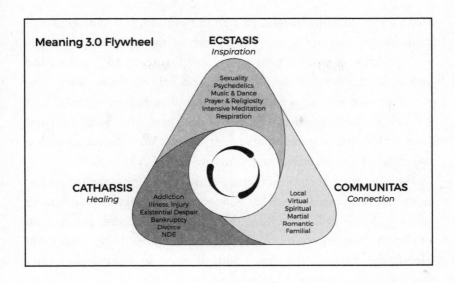

three *ecstasis*, *catharsis*, and *communitas*. While they go by different names, their role supporting human flourishing is essential. They are how we wake up, grow up, and show up. Again and again, for as long as it takes.

Let's take them one at a time.

Inspiration serves as an essential counterweight to the crushing "life's a bitch and then you die" monotony of existence. "There is but one truly serious philosophical problem," Albert Camus cheerily proposed in *The Myth of Sisyphus*, "and that is suicide." When our day-to-day grind threatens to overwhelm our will to go on, Inspiration can give us a moment where it all makes sense, a chance to lay our burdens down and stand tall. If only for a moment, we have our reason for being.

Studies show that experiences of awe can relieve stress, improve life satisfaction, decrease physical pain, and alleviate depression. It's so central to our well-being that even our primate cousins are in on the act. Packs of macaque monkeys have been observed overlooking food, fighting, and fornicating to gaze at an especially gorgeous sunset over the savannah. People who experience reliable access to peak states report having greater overall life satisfaction than those who don't.

And it's not just fleeting inspiration that happens in peak states of awe and wonder. Sometimes it's the information coming into focus that's really valuable. Insight, pattern recognition, and lateral connections all spike when the neurophysiology of these experiences comes on line. Our inner critic goes quiet; norepinephrine, dopamine, and endocannabinoids sharpen our focus and help us draw conclusions we might not have seen before. Brain waves shift from agitated beta frequency to slower, more reflective alpha, theta, and delta states and bypass the normal gatekeepers of our mind. We find ourselves less distracted, more attentive, and more inventive in these states.

Peak states are such powerful experiences that everyone from mystics to action sports athletes has gone to extreme lengths to taste more of them. Some seek them from the stillness of a meditation cushion or the soothing repetition of a potter's wheel, while others find them among the throngs on a dance floor or hurtling down a mountain. But the inner experience is similar.

"There are moments that stand out from the chaos of everyday as shining beacons," University of Chicago professor Mihaly Csikzentmihalyi writes. "In many ways, one might say that *the whole effort of humankind through millennia of history has been to capture these fleeting moments of fulfillment* and make them a part of everyday existence" [emphasis added]. Peak experiences cut through the noise and distraction of everyday living and remind us of what matters.

addiction?

Healing—the second core nutrient we all require. "The world breaks everyone," said Hemingway, "and afterward many are strong at the broken places. But those that will not break it kills." It's a hard hand we're dealt, playing this monkeys-with-clothes game.

On the one hand, we are blessed with complex abstract consciousness capable of divining the orbits of faraway planets and penning sonnets that make us weep. And on the other, life is cheap, violence and cruelty abound, and precious little of this brief experience of being alive makes a whole lot of sense. "Man is literally split in two," Pulitzer Prize–winning anthropologist Ernest Becker acknowledged, "he has an awareness of his own splendid uniqueness in that he sticks out of nature with a towering majesty, and yet he goes back into the ground a few feet in order blindly and dumbly to rot and disappear forever."

Reconciling this "red in tooth and claw" Law of the Jungle with our glimpses of the Sublime isn't guaranteed. Feeling torn between those two truths causes much of our suffering.

Nearly one in ten of us will be diagnosed with post-traumatic stress disorder in our lifetimes. The rest of us suffer micro-PTSD nearly all the time. Having a way to digest our grief, rather than choke on it, becomes essential. As Bessel van der Kolk writes, our bodies really do keep the score. Our nervous systems accumulate stressors until we're fibrillating messes. Once we're in a hijacked state, we are less perceptive, resilient, and resourceful. We are then more likely to stumble and make things worse. Hurt people, the old joke goes, hurt people. It would be funnier if it weren't so true.

Whether it's the absolution of Catholic confession, the ritual forgiveness of Jewish Yom Kippur, or the cathartic suffering of a Lakota Sun Dance ceremony, religion has always provided ways for us to mend and atone. Reset the Etch A Sketch. There's too much tragedy in the human experience to process it all unaided. Without some way to wipe the slate clean, our lives become mired. When we have cultural processes that hold us up while we suffer, we can transform that suffering into something profound. "Grief is praise," explains poet and Mayan elder Martin Prechtel, "because it is the natural way love honors what it misses."

Connection—the third essential quality that faith has always conferred upon believers—is connection to community. Those social ties, that sense of camaraderie and support, are critical to tribal primates like us. There are decades of research that connects longevity and well-being to the richness of one's personal social network.

We find ourselves living a paradox these days. While we are superficially more hyperconnected than ever (think of people you know who have maxed out their five-thousand-person "friend" count on social media), we are more isolated than ever. From our families of origin, from our neighbors, and from ourselves.

"While technology promises to connect us, it can also isolate," Vivek Murthy, the former U.S. surgeon general, writes in *Together: The Healing Power of Connection in a Sometimes Lonely World*. "While we increasingly have the opportunity to pursue our individual destinies, we can put our own goals ahead of our relationships and community; and despite all of the progress we have made in how we talk about mental health, we are still ashamed of feeling lonely."

Murthy wanted to find what lay at the heart of our current crisis, so he traveled the country interviewing people. Isolation, he concluded, is a "root cause and contributor to many of the epidemics sweeping the world today from alcohol and drug addiction to violence to depression and anxiety. . . . But, at the center of our loneliness is our innate desire to connect. We have evolved to participate in community, to forge lasting bonds with others, to help one another, and to share life experiences. We are, simply, better together."

The technical term for this kind of togetherness—the profound and healing kind—is what University of Chicago anthropologist Victor Turner calls *communitas*. It means a merging with the collective that transcends our personal separation. Quakers call it a "gathered meeting"—a collection of souls sharing a connection of spirit. Keith Sawyer at the University of North Carolina at Chapel Hill calls it "group flow"—that experience shared by sports teams and jazz bands alike—where individual decision-making merges with a collective intelligence. That experience, Sawyer noted, is so profound that it is up to three times as rewarding as an isolated peak experience.

And here's the thing about these three core elements—Inspiration, Healing, and Connection—they function much more like spokes on a wheel than rungs on a ladder. They don't reveal themselves in a fixed progression or sequence. But once you engage one, the other two often follow. They make up the cycle of our lives.

Regardless of which branch we enter through—whether it's deep healing, powerful inspiration, or committed connection, this three-legged process is more or less how living gets done. Life is irreducibly tragic—we know that much. That's where healing becomes so essential—it gives us a chance to patch our bones and mend as we go onward. But occasionally, it's undeniably magic—and that's easier to forget. That's what inspiration does: It reminds us that there's beauty and perfection around us, if we only remember where to look. When we find ourselves whipsawed between those two poles, we have to laugh together at the Full Catastrophe that is our mortal lives. Then it's Comic too. That's what connection does—it gives us a chance to share the burden and absurdity of life with others.

If we couldn't weep, worship, and laugh, we wouldn't be able to bear witness to this crazy ride. So that's what we're shooting for: a way to wake up, grow up, and show up. Just in time.

*   *   *

Now it's time to combine our IDEO-inspired design process into a practical protocol.

To recap: A viable candidate for Meaning 3.0 will need to fulfill the pro-social functions of traditional 1.0 Faith—**Inspiration, Healing,** and **Connection.** And, to stand a chance of helping the world, it needs to fulfill the inclusive promise of 2.0 Modernism, and be **Open Source, Scalable,** and **Anti-fragile.**

But delivering on both of those requirements isn't easy. If it was, we wouldn't be suffering from so much existential dread, trauma, and isolation. There are some tools that reliably check all of these boxes, but we've been overlooking them.

In the same way that culture sits upstream from politics, biology sits upstream from psychology. That means in the war for hearts and minds, we should be paying much more attention to our bodies and brains.

The closer to our primitive survival circuitry we are working, the simpler, more powerful, and more reliable those interventions can be. "Give me a lever long enough," Archimedes famously said, "and I can move the world!" The evolutionary imperatives of our bodies are the longest lever we have to try and move the world.

Four of the most potent and accessible physical drivers to shape consciousness and culture and help us build Meaning 3.0 are:

Respiration—We are hard-coded to ensure our oxygen supply remains constant, so modulating breathing is one of the surest-fire ways to shift physical and psychological states.

Embodiment—The core regulators of our parasympathetic and sympathetic nervous system play an enormous role in our health, well-being, and stress resilience. They are the metronome of our physiology that sets the rhythm of our lived experiences.

Sexuality—If we do not procreate we die. So there are tons of neurochemical drivers baked into our systems to ensure we do. Understanding them allows a powerful reorientation to this central life-giving activity.

Substances—Humans, and most other animals, routinely seek to shift states as part of their learning, growing, and mending. Ron Siegel at UCLA has even gone as far as calling the intentional pursuit of intoxication a "fourth drive—a desire to feel different, to achieve a rapid change in one's state" that is "as much a part of the human condition as sex, hunger, and thirst."

To those four we can add the most ancient and effective amplifier of experience:

Music—From ancient fireside chants to cathedrals to chain gangs to concerts, music has accompanied us on the journey of human civilization. It not only "soothes the savage beast"; it shapes our physiology, sense of connectivity, and capacity for awe.

Because each of these Big Five are so central to human biology and consciousness, even small tweaks can yield large gains. By focusing on our bodies rather than more complex or expensive technologies, we stand a better chance of meeting our design criteria for crafting Meaning 3.0 of Open Sourcing (anyone can begin tinkering—no expensive medical devices or VR headsets required), Scalability (nothing is cheaper or more accessible than our own bodily function), and Anti-fragility (once we master these tools we expand our resilience, and no one can take them away).

Respiration, embodiment, sexuality, substances, and music supporting inspiration, healing, and connection.

It's a simple protocol, echoed across the world for thousands of years. If you examine any traditional religion, you will find evidence of these drivers at work. The emerging field of neuroanthropology, where we examine not only customs and rituals but the functional physiology beneath them, gives us new understandings of ancient practices. And once we reverse-engineer these examples, we can use what we've learned to create even more effective versions. That's culture architecture in action. We can strip out any mythologies that no longer serve us, but keep the technologies that actually do.

Crypto-Puritans, Straight-Edgers, and Lizard Brain F*ck Monkeys

Even a quick glance at this road map might trigger skepticism, judgment, or unseemly enthusiasm. After all, there are lots of cultural taboos and customs informing our relationship to these topics— especially our relationships to our bodies, sexuality, and substances (at first glance, breathing and music seem less controversial, but they, too, have their issues).

Rather than shy away from these topics because they are controversial, we should take it as a sign that we're on to something important *that they are so controversial*. Taboos, after all, don't arise unless there is something powerful at stake. Virtually all societies strictly channel access to "techniques of ecstasy," to borrow Mircea Eliade's memorable phrase, into approved forms. Sex for procreation but not for recreation. Intoxication for stress relief but not for epiphany. Music to reinforce Apollonian order (like army marches and church hymns) but not for Dionysian revels (like Elvis and the Grateful Dead).

No civilization worth its salt hasn't tightly prescribed access to these five forces. Otherwise nothing remotely "civilized" would ever get done. Way back in Old Testament days, Moses scarpered up Mount Sinai, leaving his people to their own devices for forty days and forty nights. When he came back down, he found his kinsmen off their faces on a sexy, boozy bender. Moses literally threw the book at them—smashing the Ten Commandments, filled with thou-shalt-not-covet-this-or-that—to the ground. And so began the process of corralling a bunch of desert pagans into upstanding pillars of Western civilization. It hasn't stopped since.

How else do you think the nineteenth-century Mormon Church managed to settle and irrigate the deserts of Utah? Carousing and cavorting, drinking and fornicating, rocking and rolling—all these things were categorically off the table for the Latter-Day and Saintly devout. By channeling all of that pent-up energy into ditch digging, the Mormon elders were able to turn a desert into the Garden.

So let's return to our initial question: WWID? What would Meaning 3.0 look like if built from design thinking like IDEO? Even though this is potentially volatile terrain, we'd be remiss to miss the power and potential of our evolutionary drivers. We're all different in how comfortable a clear-eyed look at this content will make us. In general, though, our responses will roughly align with one of three personality types: the Hedonist, the Conformist, and the Purist. Understanding the strengths and weaknesses of each position should give us a helpful handle on finding our way forward.

The Hedonist, when confronted with the chance to optimize ecstatic experience, is generally *all in*. Their challenge isn't willingness to try new and potentially pleasurable things, it's in knowing when to stop. "Beware unearned wisdom," Carl Jung once cautioned. Hedonists are up to their ears in it. They are governed by the maxim "if it

Ecstatic Personalities

	HEDONIST	CONFORMIST	PURIST
Core Identity	Sensation Seeker	Rule Follower	Identity Protector
Catch Phrase	If it feels good, do it	If it's what the doctor ordered	My body is my temple
Missing Link	Brakes	Steering	Gas
Substance of Choice	Cocaine, Champagne & Reefer	Ambien, Adderall & Alcohol	Wheatgrass, Elixers & Cacao
Achilles Heel	Addiction	Compliance	Pride
Resistance	You're not the boss of me	But who would I be if I did that?	I don't need those crutches
Core Value	Full range of experience	Advice of experts	Sanctity of mind and body

Hedonic Engineering

feels good, do it." Sex, drugs, and rock and roll are very much in their playbook, and they often overdo it. Infidelity and addiction are their Achilles' heels. Brakes (to slow their pursuits) are their missing link. Lizard Brain Fuck Monkey could be their nickname.

The Purist, when presented with novel techniques of ecstasy, especially those that involve wild abandon, often shuts down. They tend to prefer the "earned wisdom" of meditation, yoga, or prayer to the potentially reckless or debauched. They are likely to view more volatile approaches to transformation with suspicion, considering them cheating or a shortcut. Wheatgrass and elixirs are their substances of choice. Their catchphrase is "my body is my temple." Pride is their Achilles' heel. Gas (to accelerate their growth) is their missing link. Crypto-Puritan could be their nickname.

The Conformist, surveying the list of our Big Five, wouldn't necessarily know what to think. They tend to defer to established authority—medical, legal, or religious—to tell them what is within and beyond the pale. They might not give a second thought to three cocktails each night, backed with an Ambien chaser, but blanch at a joint getting passed around at a party. They could willingly have their child on a methamphetamine for their ADD, or their spouse on a benzodiazepine for anxiety, but consider psychedelic therapy frightening. "If it's what the doctor ordered" might be their catchphrase. Compliance is their Achilles' heel. Steering (out of the ruts of consensus opinion) is their missing link. Straight-Edge is their nickname.

So as you read these personas, note which one has felt most true for you in your life. Notice how they have both helped and harmed your own attempts to experience Ecstasis (peak experience and awe), Catharsis (deep healing and integration), and Communitas (profound connection with others).

We can't get sidetracked in sensation-seeking like a Hedonist might. Nor can we turn our noses up at approaches that don't fit our idealized identity as a Purist might. And we can't ignore novel solutions that might bring powerful benefit as a Conformist might.

While they all have blind spots, each of these orientations holds a core value that the others would do well to incorporate. The Hedonist values sucking the marrow out of life and pursuing the fullest range of experience possible. The Purist values the sanctity of mind and body. The Conformist values expert advice and evidence.

If we can integrate these three orientations, we will be stronger and more effective. We can become something more than any of them—Hedonic Engineers—technicians of the sacred. We can remember who we are through sublime peak experience, we can mend where we're broken through cathartic healing, and we can choose to connect—as couples, communities, and citizens.

That's the challenge in front of us: to engineer Ecstasis without the Crave (of addiction to altered states), prompt Catharsis without the Cringe (of indulgent self-help), and create Communitas without the Cult (of unreliable leaders and followers). That's a Meaning 3.0 worth living into. It cannot replace a thousand personal and collective decisions and actions that we all must make on the road ahead. But it might give us a chance to recapture our own rapture in time to do what we must with conviction and courage together.

PART II

The Alchemist Cookbook

I went to the Garden of Love,
And saw what I never had seen:
A Chapel was built in the midst,
Where I used to play on the green.

And the gates of this Chapel were shut,
And *Thou shalt not.* writ over the door;
So I turn'd to the Garden of Love,
That so many sweet flowers bore.

And I saw it was filled with graves,
And tomb-stones where flowers should be:
And Priests in black gowns, were walking their rounds,
And binding with briars, my joys & desires.

—William Blake, from *Songs of Experience*

In 1971, an expat English teenager named William Powell holed himself away in the New York Public Library and began unearthing homemade recipes for everything from pipe bombs to surveillance tactics to bathtub LSD. He compiled them into a slim, 160-page manifesto titled *The Anarchist Cookbook* and published it with the only editor who'd take him.

The Anarchist Cookbook read like what it was, equal parts Boy Scout handbook, Spy vs. Spy manual, and Che Guevara fan fiction. Powell had hoped the volume might empower "the silent majority" who could use these recipes to fight for freedom and justice against the faceless forces of tyranny. It didn't turn out as planned.

The book was promptly banned, and monitored by J. Edgar Hoover's FBI, the CIA, and other intelligence agencies. Young Powell got spooked and renounced the book, but that did nothing to stop its underground following. On the way to selling over two million copies over multiple printings, it became the most stolen library book of all time.

Part Two of this book shares none of the violent and anarchic tendencies of its predecessor. Instead it deliberately inverts its approach: learning how to blow yourself (rather than others), sky high with common household materials. This time the aim isn't revolution, it's transformation. It's not about harming others, it's about helping ourselves. But the goal—to level the playing field for a silent majority of people willing to take a stand for freedom and justice against the faceless forces of Misrule—that much remains true.

So do the cautions. *The Anarchist Cookbook* was catnip for miscreants. It ended up in the hands of bomb throwers and lone shooters as often as dedicated activists. This Alchemist Cookbook is equally volatile. The recipes that follow can be exploited by governments and sociopaths, as easily as by saints and sages.

* * *

Our task is to understand the potentials in this alchemical cookbook one ingredient at a time. Easiest to hardest. We'll begin exploring one of the least controversial but most powerful tools we have at our disposal—breathing. Tweaking the rate and depth of our breathing, and even swapping out the gases we're breathing, can have profound effects on consciousness.

From there, we will continue our survey of transformative techniques with physiology. Pleasure and pain can get hot-wired to powerfully shift states. Dopamine and endorphins feel awesome and make us hurt a little less. The vagal nerve and endocannabinoid system seem to play some interwoven role in regulating our autonomic nervous system in ways that we're only just beginning to understand.

Then we'll look into music, which when intentionally programmed, creates sonic and lyrical states that transport us and connect us. More than almost any other intervention, it can color our surroundings and experience. Music is the wallpaper of our minds.

Then we will visit the role of drugs in sacred contexts. It's a touchy topic for some, but as we will see, there are plenty of examples in the past and present to inform how we might move beyond placebos and into sacraments that actually work.

Finally, we will consider sexuality and its role in culture and consciousness. The neurochemistry of lust, attraction, and bonding plays a powerful role in shaping our consciousness. Orgasm does all sorts of healthy things for our hearts, minds, and relationships. This one is charged enough that we will devote two chapters to it, in hopes that the argument is disarmingly persuasive.

Alchemy, often thought to be the pursuit of turning lead into gold, has another, less common meaning. For thousands of years adepts have tried to turn the lead of our mortal lives into the gold of realization. In the Greek and Judeo-Christian traditions, that achievement took the name *anthropos*—integrated, balanced Vitruvian Man.

Today, we don't need to make it sound so mysterious or exceptional. Consider this Alchemist Cookbook a collection of recipes to turn the dross of our half-baked existence into the gold of HomeGrown Humans. People taking a stand for this planet, these bodies, this lifetime. All of us, or none of us.

CHAPTER 5

Respiration

Everything in heaven and earth breathes. Breath is the thread that ties creation together.

—Morihei Ueshiba, founder of Aikido

Into the Mystic

A long, long time ago, a village elder of the Anangu people sat down next to a giant sandstone rock. They put their lips to the mouthpiece of a wooden tube and began to play. Some early European settlers called that instrument an "ulbura trumpet." Today it's more commonly known as a didgeridu, after the warbling, buzzing tones it makes.

Then as now, it created an almost otherworldly droning sound, overlaid with acoustic squiggles and pulsations. On and on it went, a sonic prayer to Uluru (briefly known as Ayers Rock), the giant stone monolith standing behind the elder. On and on it went, vibrating out to the Milky Way and the stars above, and to the Ancestor Beings, never stopping. Eventually, the musician was drawn into a trance connecting them to the minds of their ancestors. No longer playing the didgeridu, but rather being played by the instrument itself, they surrendered into the Dreaming.

"Ancestor-mind . . . is all about deep engagement, connecting with a timeless state of mind or 'alpha wave state,' an optimal neural state for learning," Tyson Yunkaporta, a member of the Apalech Clan and professor of Indigenous Knowledges at Deakin University in Melbourne, writes. "It is characterised by complete concentration, engagement and losing track of linear time. Ancestor-mind can involve immersive visualisation and extra-cognitive learning such as revealed knowledge in dreams and inherited knowledge in cellular memory."

The elder kept their song going through a special technique known as circular breathing. It involves puffing out a cheek to hold extra air and then, just as you take a breath, you "squirt" that stored air through the instrument. The result is a nonstop delivery of sound as you learn to breathe in and out almost continuously. Trumpet and wind instrumentalists use it sometimes, but no one has mastered this technique as thoroughly as the first nations of northern Australia.

While the didgeridu counts as among the most ancient and simple instruments on record, its role as a trance-inducing tool is surprisingly complex. The frequency of the didgeridu typically ranges from 60 to 100 Hz. "This tone generation, modulated by lip vibration," Krzysztof Izdebski, a professor at the San Francisco Conservatory of Music, writes, "is supported by circular breathing, allowing for an uninterrupted length of sound generation. Inhalation introduces sound pulsation . . . including conscious . . . vibration, all used to enrich both the sound and the artistic meaning of the played sequence."

Those "conscious vibrations" do something else as well. They release a potent neurotransmitter that alleviates stress, prompts a shift in physiological states, and enhances access to trance consciousness. Scientists at the Karolinska Institutet in Sweden have found that nasal breathing results in 15 to 30 percent better oxygenation than mouth breathing. And if you vibrate the nasal cavity while doing it, as didgeridu players do, it boosts nitric oxide by up to *fifteen* times.

Nitric oxide is a powerful molecule that crosses the blood-brain barrier and takes us from vigilant and stressed into calmer, more resourceful states. According to Harvard's Herbert Benson, "molecular studies have shown that the calming response releases little 'puffs' of nitric oxide, which has been linked to the production of such neurotransmitters as endorphins and dopamine." Benson discovered that the transition from waking consciousness to peak states is triggered by a flush of nitric oxide through the nervous system. It works as a signaling molecule, sending information back and forth between parts of the brain that don't normally communicate, dialing down stress responses and dialing up deep relaxation and connection. He calls nitric oxide the "spirit" or catalyst of the peak experience.

The boost in nitric oxide that the didgeridu creates has all sorts of general health-giving benefits as well—ranging from lessening breathing difficulties like asthma and sleep apnea to reducing mental stress. One study found that "didgeridu sound meditation is as effective as silent meditation for decreasing self-perceived negative arousal, tiredness, and energy and more effective than silent meditation for relaxation and acute stress."

Most recently, doctors at the Swedish Institute for Infectious Disease Control have found that what makes didgeridu playing so healthy might even help with acute respiratory viruses like COVID. "Our results demonstrated that [nitric oxide] specifically inhibits the replication cycle of SARS CoV, most probably during the early steps of infection, suggesting that the production of nitric oxide . . . results in an antiviral effect."

Sitting around a campfire at the foot of a sacred site like Uluru, that aboriginal elder was able to play themselves into a trance and enter Dreamtime. In that mythic space, out of regular time, elders connected with the sacred song lines of their lineage, and communed with their ancestors "born out of their own Eternity." And while there's profound impact from set and setting, culture and context, their access to Dreamtime was underpinned by something as simple as an unusual circular breathing pattern, vibration of the sinus cavity, and the overproduction of a key neurotransmitter.

All of which is to say that an act as simple, essential, and largely unconscious as breathing can have profound effects on our bodies and brains. By adjusting the rate, depth, and rhythm of our respiration, we can meaningfully change how we feel, how we heal, and what we see.

The Gospel of Gasp

These days, breath work is having a bit of a moment.

Yoga studios, spartan training camps, and podcasts are constantly talking about breath work and biohacking. Top teachers hop from Tulum to Bali, from Brooklyn to London, delivering transcendence as they go. It's become an increasingly trendy way to spend a Friday night.

But survey this scene and you'll realize that everyone's method is slightly different. Some of the instructions can feel downright confusing. Others are handed down solemnly, like holy writ—the Gospel of Gasp. At its simplest, though, breathing is something we all do. It's something we've always done. From the first moment we come into this world, until the last moment we leave it.

Whether it comes wrapped in spiritual, martial, or athletic language, breath training boils down to three things: oxygen, nitrogen, and carbon dioxide. Varying the rate, depth, and rhythm of our breaths changes the ratios of the three gases that make up our atmosphere. In turn this affects how our bodies and brains perform and how our hearts and minds feel. That's pretty much it.

Take a deep breath right now. Hold it for as long as you can. Feel those first spasms in your belly or swallows in your throat. Keep going until you have to let it out. Notice how long that was. Most untrained efforts clock in somewhere between thirty and ninety seconds. That's what's known as your "static apnea" score—a fancy term for holding your breath. By the end of this chapter yours should double.

Now ask yourself, why did you have to breathe when you did—why couldn't you have gone longer? Most people would reasonably conclude, "I was running out of air." And by that they'd probably mean, running out of oxygen. Except that's not what just happened. You had plenty of oxygen left. What gave you that insistent, increasingly unpleasant "air hunger" was actually a buildup of carbon dioxide (CO_2). Think of it as Nature's early warning system. It saves us from cutting things too close and coming up snake eyes in the oxygen-to-the-brain game.

This time, take another deep breath, but then let it all out. Pinch your nose with thumb and forefinger and see how long you can hold your breath with empty lungs. This will measure your CO_2 tolerance. Rather than white-knuckling this one, just take it as far as that first involuntary breath movement (IBM). Note your time. It was likely much shorter. Starting scores range from twenty to forty seconds. Elite athletes can comfortably hold for sixty to ninety seconds or more. It's a good indicator of VO_2 max and aerobic fitness.

It can also be trained. Because "air hunger" caused by CO_2 buildup is such a panic-inducing experience, and because they spend a lot of time underwater where panic would be deadly, Navy SEALs train with a technique called box breathing. We can too. Start with a five-second inhale, then hold for five seconds, exhale for five seconds, then hold for five seconds again. That's your box. When you have the hang of it, extend to ten- or fifteen-second intervals. It gets harder. And the hardest is typically that fourth side, after you've exhaled completely, and are testing precisely how well you can manage your CO_2. The more we can familiarize ourselves with the edges of our physiology, the more control we have at the edges of our psychology.

Now that we've practiced managing the discomfort of excess carbon dioxide, we can game the system a bit. By artificially lowering the amount of CO_2 in our bloodstream, it takes longer for us to feel that first IBM. Take a big lungful of air, and exhale forcefully like you were blowing out the candles on a birthday cake. Keep doing this for fifty repetitions, filling your belly and breathing strongly out through pursed lips. You might feel tingling in your face or fingers. Keep it up, and you might even experience involuntary hand contractions. That's because hyperventilating has changed your blood pH to alkaline. You've also blown off a lot of carbon dioxide, which lets you hold your breath for longer before feeling the urge to inhale again.

While you're still in tingly alkalosis, retest how long you can passively hold your breath again now. Exhale slowly, inhale fully, and hold. Now that you know those early urges to breathe are still well within your comfort zone, and you've just lowered your baseline CO_2 by hyperventilating, you should be able to hold your breath a good bit longer. Relax anywhere you feel tension. Go quiet and sit in the center of your attention. Hold it until you truly can't anymore. How did you do? Many people report improvements from their baseline score between 25 and 50 percent.

(Important: While free divers use this technique to maximize their time underwater, it can lead to shallow water blackout drowning because they have overridden their bodies' natural safety system. Do not do this in water without trained supervision and safety protocols.)

Hopefully you're feeling more comfortable managing your CO_2. The next step is to slow our oxygen burn. We can do that by dropping our heart rate. Faster heartbeats guzzle more gas. Vagal breathing, where we double the length of our exhales to our inhales, signals to our bodies that all is right with our world and engages our parasympathetic system. Ten-second exhales, followed by two-second holds, followed by four-second inhales work well.

Andrew Huberman, a neuroscientist at Stanford University, has discovered that if you soften your gaze to the edge of your vision (letting your eyes drift to ten and two on the clock), and breathe through your nose while humming, you can get an even deeper relaxation response. And if on the final phase of your inhale, you vigorously sniff in additional air, it can "pop" open your alveoli (the tiny sacs in your lungs) for more oxygenation. Practice this vagal breathing for five minutes and gently check your pulse. It should be 10 to 30 percent lower than your normal resting rate.

While this technique was developed by free divers so they can consume as little oxygen on their dives as possible, it works well in traffic, before public speaking, or among rowdy children. The old adage "Before you respond in anger, slow down and take a few deep breaths!"

is a folk version of this same basic approach. Adding nasal breathing, humming, and a softened gaze only adds a layer of science onto that foundation.

Holotropy

Now that we have a basic grasp of the chemistry of breath, let's take a quick survey of the ways we can put these gases to work. By changing the rate, volume, and depth of our respiratory patterns, we can shift the ratios of oxygen, carbon dioxide, and nitrogen to profound effect. The subjective experience can range from relaxation to alertness to transcendence.

Despite a host of complicated names and specific techniques, all of these different breathing practices break down into roughly three categories: acceleration, brakes, and steering.

Acceleration—These are any practices that look to energize or "upregulate" our nervous system. Think of a swimmer huffing and puffing and swinging their arms as they step up onto the blocks at the Olympics, or a high-altitude mountaineer pursing their lips to improve air exchange in their lungs as they climb Everest.

Brakes—These are exercises that look to de-stress or "downregulate" our nervous system. Think of a nervous performer taking slow, deep breaths before walking onstage, or the free divers' vagal breathing technique we just discussed.

Steering—These techniques aim to shift consciousness from waking-state normal to a more meditative, contemplative, or shamanic experience. Think of a kriya yogi alternating breaths out of each nostril while chanting a mantra, or a transcendent breath work session.

We've briefly covered the mechanics of acceleration and braking. Let's take a closer look at steering and how to blend all three techniques to create the fullest experience possible.

Czech psychiatrist Stanislav Grof is one of the modern pioneers of transcendent breath work, but he came to it by necessity rather than by choice. When the federal government made LSD illegal for medical research in 1968, the Johns Hopkins researcher was forced to hunt for a legal substitute that offered the same potent combination of healing and state-shifting experience. After some experimentation he discovered what he came to call holotropic breath work (literally "to move toward wholeness")—a rapid breathing technique that builds on the "blow out the birthday candles" hyperventilation exercise we tried earlier and extends it for as long as three hours.

To this technique Grof added stimulating music meant to drive the pace of the experience. The brain, subjected to this extended overbreathing, begins to experience chemical changes in regions that govern visual processing, proprioception, and memory. Some people lose connection to the default mode network, which can lead to experiences of ego death, followed by an immersion into cathartic non-ordinary states of consciousness. Research has shown improved outcomes for a number of treatment-resistant conditions like schizophrenia and manic depression.

If you want to try a simple version of state-shifting breath work, and you don't have any preexisting medical or psychological contraindications, you can find a partner to spot you. Lie down in a quiet, comfortable spot on the floor. Set a timer for one hour. Find high-quality headphones and an eye mask to intensify the experience and choose an intentional playlist of powerful, evocative music. Turn it up as loud as is comfortable. Breathe as fast as possible as deeply as possible for as long as possible. See what happens.

You may experience the tingling and crimping we mentioned before as alkalosis kicks in. You may find yourself drifting into a daydreamy state, or possibly something more intense or meaningful. Whatever comes up, allow it all to come and go.

If not enough is happening, you can hit the accelerator by breathing faster and deeper. If too much is happening, you can tap the brakes by slowing down your pacing. Change the selection and volume of music to steer your subjective experience. When your session is complete, do a body scan and notice how and what you're feeling. Feel free to journal or voice record any thoughts or insights you had, or discuss the experience with your spotter.

Over decades of sessions, Grof logged thousands of participants' reports and noticed something interesting. In a reverse of the famous Good Friday experiment at Harvard where seminarians on psilocybin mushrooms had experiences indistinguishable from mystical states, participants in holotropic breath work often had experiences just as profound as those Grof had noted with LSD therapy. All of the transcendence, none of the drugs.

Patanjali, the founder of modern yoga, said, "Breath is the umbilical cord to the universe!" Once you understand the basics of acceleration, brakes, and steering, respiration can take you wherever you want to go. To infinity, and maybe even beyond.

(Stan Grof is an adviser to a study the Flow Genome Project is co-leading at Johns Hopkins to validate holotropic breathing for veterans with treatment-resistant PTSD, following the protocols that MAPS [Multidisciplinary Association for Psychedelic Studies] researchers used for the same population, but using breathing techniques in place of MDMA. For anyone interested in learning more about this study, please go to www.recapturetherapture.com/PTSD.)

Respiration Styles

PATTERN	MECHANISM	ACTION
Slow Deep, Smooth & Symmetrical	Full air exchange Improved oxygenation Down regulation	Stress management Attention training General health
Hyperventilation Rapid, Deep & Sustained	Alkalosis Reduced CO_2	Free diving preparation Psychological introspection Trauma work
Vagal Breathing 10:4 Exhalation:Inhalation	Down regulation of nervous system Increased vagal tone Decreased heart rate	Free diving preparation Stress management
Box Breathing Even Duration Inhalations, Exhalations & Holds	CO_2 Tolerance Down regulation of Fight/Freeze response	Stress management Mindfulness training
Pressure Breathing Pursed Lipped Exhalation	Increased cardio-vagal tone Oxygen saturation	Mountaineering COPD Anaerobic sport
Nasal Breathing with Vibration	Boosted oxygenation Nitric oxide production Down-regulation	Endurance sport training Circular breathing Flow state precipitation

The Pulmonauts

A couple of years ago I found myself on a boat in the Bahamas with world champion free-dive coach Kirk Krack. In addition to training world champions Mandy-Rae Cruickshank and Martin Stepanek, Krack has helped Tom Cruise prepare for underwater stunts in *Mission: Impossible*, given golfer Tiger Woods performance tips, and coached magician David Blaine for his world record breath hold attempt on *The Oprah Winfrey Show*.

That day, he was leading us through a series of preparations for free diving—where you swim as deep underwater as you can without any additional tanks. Wearing wetsuits and paired up with a partner, we were learning the basic ten second (exhale): two second (hold): four second(inhale) vagal breath prep, followed by fifty hyperventilations. Then we'd relax fully into a facedown floating breath hold. Every couple of minutes, we were supposed to signal our partner, to make sure that we were still lucid, while they counted out the seconds on the clock.

It was incredibly quiet in that space. Floating with your face immersed in cold water triggers the mammalian dive reflex, which further lowers your heartbeat (and with it, your oxygen burn rate) and shunts blood from your periphery to your core. It felt womblike. No thoughts, just sensation. The minutes ticked by: two, three, four.

Any muscle tension burns more oxygen, Krack advised, so we relaxed and then relaxed even more. A little involuntary urge to breathe, easily overcome. Five minutes. Five and a half minutes. Six minutes. Longer.

When we finally surfaced, it felt like no time had gone by, or hours had. It was hard to tell. But I was fairly certain that this was the closest thing I'd ever experienced to a full-body meditation.

For me, sitting on a cushion trying not to think about my thinking hasn't ever worked out. Give me a paddle to stroke in the water, or ski poles to push, or bike pedals to spin in circles, and I have a far better chance of getting to mindful mindlessness. I've always needed to get into my body to get out of my head.

But the breath holds of free diving checked all the boxes essential for flow states—Deep Embodiment, High Consequence, and Rich Environment. It was a perfect way to put body and mind into effortless neutral.

As we took turns practicing our maximum holds, Krack kept sharing stories—of epic record dives and of his celebrity trainings. He started telling us about magician David Blaine's preparation for his world record attempt on *The Oprah Winfrey Show.* "The record for unassisted static apnea," Krack told us, was eight minutes and fifty-eight seconds. "But if you go 'gas-assisted,'" he continued, "you can more than double that."

Blaine had practiced his breath-hold technique for months before his record attempt, fasted so his stomach was empty, and engaged in "lung packing," where he'd gulped down an additional liter of air into his already full lungs. But the real game changer was breathing pure oxygen for twenty-three minutes before submerging. Once he clambered into that giant plexiglass box at Manhattan's Lincoln Center and went under, he was able to milk his supersaturated red blood cells and hold his breath for seventeen minutes and four seconds, a new world record.

Hearing Krack tell that story and casually mention "gas-assisted" breath practices stuck with me. If my simple breath-hold experience of a few minutes had given me one of the easiest access points to a quiet mind that I'd ever experienced, what would extending that feel like? Doubling or even tripling the length of time in the void of not-thinking?

And while I have a ton of respect for free divers, their meditation is an extreme and unforgiving sport. Even the best often die. What if there was a version that more of us could experience? Could we take the building blocks of free diving—the ability to slow down heart rate, blow off carbon dioxide, super-oxygenate and pack lungs, hold breath, and drop deeply into the zone—and bring it back to dry land?

As soon as we got back from that trip I began researching. We've already noted that all shifts in respiratory states stem from tweaking the ratios of three atmospheric gases. David Blaine's example shows the power of temporarily supersaturating lungs and red blood cells with pure oxygen. But what about the other two—nitrogen and carbon dioxide? Was there anything to be gained from tweaking them?

If free divers are minimalist pulmonauts (literally "voyagers of breath"), making do with just fins and a mask, then their cousin SCUBA divers are the maximalists, tweaking gas blends for every occasion. The two biggest challenges for especially long or deep SCUBA dives are nitrogen narcosis—an intoxicating state caused by that gas under pressure—and decompression sickness, or "the bends," caused by ascending too quickly.

Increase the percentage of oxygen in your tank and you can come to the surface faster without risking the bends. Those tanks are called hyperoxic (meaning "extra oxygen") blends. Decrease the amount of nitrogen by swapping it out for another inert gas, like helium or hydrogen, and you limit the likelihood of getting narcosis on a deep dive.

Nitrogen narcosis—sometimes romantically called "the Rapture of the Deep"—is a pernicious enemy. It sneaks up on you as feelings of calm, confidence, even euphoria. For those who love their time underwater, it can seem like a positive confirmation of the whole reason you dive. Until it isn't and kills you. Divers call it the Martini Effect, and they have a rule of thumb that for every ten meters you dive below twenty meters, it's the equivalent of knocking back one stiff cocktail. Go too deep and you'll feel drunk. You'll forget safety and procedure and risk an accident or worse. Notice the symptoms and you can manage them and return to shallower waters where they subside naturally.

That's why divers sometimes train on dry land by substituting nitrogen for nitrous oxide. Breathing a blend of oxygen and nitrous oxide (similar to what dentists use), they can practice managing themselves under the influence and disorienting effects. With this cousin of the nitrogen family, you can experience some of the rapture, without risking the deadly deep. The specific neurochemistry of this effect is interesting enough that we will return to it later in the chapter.

SCUBA divers have effectively solved for the side effects of breathing oxygen and nitrogen under pressure by changing the blends in their tanks. What about carbon dioxide? I'd always assumed that CO_2 was effectively a waste gas that you were trying to minimize so you could do more with a given lungful of air. Then I learned about Soviet physician Konstantin Buteyko's research about increasing CO_2 levels to boost available oxygen in the blood. Buteyko advocated for a "Goldilocks Zone" of not too much and not too little CO_2 for optimal health and performance. That's why when someone is having a panic attack and hyperventilating, you give them a paper bag to breathe into. It helps them rebalance the amount of CO_2 in their blood and bring them back into equilibrium. That's also why deep "yogic" belly breathing can be counterproductive—you can end up overbreathing, blowing off too much CO_2 and paradoxically reducing your available oxygen levels.

But what happens if we push well past Goldilocks? We know that hyperventilating blows off CO_2 and creates a shift in blood alkalinity, along with possible shifts in consciousness. What about the other direction? What happens when you radically *increase* CO_2?

At first my research didn't turn up much, but then I accidentally stumbled on something intriguing. Roger Walsh, an MD/PhD professor at the University of California–Davis, and one of the founders of the field of transpersonal psychology, had sent me his book *Higher Wisdom*. In it, he'd interviewed many of the original pioneering psychedelic researchers from the late '50s and early '60s and captured their stories for the coming generations. This was a time when Sandoz's finest LSD-25 was being used in all sorts of hard-to-imagine studies—from treating schizophrenic children on UCLA's pediatric ward to serving as pain relief at oncology clinics. Stan Grof's original research in Hungary, combining strobe light visual entrainment with galvanic skin response and EEG measures (along with heroic doses of LSD), makes our current psychedelic "renaissance" look downright quaint. These academics were curious, fearless, and going for it.

But what really caught my attention was the recurring mention of Meduna's mixture. Named after Ladislas Meduna, a Hungarian neuropathologist and colleague of Stan Grof's, this gas blend was a mixture of carbon dioxide and oxygen. Ranging in concentration, the most common carb-oxygen or carbogen blend was 70 percent oxygen and 30 percent carbon dioxide.

Meduna, one of the pioneers of convulsive therapy, had first experimented giving schizophrenic patients the gas to see if it could prompt grand mal seizures that could help with their condition. It was the respiratory equivalent of electroshock therapy. Give a patient 70/30 carbogen to breathe and something interesting happens. Even though they're enjoying three and a half times the oxygen of regular air, they're also registering seven and a half times the carbon dioxide of exhaled breath. So despite having more life-giving O_2 than they could ever need, their brain tricks them into the acute and not altogether enjoyable experience of dying of suffocation—often to the point of prompting a disembodied altered state.

While Meduna's interest in carbogen as a convulsive therapeutic never really panned out, Grof and other psychedelic therapists found it helpful screening LSD patients for "abreaction"—or the triggering of a past trauma. If you read the accounts of patients who took the Meduna test before passing the Acid Test—several of them reported that the carbogen experience provided more profound breakthroughs and insight than the subsequent psychedelic session.

That got me thinking. LSD is one of the most powerful mind-altering substances ever discovered, and if modulating the ratios of the air we breathe could produce comparable insights, that seemed worth looking into. Initiating a crisis state like carbogen prompts, followed by a rapturous release like nitroxygen delivers, could produce a meaningful body/brain reset—all by rejiggering a couple of atmospheric gases. Now that we had a sense of what tweaking oxygen and carbon dioxide could do, it was time to explore the possibilities of nitrogen and a couple of its derivatives.

How the West Was Fun

Nitrous oxide is an inorganic compound that's been off-gassing from the atmosphere, soil, and oceans for eons. It's one of the more interesting members of the nitrogen family. While only a slight variation of the inert nitrogen that makes up roughly 80 percent of the air we breathe, this oxide has a fundamentally different effect on our nervous system. Nitrous soothes nerves and eases pain but also gives rise to experiences stranger—and potentially more therapeutically useful—than most Schedule I substances.

Today, we have new insights from the field of neuroscience into why it does what it does. So in our survey of respiration and the potent impact it can have on our bodies and brains, we'd be remiss if we didn't discuss exactly what happens when you take two atoms of nitrogen, bond them to one atom of oxygen, and inhale deeply.

* * *

On October 14, 1833, *The Albany Argus*, a small-town paper in upstate New York, published a curious quarter-page advertisement on behalf of the local museum. It invited loyal patrons to attend an exhibition by a "Dr. Coult of New York, London and Calcutta" on the effects of "Exhilarating Gas." This substance, the ad proclaimed, produced the "most astonishing effects on the nervous system," ranging from laughing and dancing to wrestling and boxing. It went on to assure prospective attendees that Dr. C. was a "practiced chemist so no fears need be entertained of inhaling an impure gas" and that ladies and gentlemen "of the first respectability" had all enjoyed its "highly pleasurable effects without debilitation." The advertisement closed with a zinger: "Those persons who inhale the gas will be separated from the audience by means of a net so that spectators . . . *will be perfectly free from danger.*" Admittance was only 25 cents.

Two weeks later, Dr. Coult appeared before a packed house. Nervous volunteers of both sexes stepped up to inhale from his contraption, tackling each other, shouting out epiphanies, and dissolving into giggles. Townsfolk could talk of nothing else for weeks. But it turned out that "Dr. Coult of New York, London and Calcutta" wasn't a practiced chemist at all—not that anyone really cared. He was a nineteen-year-old kid from next-door Massachusetts. In fact, Coult wasn't even his real name. It was *Colt*. Samuel Colt, the man who'd go on to become the most famous and wealthy entrepreneur of his age.

A few years before his Albany visit, Colt had been expelled from Amherst Academy. His father, figuring his unruly son could do with a "hands-on" education, signed him on as a ship's boy on voyages that included the aforementioned stops in London and Calcutta. According to his later memoirs, Colt became fascinated by the ship's wheel and how "regardless of which way the wheel was spun, each spoke always came in direct line with a clutch that could be set to hold it." It gave him the idea to transpose that mechanism to a pistol, creating a revolving barrel that could hold multiple bullets at a time. While at sea, he whittled two prototypes out of wood. But when he returned home, his father was unimpressed with the concept. If he wanted to take his idea to market, Samuel realized, he'd have to raise the funds himself.

Which is when the enterprising young inventor conceived his alter ego, "Dr. Coult." In less than two years of hosting exhibitions like his sold-out stand in Albany, he raised the seed capital to secure the patents for what became the iconic Colt .45. That fast-action pistol turned the tide for the Texas Rangers against the Comanches and sat on the hip of every sheriff, gunslinger, and cavalryman from Deadwood to Little Bighorn. Laughing gas, a simple combination of two common elements, prone to producing curious effects in those who breathed it, ended up bankrolling "the Gun that Won the West."

As we'll see, Colt's story isn't even the strangest in the annals of nitrous oxide.

* * *

Nitrous oxide had been known to experimenters for some time before Colt latched on to it. The gas was first synthesized in 1772 by the English chemist Joseph Priestley. A few decades later, James Watt, of future steam engine fame, invented a machine to produce "Factitious Airs." In 1800, Humphry Davy published his definitive work *Researches, Chemical and Philosophical*, which correctly identified the gas as a possible pain reliever useful in surgery and coined the name that stuck: laughing gas.

For the first half of the nineteenth century, it enjoyed popularity at "laughing gas parties" for the British upper class. Socialites gathered at country estates and London town houses to take turns inhaling the vapors and enjoying each other's reveries and insights. The poets Samuel Taylor Coleridge and Robert Southey took part, as did Peter Roget of *Roget's Thesaurus* and Thomas Wedgwood, son of the famous potter.

As these parties crossed the Atlantic, Samuel Colt capitalized on the trend. But it wasn't until forty years after his Albany exhibition that nitrous oxide truly met its match in someone who could get past the laughs and see its potential as a tool of serious insight.

Harvard psychologist William James was first introduced to the gas in the 1870s and found it instantly illuminating. At the time, he was battling back from a serious depression that had nearly cost him his career and life. Trained as a physician but increasingly drawn to philosophy and religion, James subscribed to a school of thought known as pragmatism. This worldview hinged on the stark idea that there are no universal truths or constants in the world, only more or less practical working assumptions. His initial experiences with nitrous oxide freed him from his rather bleak materialism and emotional despair. He became, by his own description, a rational mystic.

"I strongly urge others to repeat the experiment. . . . With me, as with every other person of whom I have heard, the keynote of the experience is the tremendously exciting sense of an intense metaphysical illumination. Truth lies open to the view in depth beneath depth of almost blinding evidence. The mind sees all logical relations of being with an apparent subtlety and instantaneity to which its normal consciousness offers no parallel."

Those insights made such an impact that scholars separate James's writings into clear "before laughing gas" and "after" categories. He admitted in his 1902 *Varieties of Religious Experience* that "my impression of its truth has ever since [experiencing nitrous oxide] remained unshaken. It is that our normal waking consciousness . . . is but one special type of consciousness, whilst all about it, parted from it by the filmiest of screens, there lie potential forms of consciousness entirely different."

That conviction catalyzed his work as arguably America's greatest philosophical mind. James's forays into nitrous spawned two of his key contributions to academia: the first that direct experience is more valuable than religious doctrine or dogma and the second that there is no singular and absolute truth—only a multitude of perspectives.

This mystical pluralism foreshadows much of what we are still exploring over a century later and gives us a tantalizing hint of what we are searching for in this book: a way to harness the peak experience of lowercase "rapture," without veering into certainty and dogma. James just beat us to it.

Despite the inspirational benefits that James received from his explorations with the gas, he had a persistent problem—how hard he found it to hang on to its quicksilver insights. "Only as sobriety returns," he lamented, "the feeling of insight fades, and one is left staring vacantly at a few disjointed words and phrases, as one stares at a cadaverous-looking snow peak from which sunset glow has just fled, or at a black cinder left by an extinguished brand."

Because of this persistent gap between what he could glimpse and what he could retain, and his fear that his colleagues would mock his flights of fancy as "unscientific," James discontinued his use of the substance. He spent the rest of his career trying to map with reason what he had first discovered in the realm of revelation.

James wasn't the only prominent explorer to find those insights hard to hang on to. It happened to Winston Churchill too, quite literally, by accident. While on a 1931 speaking tour of New York, Churchill got run over on Fifth Avenue. He had forgotten that traffic went the other way in the United States and exited his cab straight into an oncoming car. He was rushed to Lenox Hill Hospital, where Dr. Charles Sanford, one of the very few physicians specializing in anesthesiology in the early 1930s, was on duty. In what may have been one of his first encounters with the gas—but clearly not the last—Churchill experienced something remarkably similar to what James had before him.

"With me, the nitrous oxide trance usually takes this form," Churchill later told the *Daily Mail*, "the sanctum is occupied by alien powers. I see the absolute truth and explanation of things, but . . . it is beyond anything the human mind was meant to master." With typical dark humor, he went on to note, "depth beyond depth of *unendurable* truth opens. I have therefore regarded the nitrous-oxide trance as a mere substitution of mental for physical pain."

Despite the public revelations of academics and statesmen like James and Churchill, the mysteries of nitrous oxide remained largely underground. The notion that the gas's genius always disappeared on return to sobriety led most observers to dismiss it as a tool of serious inquiry.

By the end of World War II, "laughing gas" had established itself as a benign and commonplace anesthetic. From dentist chairs to doctor's offices to birthing rooms, the compound was used to calm the nerves of kids getting fillings, soothe the pain of mothers delivering babies, and ease the minds of patients sedated for surgery. The World Health Organization found it so useful it even placed it on its *List of Essential Medicines*. "It is a cerebral depressant and produces light anesthesia without demonstrably depressing the respiratory or vasomotor centre," the WHO explained, acknowledging rather blandly, "induction is rapid and not unpleasant *although transient excitement may occur.*"

Since then, nitrous oxide has gone on to play a somewhat schizoid role as a harmless sedative administered by white-coated professionals and as a casual diversion for those seeking its "transient excitement"— often to the point of abuse. In 2016, the Global Drug Survey reported that the United Kingdom had the highest instance of illicit use of all nineteen countries studied. Overall, nitrous oxide now ranks as the seventh most popular recreational drug in the world.

In the United States, *The Village Voice* investigated the Nitrous Mafia—a gang of ruffian black marketers who traveled the music festival circuit selling giant balloons of "hippie crack" to eager concertgoers. "It's an instant rush of pure euphoria," fan Justin Heller told the *Voice*, "but it only lasts for 30 seconds or a minute, and then you want it back." When asked why he chose to partake, another enthusiast explained, "Because nitrous is the best orgasm I've ever had in my life."

Between these two poles—helpful anesthetic or mindless diversion—the most interesting thing about this substance keeps getting forgotten. From Samuel Colt proclaiming it "the highest of all possible heavens" to William James noting its "intense metaphysical illumination" to Winston Churchill acknowledging it as the "absolute truth and explanation of things," we've overlooked the most obvious question, again and again.

What were all those gas-drunk explorers actually laughing about?

To be sure, it's not the high-pitched giggles that helium provides. It's not the goofy euphoria of cannabis or even the spill-your-drink buzz of a few beers. If we are to take the accounts of early explorers at face value, the laughter of laughing gas comes from nothing less than sheer gobsmacked amazement. Perhaps the only rational response to nearly instantaneous revelation.

With nitrous oxide intoxication, the mechanism of action is fundamentally different from the disinhibition of alcohol or other common inebriants. For starters, nitrous oxide triggers three of the six neurochemicals central to almost all non-ordinary states of consciousness—norepinephrine, dopamine, endorphins (the other three are anandamide, serotonin, and oxytocin). That alone is more than enough to qualify it as a "molecule of interest" in our investigation of state-shifting tools.

Its *anxiolytic*, or antianxiety, qualities stem mainly from its bonding to dopamine and benzodiazepine receptors (think Valium and Xanax); its *analgesic*, or pain-relieving, properties come from the endorphins or opioids it releases (think morphine or OxyContin). We're carefree and pain-free, and feel *awesome*. That combination puts nitrous oxide squarely in the ranks of go-to comfort drugs but doesn't explain how it inspired Samuel Taylor Coleridge's poetry, William James's philosophy, or Winston Churchill's reveries.

Fortunately, in the last ten years, we've learned more about the biological and chemical underpinnings of the nitrous experience than we'd gathered over the past two centuries.

The Amazing Nitrogen Family

As we track down what the World Health Organization so blandly described as the "transient excitement" that nitrous oxide produces, there are a few more links to connect. They bring us all the way back to William James's stomping grounds at Harvard Medical School. There, Herbert Benson, whom we met earlier, became the leading authority on the body's biological response to peak experience. His quest led him to a deep study of the nitrogen family and nitrous oxide's kissing cousin, *nitric* oxide. This neurotransmitter carries away stress chemicals from the brain and serves as a vasodilator in the body—Viagra, which directly boosts nitric oxide production, makes use of this tidy little side effect.

Nitric oxide (NO), identical to nitrous oxide (N_2O) but for one nitrogen atom, is, according to its foremost researcher, "the catalyst of physical, mental, and even spiritual experience." That's tantalizingly close to the subjective reports of nitrous users through the centuries. And here's where it gets really interesting: once inside our lungs and brains, the two gases behave similarly. When a user inhales nitrous oxide, enzymes in the brain break it down *into nitric oxide*. It then zips across the blood-brain barrier and up and down our spinal column, faster than thought.

Just across town from Benson's lab, researchers at MIT have discovered a neuroelectrical explanation for some of this molecule's unique effects. As reported in the journal *Clinical Neurophysiology*, Dr. Emery Brown found that when subjects were tracked with an electroencephalogram (EEG) while inhaling a fifty-fifty gas blend of "nitroxygen," something fascinating happened to their brain waves. They shifted from high-frequency beta waves (12.5–30 HZ—the kind normally associated with alert thinking) into extremely low-frequency delta waves (0.1–4 Hz—the kind normally associated with deep and dreamless sleep). And there was another unusual thing about those readings: the amplitude, or height, of those delta waves was *double* what they normally are when we're sleeping.

"We literally watched it and marveled because it was totally un-expected," Brown told *MIT News*. *"Nitrous oxide has control over the brain in ways no other drug does"* [emphasis added]. That's a pretty bold statement coming from a world-class researcher with access to an unlimited medicine cabinet.

This was such an unexpected finding because in EEG research, delta waves are very much the redheaded stepchild. Sleep researchers pay a bit of attention to them, but not nearly as much as they do to REM cycles, the rapid eye movement where most dreaming happens. Waking EEG studies tend to focus on beta waves—where we do most of our problem-solving and cogitating—or alpha and theta frequencies—where, if we're lucky or skilled enough, we experience flow states, hypnagogic states (those moments in-between waking and dreaming), or deep meditative states. But waking delta? That's an underreported story. And it just might hold the key to unlocking nitrous oxide's secrets.

"If you see slow EEG oscillations," Brown says, "something has happened to the brainstem." Without those excitatory signals from our brain stem lighting up higher brain functions, you usually fall unconscious and into deep delta-wave sleep (or anesthesia). Except with nitrous oxide, you *don't fall asleep*. You're awake and aware of the experience. You even have some ability to steer. It's like backdoor lucid dreaming.

Brown's team uncovered another detail, one that explains why James and Churchill both experienced sudden insight followed by frustrating amnesia. The delta waves only last a few minutes, after which the brain returns to normal. "These slow-delta oscillations begin approximately 6 min after the switch [to breathing 50/50 nitroxygen] and last from 3 to 12 min," Brown explained, "before returning to the beta and gamma oscillations." Even with continued exposure to the gas, that three-to-twelve-minute window of waking delta is all you get, before brain activity adapts and normalizes.

Brown hypothesizes that nitrous molecules exert this remarkable control by binding to receptor sites in the thalamus and cortex. This knocks out arousal signals from deeper down in the brain, allowing a full system reboot. Delta-wave activity has also been shown in DMT and ketamine states—both experiences renowned for their other-worldliness as well as their access to robust amounts of salient information.

A new Stanford study published in *Nature* has shown that the dissociative or otherworldly effects of delta-wave EEG activity correlate directly with the antidepressant effects of ketamine therapy. "This state often manifests as the perception of being on the outside looking in at the cockpit of the plane that's your body or mind—and what you're seeing you just don't consider to be yourself," Karl Deisseroth, the lead author, said. When this team was able to use electrical impulses to stimulate patients' brains into delta frequencies, they had that same dissociative experience, even without the drugs. And those moments of "being on the outside looking in" appeared to alleviate depressive symptoms. More delta, in other words, less blues.

Another recent study has shown an additional positive element of delta-wave activity. In a sleep study researchers found that only during slow-oscillation delta waves is the intracranial pressure (ICP) low enough to allow cerebrospinal fluid to come in and "wash" the brain tissues of beta-amyloid plaque. If you sleep poorly, or don't get enough delta-wave cycling, the research shows you're at a higher risk for early-onset Alzheimer's and a host of other neurodegenerative conditions.

Regardless of what method we use to get there—ketamine, meditation, brain stimulation, or nitrous oxide —once we find ourselves in a waking delta-wave EEG state, the results are often profound. Delta waves, it's becoming clear, can mend our brains, spark our minds, and soothe our souls.

* * *

Taken together, the MIT, Harvard, and Stanford studies go a long way to explaining what William James was marveling about all those years ago. Up until now, we've had only the halting accounts of users who, while insisting that *something* profound occurs in the spaces afforded by the gas, were never exactly sure what it was or why it kept happening. As James lamented, "one is left staring vacantly at a few disjointed words and phrases."

But today, we've got more tools in our kit. The fields of comparative religion, optimal psychology, and neuropharmacology that James himself inspired give us more precise language and frameworks to interpret these experiences with. Voice recordings and medical measurements allow us to capture more of the fleeting and dreamlike insights that slipped through his fingers so long ago.

Nitrous oxide knocks out conscious processing, accelerates pattern recognition, and boosts the signal of how fast we can think, dramatically. And it does it for anyone with enough wherewithal to retain what they learn. This does not make it harmless—any more than the wine served at Communion absolves us from alcoholism and organ failure if abused. But it does point a way forward when considering a move beyond "placebo sacraments" toward ones that more reliably deliver insight and inspiration.

When "Dr. Coult of London and Calcutta" decided to make a few bucks delighting bored bystanders with laughing gas, he couldn't have known that what he was peddling would exceed his own hype. By switching out the nitrogen in the air we breathe for a slight variation, we unlock worlds of information and inspiration normally inaccessible to us. And it works for people experiencing pain, anxiety, and trauma, as well as those who want to plumb the depths of the human condition. "No account of the universe in its totality can be final," William James reflected, "which leaves these other forms of consciousness quite discarded."

That's a possibility that should take our breath away.

The Breath of Life

So what would it look like to combine all of the respiratory practices we've just explored into one, integrated Vital Respiration Protocol? Warm up with box breathing to increase our CO_2 tolerances and diaphragmatic control. Master the free diver's vagal breathing to lower

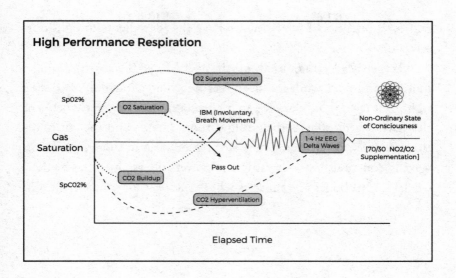

our heart rates (you can even throw an ice mask on your face if you want to induce the mammalian dive reflex). Blow off excess CO_2 with Grof's holotropic hyperventilating, supersaturate our red blood cells by pre-breathing pure oxygen, and then practice gas-assisted static apnea with a 70/30 nitrous oxide/oxygen blend, or a 30/70 carbon dioxide/oxygen blend.

If we're feeling creative, we could take a cue from the patients who found Meduna's Mixture so profound and add one more thought experiment to the practice. On that final inhalation of pure, life-giving oxygen and nitrous oxide, why not imagine it's your first gasping breath as an infant? And after you hold it for what seems like an actual lifetime, until there's no fighting it anymore, exhale as if it's your last on this earth.

By combining traditional and modern breathing techniques, would it be possible to step outside of regular time, and, like that ancient didgeridu player, access some version of Dreamtime? What are the depths of experience we can glimpse if we take the habitual and unconscious process of breathing and make it deliberate and intentional?

As we will see at the end of Part Two, this Vital Respiration Protocol can serve as a foundation for more ambitious undertakings. Combined with embodiment triggers, driving music, selective substances, and even intentional sexuality, we have the ingredients to light ourselves up.

"Oxygen: Everything needs it," the poet Mary Oliver writes, "bone, muscles, and even, while it calls the earth its home, the soul." And she's right. But it's not only oxygen that's profound. It's all the elements of the Earth's atmosphere, including carbon dioxide and the entire nitrogen family. By changing how we breathe, we can tune the dials on waking consciousness—as easily and powerfully as any other method we have. Our bones and muscles will thank us. Our souls might too.

CHAPTER 6

Embodiment

For most of Western history, since Aristotle and Augustine, we have valued head over heart, cognition over emotion. Our bodies, filled as they are with hungers and desires, have been seen as unreliable servants compared to the masters of our minds.

That bias only became more entrenched over time. Today our increasingly abstracted and digital lives have left us wandering around like disembodied heads on sticks. It's no wonder modern life can feel so disjointed and dejected.

But that's been changing recently.

An emerging field of embodied cognition has begun mapping exactly how intertwined our feeling and thinking really are, and how connected our feeling is to our healing as well. Bessel van der Kolk, a psychiatrist who has held appointments at Boston University and Harvard University, has been one of the pioneers establishing the connection between physiology and psychology. In his book *The Body Keeps the Score*, he argues that trauma has a physical signature that has to be released if we are to heal.

Lisa Feldman Barrett, a psychologist at Harvard Medical School and the author of *How Emotions Are Made*, has dismantled much of neuropsychology with her theory of constructed emotion. She suggests that well below conscious emotions lies our interoception, which is literally our guts trying to guess what's going to happen next and prepare us accordingly. If we can manage our interoception, Barrett suggests, we can take more responsibility for our emotions too.

These researchers and hundreds of others are giving both proof and permission for us to reconnect our bodies and brains. From breathing, to moving, to meditating, to biofeedback, there are increasingly varied ways for us to discharge trauma and heighten integration, and none of them requires lying down on a couch to talk about it.

Beyond these academics, there are some even stranger things going on in the field of embodied cognition. They can give us a sense of how powerfully our physicality shapes us, and how we in turn can shape our physicality. Rather than trying to tame or transcend our bodies, as Aristotle and Augustine might have encouraged, we can learn to inhabit them fully, and without apology.

Make It Hurt So Good

> *Nature has placed mankind under the governance of two sovereign masters, pain and pleasure. It is for them alone to point out what we ought to do, as well as to determine what we shall do.*
>
> —Jeremy Bentham

This is one of those real-life stories that has too many twists to sound believable. So I will tell it straight, the way I heard it. It involves a Bengali German noblewoman turned federal agent, her conservative intelligence operative husband, real-life vampires, underground sex clubs, and, ultimately, the traumatized first responders of 9/11. Along the way, it will give us some insight into the power of the body to heal the wounds of our hearts.

It started last year, when I'd been invited to the Harvard Club in New York to speak about a book I'd just written, *Stealing Fire*. The imposing stone façade of the 134-year-old club is a monument to exclusivity, even in midtown Manhattan. It's a New World Hogwarts for the culturati, complete with moth-eaten animal mounts, dusty portraits, and a stuffed elephant on the staircase.

After I gave my talk I was invited to dine with the event sponsor, a Harvard alumna named Nermin Ahmad, a retired Navy SEAL, and the widow of one of Bernie Madoff's sons. The wine flowed and the conversation with it. Inevitably, someone asked what I was working on next. I shared the outlines of the breath work and PTSD research project the Flow Genome Project is working on with Johns Hopkins.

"Ah!" said Nermin, with a mischievous glint. "Then I should definitely tell you about the time my husband and I went undercover in the vampire community."

That concluded small talk for the night. Someone topped up our glasses, and we settled in.

Nermin told us that right after 9/11 she'd worked for the Department of Homeland Security, first in Washington, D.C., on the anthrax scare, then in New York City, where she took on an additional freelance assignment: infiltrating the New York underground to track domestic terror cells.

The first briefing? Vampires. Not *True Blood* cosplay wannabes, but as close to the real thing as you could get: flesh and blood (and actual fangs). "My husband and I were intrigued," she explained. "What is this vampire community? What makes them up? . . . Is it another cult? Was it a way of getting money out of rich children? Is it used to control people? Do they have a political intent?

"Our analysis was that there were about seventy-five thousand self-proclaimed vampires in New York City at the time. . . . Many turned out to be the door people for bars and restaurants with a night scene. It was interesting to look at them. One moment they'd have regular teeth, the next moment, they'd have fangs."

About those fangs.

One of the key figures of this movement was Father Sebastiaan, "a gentleman and dentist who'd made a lot of money as the creator of retractable fangs for the vampire community." Apparently there was quite a bit of demand. He sold them at a premium to vampires in the United States, Germany, Scotland, and England.

It wasn't all fancy dress and fake teeth. "The vampires did drink plasma," Nermin admitted. "They'd have a 'rebirth' every year where a vampire goddess submerged from a bathtub full of plasma, and everyone would drink the remaining plasma, in the bath. We were there solely as guests," she clarified when she saw the looks on our faces.

Every Friday night for the better part of two years, Nermin and her husband would find their way to downtown hotspots—kinky cabaret dinner clubs like La Nouvelle Justine and Lucky Cheng's. Despite their original assignment to infiltrate a suspected terrorist cell or possible Satanic cult, Nermin and her husband found themselves struck by the raw humanity of this subculture.

"After two years we decided the vampires were no risk to society," Nermin explained. Her husband did file a briefing on them but clarified they were no threat to civil society. "We actually grew to be quite fond of these communities. They were amongst some of the kindest, most welcoming people I'd ever known and they really kind of wrapped their souls around me."

While adventurous tourists could walk into those clubs, sit down, and be titillated by the campy performances, those venues also served as a discreet rally point for a more serious core community. "Most of these restaurants were equipped with underground dungeons and secret tunnels that connected them. There was also the Hellfire club nearby [with a hard-core BDSM (bondage, discipline, and sadomasochism) scene]," Nermin said.

She and her husband noticed an unexpected and entirely different population drawn to Justine's and the Hellfire Club. Firefighters and paramedics who'd recently survived the tragedy of the Twin Towers started showing up in surprising numbers. From a group of people who couldn't seem to get enough blood to those who'd seen way too much of it, the BDSM world seemed to be serving a purpose beyond thrill seeking.

"As I began to taper off [our research of the vampire community] we noticed that an increasing number of first responders had survivor's guilt," Nermin said, "and a call went out to professional dominatrixes who were willing to train with them, to be available to give what I called 'a concerted beating.' It's not beating someone till they cry. It's beating someone in a way that allows their soul to release, so it's beyond crying.

"It's coming to terms with the very basic self. It's not seen as sadistic, it's seen as curative. I was curious, are they just bullshitting?" she wondered. "Is this just an extreme form of sadism or is it actually something that could be useful?"

Nermin asked some of these NYFD members what drove them to seek out these intense experiences. "Many of the first responders were experiencing survivors' guilt and actually found relief through the floggings," she said. "They had earned the right to be happy and alive again."

Since she had never witnessed a mass casualty event or BDSM, Nermin was searching for a way to understand. Her husband, who'd served in Europe during World War II, "got where they were coming from and that this wasn't a bad thing or wrong thing. This was a way of dealing with PTSD by going into yourself to get over the guilt feeling. . . . *If you can solve it by yourself, you have a better cure for it*" [emphasis added].

He shared with his wife that the hardest part of survivor's guilt is second-guessing those moments where you could've done something different. "When you watched your friends being killed or dying and you wonder if you could have saved their lives. And the need to be affirmed that you had a right to be alive when they weren't. Most of them just needed to weep in a safe place."

Based on my limited understanding of whips, leather, and dungeons, it had always seemed there was an erotic, almost lurid component to what was going on in BDSM. But in this situation that wasn't the case. "There was never sex in any of that," Nermin explained. "First of all, explicit sex, orgasmic release for a female or a male, is illegal in New York in any place that serves alcohol. And second, these guys didn't get aroused from the beatings. They were naked, so you could tell."

So what was going on here? What was happening to provide such

profound experiences of healing, of moving beyond random traumatic pain, by deliberately inflicting even more pain? It was more
than simple atonement or punishment for survivor's guilt. And it was
the polar opposite of most approaches to trauma—which usually
go to great lengths to lessen rather than intensify painful feelings on
the road to healing.

If what those grieving first responders said was true, it offered "a
coming to terms with the very basic self," a "soul release." But how was
this happening?

*   *   *

A decade after the underground scene in Manhattan had run its
course, researchers at Tilburg University in the Netherlands did some
empirical studies that confirmed Nermin's earlier reporting. The
Dutch researchers surveyed a thousand practitioners of BDSM to determine if participants were more or less mentally healthy than the
regular population. The prevailing assumption was that people drawn
to these communities and practices were somehow damaged goods
and were reenacting compulsions from earlier trauma. As recently
as 2014, if you were found out to be a BDSM player (as they call
themselves), you could be denied custody of your children in divorce
proceedings.

The Tilburg study turned up some interesting results. Specifically,
when measured against the Big Five Personality Traits (often referred
to as the OCEAN scale, for Openness, Conscientiousness, Extrover-
sion, Agreeableness, and Neuroticism), the researchers found that
people who took part in BDSM were less neurotic, more open, more
conscientious, and more extroverted than the control group. They
were also less sensitive to rejection and reported a higher sense of well-
being. Agreeableness, however, was unaffected, as the subjects skewed
toward salty.

But something within the experience of focused pain and deliberate loss of control appeared to have a health-giving effect. These
people weren't broken—whatever they were doing was leaving them
healthier than normal.

Another researcher, social psychologist Brad Sagarin, wanted to get past subjective self-reporting into the neurobiology of the kink experience itself. First, Sagarin confirmed what practitioners already knew—that engaging in the practice of focused pain, combined with surrender of physical and emotional control, led to a reliable change in consciousness. For many, this was the central motivation driving their practice. "We do get these descriptions of a kind of dreamy, floaty, pleasurable feeling," Sagarin says. "People lose the distinction between themselves and their partner, between themselves and the universe . . . people's executive function capabilities get temporarily reduced and one of the pleasurable side effects of that is the altered state that people find themselves in."

Sagarin hypothesizes that transient hypofrontality, where activity in the dorsolateral prefrontal cortex decreases (and with it, the executive function of the conscious self), is a key part of the experience those New York first responders were seeking. "When that area of the brain gets down-regulated," Sagarin told *The Atlantic*, "we can lose the distinction between ourselves and the universe." That's the anatomical explanation—the most complex parts of our brains shut down and we experience that as relief from distressing thoughts and memories.

But there's also a chemical element that comes with it—a flooding of norepinephrine, cortisol, endorphins, dopamine, and anandamide. They share considerable overlap, Sagarin notes, "with the euphoric and dissociative experience of endurance runners, [mountaineers], meditators, and individuals under hypnosis."

So while the first responders sought out relief in dungeons, everyone from ultramarathoners to CrossFitters (who engage in grueling workouts) to Vipassana meditators (who must undergo nine days of excruciating seated meditation) are all looking for the same end result. "It's because of this lack of blood flow and neuronal signaling that marathon runners and kinksters will find themselves in an altered state of consciousness," says Sagarin, "one that's usually described as dreamy and pleasurable."

* * *

Harnessing pain to shift mental state has well-documented antecedents in many religious traditions. The traditional Lakota Sun Dance
ceremony, a grueling initiatory rite involving fasting and suspension
from body piercings until the flesh tears away, is a well-known, if
romanticized, example. The 1970 film *A Man Called Horse*, starring
Richard Harris (of King Arthur in *Camelot* and Albus Dumbledore
in *Harry Potter* fame), exposed the popular imagination to this secretive practice.

There are comparable practices around the world. In Scandinavia,
the priests of Odin used to endure horrendous suffering in imitation
of their god, who hanged himself for nine days and nights on the
Cosmic Tree. The followers of Mithras observed a secret initiatory
ritual from boyhood to manhood that involved trance, flogging, sleep
deprivation, and other classic techniques of state induction. The Spartans held a Feast of Flagellations at the altar of Diana, where boys
were beaten nearly senseless by the gathered crowds (and expected to
endure their punishments silently as an honor to their families).

To this day, the Penitentes of northern New Mexico annually re-
enact the passion of Jesus of Nazareth—shouldering heavy wooden
crosses, wearing crowns of sharp thorns, and submitting to floggings
with brine-soaked whips. A few are even chosen for the honor of being tied up on crosses and symbolically crucified on Good Friday.

Privation, pain, and suffering have an ancient, if counterintuitive,
relationship to healing. Long before the firefighters of New York
found their way to redemption through underground clubs, devotees
have been purposefully harnessing these techniques to decouple what
they are feeling physically from what they experience emotionally.

As far as we know, humans are the only animal wired up this way.
Pain is a uniquely human indulgence. Spicy foods, roller coasters, and
horror movies aren't pleasant on the surface. Perversely, we love them
all the more because of it. Scientists have tried and failed to mimic
our preference for spicy peppers in rats. Animals can be trained to
self-harm to get a reward but only with positive reinforcement like
food. "Generally, when an animal experiences something negative, it
avoids it," explains Paul Rozin, of the University of Pennsylvania. "If

an animal took a roller coaster it would be scared, and it would never go again."

We appear to be unique in the animal kingdom in discovering you can hot-wire pain to experience pleasure and even healing.

* * *

Beyond the neurophysiology of these experiences, they share another common trait: virtually all of these communities—from vampire undergrounds, to Sun Dancers, to Penitentes—have been misunderstood, feared, and suppressed by the larger societies around them. Something about the strange power in these observances unsettles those who'd like to maintain monopolies on the use of painful punishment or direct access to spirituality (or both).

In the fourteenth century, the Catholic Church condemned a brotherhood of flagellants in Spain and Italy as a cult. The friars, it seems, had taken the Church's exhortation "to live a Christ-like life" further than was comfortable. The U.S. government banned indigenous observance of the Sun Dance in the 1890s because they were afraid that it would incite a spiritual revival and uprising. The only reason I was able to write about the 9/11 first responders in New York was that their community was infiltrated by paid informants during the War on Terror.

* * *

And yet one thing is constant across these practices and the communities that keep them. While we cannot manage the amount of pain that comes to us in these lives, if we choose to meet it on purpose and with intention, it can hold the key to healing.

Perhaps the most poignant expression of the power of transformative suffering is the Tibetan Buddhist practice of Tonglen. In most contemplative disciplines, the subject either tries to cultivate positive feelings like equanimity or compassion or they seek stillness and emptiness. But in Tonglen, you do the exact opposite: You steer into the skid of your suffering, and the suffering of the entire world.

You visualize your own pain and grief as black, sticky tar or smoke,

and picture inhaling it into your body. Then as you exhale you transform it into white light and love. Once you can handle metabolizing
your own pain, you extend your focus outward to your friends and
family, then to your community and country, and ultimately to the
entire world. You literally learn to treat our collective suffering as the
raw material for fueling love.

After the global success of her book *The Color Purple*, Alice Walker
experienced the death of her mother, a debilitating battle with Lyme
disease, and intense backlash for her unflinching portrayal of domestic violence in the African American South. While she was broken
and suffering she struck up a friendship with the Tibetan Buddhist
teacher Pema Chodron. "It was Tonglen, the practice of taking in
people's pain and sending out whatever you have that is positive, that
helped me through this difficult passage," Walker shared. "In my experience suffering is perennial; there is always suffering. . . . I used to
think there was no use to it, but now I think that there is."

Chodron, deeply acquainted with personal heartache herself, replied, "We can take that very moment and flip it. The very thing that
causes us to harden and our suffering to intensify can soften us and
make us more decent and kinder people. That takes a lot of courage."

So whether first responders transmuting psychological pain by
cultivating physical pain, or Sun Dancers and Penitentes seeking
connection to the Divine through agony, to Walker and Chodron
meditating on all of our shared suffering as a way to make sense of
their personal grief, we have a way forward. And it's through the paradox that by embracing our suffering, we end up suffering less.

Or as Walker puts it, "My heart's been broken so many times, it
just swings open wide now, like a suitcase."

Bliss Comes from Within

A few years ago Jordan Peterson, scourge of progressives and adopted
patron saint of the alt-right, wrote a self-help book called *12 Rules for
Life*. In it, he told the story of lobsters, serotonin, and the need to assert

oneself or be dominated by those who do. Wimpy lobsters, Peterson maintained, experienced depleted serotonin after getting their asses kicked. This made them even more subservient, prompting more ass kickings. The solution for our downtrodden crustacean cousins (and for the twentysomething males who latched on to Peterson) was to take their fight to the world.

"Look for your inspiration to the victorious lobster, with its 350 million years of practical wisdom," encouraged Peterson. "Stand up straight, with your shoulders back." The lobster meme stuck, showing up on bumper stickers, social media posts, and T-shirts for his adoring fans. Marine biologists cringed at his appropriation of crustaceans, noting that our last shared ancestors were ancient sea worms and that there was a lot of variance in how serotonin has informed animal behavior since then.

While Peterson's attaboy moralizing may not have held up to scientific scrutiny, he wasn't wrong to scour the sea floor for insights into the human condition. He was just looking under the wrong rocks. And he was two hundred million years too late.

Sea sponges are among the most primitive and ancient invertebrates, showing up in the fossil record over 550 million years ago. Recently biologists have confirmed they have receptors for a little-known set of neurotransmitters called *endocannabinoids*. Receptors for these signaling molecules have been found in all more complex vertebrates too. They are ubiquitous and central to the nervous systems of virtually all life on earth (and under the sea). But we still wouldn't know the first thing about the endocannabinoid system of the sea sponge, or its central role in human health and well-being, if it weren't for the stoner son of a famous U.S. senator.

First, some backstory.

In 1964, Raphael Mechoulam, a biochemist at Hebrew University, noticed a strange gap in the medical record. Back in 1805, Prussian chemist Friedrich Sertürner had successfully isolated morphine from poppy seeds. By 1859, another German scientist, Albert Niemann, had isolated the alkaloid cocaine from coca leaves. Identifying both of these compounds led to major advances in our understanding of the endorphin and dopamine systems that govern our experience of pain and pleasure.

But Mechoulam realized no one had any idea about the chemical makeup of one of the most widespread and oldest medicines in the world—cannabis. Burnt hemp seeds show up in Neolithic European caves and archaeologists have recently confirmed that the plant originated on the Tibetan Plateau as far back as twenty-eight million years ago. By botanical accident, this hardy weed creates compounds that fit lock and key into the most ancient parts of our brains. As a result we have carefully cultivated it and carried it around the world. As Michael Pollan put it, "Cannabis pleasures our minds in order to use our feet." Despite the plant's global range and centuries of use, it occupied a lingering blank spot in the scientific record.

But back in 1964, Mechoulam didn't even know where to start. Weed was hard to come by in Jerusalem. So Mechoulam got in touch with an army buddy who was now a high-ranking police officer. He surreptitiously scored five kilos of contraband hashish—molded into 200-gram bricks the shape of shoes and branded with the logo ISTANBUL.

Mechoulam smuggled it back to his lab and used a new technique to isolate the core compounds. He found two: delta-9-tetrahydrocannabinol and cannabidiol. Or THC and CBD, as they are more commonly known these days. Inspired by his findings, he set to work banging out grant proposals.

This did not go well.

The head of the U.S. National Institutes of Health's pharmacology division rejected him outright, explaining, "Cannabis is not an American problem. It is used in Mexico and by some jazz musicians in the U.S. but that's about all." The NIH director encouraged Mechoulam to reapply for funding once he'd settled on a more appropriate area of study.

Mechoulam was understandably dejected, but then he got a lucky break. Less than a year later that same NIH administrator who had denied his funding made an urgent transatlantic call asking to speak to him. A prominent U.S. senator had recently caught his son smoking pot. Loads of it. This was before Nancy Reagan's eggs-in-a-frying-pan War on Drugs, but well after *Reefer Madness*. The politician wanted to consult with the only scientist in the world who might have any idea of the science beyond the hysteria.

The next day, the NIH official took a direct flight over from Washington, D.C. to Israel to meet privately with Mechoulam. Forty-eight hours later, he'd returned to the United States having smuggled ten grams—nearly the entire world's supply—of chemically pure THC back through the airport. The U.S. Customs agents couldn't bust him because they didn't know what they'd found.

From that moment in 1965 until today, the NIH has been discreetly funding Mechoulam's lab. Israel became the leading center of cannabis research, with Mechoulam himself publishing four books, authoring over four hundred papers, and obtaining twenty-five patents since.

Mechoulam's lab eventually found what they'd been searching for—the complex system within our brains that processes cannabinoids. By the late '80s, they'd also isolated the neurochemical that mimics them—*anandamide* (named after the Sanskrit word for bliss). But naming it the "bliss molecule" might have been underselling it.

The endocannabinoid system (or ECS) is the name for that entire physiological network. It turns out to be the largest signaling system in the body and plays a central role in regulating blood sugar, hormones, pain, reward, heart rate, digestion, metabolism, and bone growth. It protects against inflammation and serves as the communication system between the brain and all vital organs. It also appears to serve a central role in healthy child development, supporting suckling and bonding between mothers and infants, and allowing painful memories to be released. It even helps heal traumatic brain injuries.

In a 1998 study involving soldiers who had suffered blunt-force head trauma, researchers found that if medics could get cannabinoids into the patients' bloodstreams within four hours of the accident, they could meaningfully reduce the "glutamate storm" that the brain releases after impact. It's that excess glutamate that creates slurred speech, tremors, and cognitive confusion and, if unaddressed, lasting damage. The ECS was de-escalating the brain's emergency response system by getting the glutamate shock troops to stand down.

But those endocannabinoids do something even more interesting. Dr. Esther Shohami, one of the leading specialists in cannabinoids and traumatic brain injuries (TBIs), found that endocannabinoids "direct stem cells to become brain cells and contribute towards recovery." Until the past decade, most neurologists believed that stem cells were only active during prenatal development. Shohami's research shows that they help healing and growth throughout life. All stem cells are waiting for is the signal from the ECS to get back in the action.

The implications of this work haven't gone unnoticed. In 2003, the U.S. government filed a patent on cannabinoids as neuroprotectants and antioxidants. They even got the Nobel Prize–winning discoverer of dopamine to be a signatory. Meanwhile, cannabis remains a Schedule I drug, defined as *having no therapeutic value*. The government took elaborate steps to patent the direct therapeutic application of a substance they legally insist has none.

Richard Friedman, a psychopharmacologist at Cornell University, has confirmed the ECS heals our minds and not just our bodies. While everyone has anandamide coursing through their systems, some of us have a genetic variation that produces less of the enzyme that de-activates it. Like a naturally occurring Prozac, which inhibits the re-uptake of serotonin, this mutation, Friedman says, "leads to more of the bliss molecule anandamide bathing the brain."

And when that happens, the Cornell team found, people with this mutation experience "changes in the neural circuits involved in anxiety and fear. Specifically, they had greater connectivity between the prefrontal cortex, the executive control center, and the amygdala, which is critical to processing fear. . . . A stronger connection between these two brain regions is known to predict lower anxiety and greater emotional control." In short, they were happier and less anxious. They were also 50 percent less prone to addiction to cannabis and opioids.

With more of the bliss molecule coursing through their brains, they apparently felt less need to supplement with external drugs. That's important. While it's tempting to jump from all of these positive findings on the ECS to advocate for cannabis as a cure-all, it's rarely that simple. "The problem is that cannabis swamps and overpowers the brain's cannabinoid system," Friedman explains, "and there is evidence that chronic use may not just relieve anxiety but interfere with learning and memory." The difference between a tonic and a toxin, the Renaissance alchemist Paracelsus reminds us, is always the dose.

While the Israelis pioneered the research into the protective and healing role of cannabinoids in brain injury and physical trauma, the Cornell team found that benefits extend to psychological trauma as well. "The results were clear . . . *humans with the cannabinoid mutation showed enhanced fear extinction—that is, they learned more efficiently how to be unafraid*" [emphasis added].

Sufferers of PTSD cannot do this. War veterans experience the flash-bang of fireworks on the Fourth of July and are instantly catapulted back to a roadside bomb blast. Victims of sexual assault feel a hand on their shoulder in a crowded club and flash back to the night they were abused. But our endocannabinoid system can help us soften those haunting memories.

It lets us "temporarily forget most of the baggage we usually bring to our perception," Michael Pollan explains. "[It] restores a kind of innocence to our perceptions of the world . . . the cannabinoids open a space for something nearer to direct experience. . . . There is another word for this extremist noticing . . . and that word, of course, is wonder."

These compounds live in us, and they help us. The network that governs them is central to regulating our entire nervous systems, and yet, 90 percent of U.S. physicians are totally unaware of their role in health and well-being. Dr. Allyn Howlett, noted for her discovery of a key endocannabinoid receptor, suggests that endocannabinoids do "exactly what Adam and Eve would want after being thrown out of Eden. You couldn't design a more perfect drug for getting Eve through the pain of childbirth and helping Adam endure a life of physical toil."

By letting us forget our pain and heal our hearts and minds, endocannabinoids help us remember something deeper and more lasting.

We may have been thrown out of Eden, but the simple wonder of being alive is available to all of us.

And that's something those sea sponges could have told us a long time ago.

Wandering Nervously

A few years ago, the U.S. Navy SEALs discreetly reached out to Dr. Paul Bach-y-Rita, the "father of sensory substitution." They needed some help with their combat divers and found out this University of Wisconsin neuroscientist was the guy to call. For years, Bach-y-Rita had been pioneering ways for people with different disabilities to rewire their brains. Braille and white canes for blind people, Bach-y-Rita had realized, were low-tech sensory substitutions. Over time, people learned to "see" from translating bumps on a page or taps from a cane. But why stop there? he thought. What might sensory substitution using digital technology look like?

Back then, the SEALs had a different problem. Their divers weren't blind by accident, they were blind by necessity. And they needed to find a better way to see in pitch-black underwater operations when lives were at stake.

Bach-y-Rita's lab had developed a low-voltage electric tongue depressor that sent out pulses of juice into a blind person's mouth. The nerve endings on our tongues are as sensitive as our fingertips, so like a high-tech white cane, patients could learn to use signals from the paddle to orient in a 3D environment.

The SEALs hoped they could learn to "see" based on the electric tingling on different parts of their tongues. Feel a slight buzz on the left side of their mouths, they'd know to swim left. On the tip of their tongue, they'd know to swim down. On the back of their tongue, they'd need to ascend. It allowed a commander in a zodiac boat stationed well outside the danger zone to steer his divers with much more precision. They would no longer be flying blind.

Then they noticed something unexpected in their trials. When the divers resurfaced from extended night dives, they were often disoriented, experiencing nausea and vertigo. It would take them a while to regain their bearings—like the spatial equivalent of the bends. But the divers who'd been wearing the tongue paddles were fine. Something about the electrical stimulation was helping them adapt better to the strange sensations of an underwater blackout.

A few years later, one of Bach-y-Rita's colleagues in Madison got into a car accident that nearly crippled him. On a hunch, he decided to self-administer the tongue stimulation as part of his rehabilitation. It worked for him, too. He was able to cut the time that his orthopedic surgeon had slated for his recovery by half. But the question Bach-y-Rita wanted to know about both of these discoveries was how?

Fast-forward a decade and this technology is now in Phase III clinical trials. The PoNS device, as the most recent version is known, has been approved for use in rehabilitating brain injuries and multiple sclerosis. The researchers have teased apart what's going on that makes that kind of healing possible.

There's a reason that the tongue is so sensitive—it's packed with nerve endings. Those same neurons that allow us to taste food, chew, and swallow (and steer underwater) all root back to essential cranial nerves. There are ten main ones that can all be simulated via the tongue, including those that modulate our facial expressions, eating, and a host of sensorimotor functionality. They also regulate our autonomic nervous system via the vagus (or "wandering") nerve, which branches all the way down to the base of our spines.

From the surface of the tongue, it's a direct route to the brain stem, which is made up of three sections—the midbrain, the pons (hence the naming of the device), and the mellifluously named medulla oblongata, where the vagus nerve originates. It's pretty much the Grand Central Station of our nervous system. Stimulate the tongue in specific regions, and you have a direct hotline to the cranial nerves that run the rest of our bodies. And unlike consumer biohacking headsets, stimulation via the tongue goes straight to the nerves it's trying to reach instead of getting deflected by our thick skulls.

The beneficial effects of this type of translingual neurostimulation

(TLNS) go far beyond rehabilitation. Over the past twenty years, a slew of papers has shown that TLNS protects our brains, improves our movement and balance, and boosts vitality as much as deliberate physical rehabilitation or workouts. It offers what amounts to a *"bottom-up neuromodulation of global brain function"* [emphasis added].

When I asked Dr. Ryan D'Arcy, one of the world's leading neuroscientists specializing in traumatic brain injuries and the lead researcher on the PoNS trials, what's going on, he made this analogy. "The way it appears to be functioning is almost as a global-level reset of the nervous system—in the same way that if your computer is glitching out because you've left it on too long with too many apps or windows open, and then sometimes all it needs is to turn it off, and let it power back up fresh. So even if we're directly targeting only a couple of pathways like the trigeminal nerve, *what we're seeing is a global cascade triggered across a number of additional nerve pathways and bodily functions"* [emphasis added].

D'Arcy and his team are now starting to test TLNS's impact on peak performance. "Especially when combined with neuromodulation, i.e., intentional visual, movement, respiration, and balancing protocols," D'Arcy said, "we're starting to see some really interesting results." On a visit to their labs in Vancouver, I was lucky enough to serve as a guinea pig in one of those off-label trials.

We had an extra day on our calendars, and D'Arcy, who used to be a competitive mountain bike racer and big mountain skier, insisted we head up to Whistler to try out the trails. But really, it was a setup. The bikes looked more like motorcycles without motors. And the trails weren't like anything I'd ever seen. Riding the gondola to the top of the mountain, I could look down and see giant bermed tracks with ten-foot-high banked corners, huge tabletop jumps, and lots of places to come unglued. It looked like a muddy roller coaster minus the carts. We took a few warm-up runs, and I kept repeating to myself, "The sole goal is to make it to happy hour in one piece."

But sitting at the top, getting ready for our third lap, Ryan looked over to me with a grin. "Ready to get your flow on?" He handed me the PoNS device, had me put the paddle into my mouth, and cranked up the juice. It felt like I'd just gobbled a fistful of PopRocks. My cheeks puckered, my tongue stuck to the roof of my mouth, and I began drooling like a Saint Bernard. I lowered my helmet and took the lead back down the track.

Only this time, I wasn't thinking. I wasn't even steering. I was doing my best to hit the line, feel the G-forces, and surrender to the sinuous logic of the course. When I got to the bottom I turned to high-five the rest of the crew. But they weren't there yet. In the first couple of laps we'd all been banging handlebars the whole way down. This time, somehow I'd ended up a football field ahead.

For the next week when falling to sleep I'd find myself sucked back into the sensations of that run. In the same way we might startle ourselves awake, imagining we're stepping off a curb or falling down an elevator, I would feel the hypnotic oscillation between carving turns and floating jumps. I'd only ever experienced that kind of somatic hangover from powder skiing or catching waves—but this time, it was from mountain biking—and a nine-volt straight to the brain stem.

* * *

Houston, Texas—1995. Jiro Takashima had a capital "P" problem. His prostate. It wasn't working so well anymore. His doctor had given him some medications to manage the issue, but he still found himself getting up multiple times each night to pee. Trouble sleeping. Leaks. No fun.

His doctor called him into his office to give him a choice: either agree to surgery (and run a distinct risk of nerve damage and lifelong erectile dysfunction) or commit to daily digital relief from a nurse. Takashima, an accomplished mechanical engineer with several patents (and some dignity) to his name, thought, "Hey, if this is something I can do myself, I would rather not have to go into a doctor's office and have a stranger sticking their finger up my ass every week."

Utilizing some wire and medical-grade plastisol (moldable plastic clay), he started to hand-design an anatomically designed prostate massager. Over a couple of years of trial and error, he developed and tested the product on himself. "I've created something," he realized, "that is actually functional." So he filed a patent and began selling them through classified ads in the back of a Houston newspaper.

He started asking customers for feedback—nothing high-tech, just handwritten surveys. Users were having the same types of responses like, "Hey, I'm 67 years old having enlarged prostate and been looking for something like this and it's actually changing my life." Patients showed improvements between 85 to 90 percent.

Along with those handwritten surveys, Takashima's fledgling company, Aneros, started receiving testimonials asking, "I don't know if this is normal, but I had improvements on my prostate problems, but I was also having these tingling sensations." Some men were writing in, saying, "This has changed my life. I'm having what feels like female orgasms, *multiple* orgasms." Some patients were describing euphoric sensations and others were describing spiritual experiences. Reports of what users came to call the "Super O" kept coming in.

The movement spread—racking up over a hundred thousand registered members on the forum. And while Takashima's original clientele were older men suffering from enlarged prostates, the Aneros forum now comprises men of all ages. To date, it has sold over 1.5 million units. What began as medical relief for an embarrassing condition became an accidental movement for men to reclaim their sensitivity and embodiment.

The more I researched the science and read the forums, the more I was intrigued. Was it really possible that the pinnacle of psychosexual consciousness could be attained with a curiously curvy implement parked where the sun never shines? The Super O doesn't appear to be the sole result of prostatic stimulation; there's something else going on. "The distention of the rectum . . . causes the vagus nerve to fire," Princeton gastroenterologist Anish Sheth writes. "It can bring a sense of sublime relaxation." It prompts a drop in blood pressure and heart rate, goose bumps, and feelings of exhilaration.

"The vagus nerve is responsible for the regulation of internal organ functions, such as digestion, heart rate, and respiratory rate," University of Bern molecular psychiatrist Sigrid Breit writes in the journal

Frontiers in Psychiatry, "as well as vasomotor activity, and certain reflex actions, such as coughing, sneezing, swallowing, and vomiting."

Think about that—gagging, puking, sneezing, shitting, and orgasming—all of these spasms of our bodies that we equate with our most raw, revealed, even pathetic selves can also increase our equanimity and euphoria. That wide range of response is triggered by the vagus nerve that starts in our brain stem and meanders down our spine.

This effect isn't accessible solely by men. Research has demonstrated that women who have suffered spinal cord injuries can rewire their arousal circuits and learn to have orgasms through the vagus nerve, which travels from the uterus, cervix, and vagina to the brain's pleasure centers. "To some it may feel like a religious experience," Sheth offers, "to others like an orgasm, and to a lucky few like both."

* * *

The thread we've been gently tugging on in this chapter has something to do with pain and how we heal it. And it leads to the deepest structures of our nervous system—specifically the brain stem and its power to offer what neuroscientist Ryan D'Arcy termed a "global nervous system reset." It's there in Raphael Mechoulam's discovery of the centrally regulating endocannabinoid system and the tip-to-tail function of the vagus nerve that Jiro Takashima stumbled upon. It even shows up in the cross-linking of pleasure and pain that Nermin Ahmad noticed with the NYC first responders.

Once we strip off our clothing and even lop off our arms and legs, we are, after all, little more than prefrontal cortexes connected to spinal cords connected to erogenous zones. Put even more bluntly—we're worms with mouths, genitals, and arseholes. The human experience, despite all of its abstraction, complexity, and self-consciousness, is, at a biological level, unnervingly basic. And how that ancient linear circuitry works provides real insight into how we feel and heal.

Ernest Becker, author of the Pulitzer Prize–winning book *The Denial of Death*, contrasts the highest intimations of our spiritual selves with these unavoidable processes of our animal selves. "To fashion the sublime miracle of the human face, the *mysterium tremendum* . . . to do all this, and to combine it with an anus that shits! It is too much. Nature mocks us, and poets live in torture."

But where Becker waxes poetic about the human condition, he misses a potentially even deeper neurobiological truth. From our brain stem down to our root, we are wired for wholeness and even transcendence.

As we glimpse "the sublime miracle, the *mysterium tremendum*" that Becker yearns for, we find it in the most primitive convulsions of our nervous system. As much as we might dance around it, or seek to repress our core physicality, it is an essential and unavoidable part of the human experience. It's not that our animal selves lie in contradiction to our angel selves. Our animal selves are literally our stairway to heaven.

Despite his brilliant insights on so many aspects of the human condition, Becker was wrong on this one. Nature doesn't mock us. It unlocks us.

CHAPTER 7

Music

There are ten levels of prayer. Above them all is song.

—Hasidic saying

The Stomp Heard 'Round the World

Saturday, July 13, 1985. Wembley Stadium, London. Bob Geldof had a massive problem. He was trying to pull together the benefit concert to end all concerts—a global fund-raiser for the Ethiopian famine ravaging that country. It was supposed to beam out to 150 countries and raise millions in aid relief. But nothing was going as planned. Paul McCartney's microphone had crapped out for the first two minutes of the classic Beatles tune "Let It Be." U2 ran long and had to drop their anthem "Pride (In the Name of Love)." Fuses blew for the Who. Led Zeppelin—reuniting for the first time since their madcap drummer John Bonham had died—flailed, drunken and out of tune.

And with each of these mishits and wobbles, the fund-raising stalled. The donations needed for Ethiopia just weren't coming in. Phone banks sat quiet.

Then, a last-minute addition walked onto the stage. The band Queen. It didn't look good for them either. Freddie Mercury, the band's volatile but charismatic leader, had recently taken a hiatus from the group and descended into debauchery and drug use. He'd also just been diagnosed with AIDS, which in those days was an effective death sentence. Their future together as a band was far from certain.

But for the next twenty-one minutes, none of that mattered.

At 6:41 p.m. London time, the band went on. "I remember a huge rush of adrenaline as I went onstage and a massive roar from the crowd," Queen guitarist Brian May recounted. "Freddie was our secret weapon. He was able to reach out to everybody in that stadium effortlessly, and I think it was really his night."

Mercury belted out a line, *Aye-Oh!* really more of a yodeling vowel, and the audience responded—amazingly in tune. It sounded like that scene in *Close Encounters of the Third Kind* where a whole hillside in India erupts with a singsong chant. Goose bumps around the world.

Then they laid into "We Will Rock You."

STOMP STOMP CLAP. STOMP STOMP CLAP. STOMP STOMP CLAP. The opening that, to this day, gets kids and grandparents on their feet at football games and swim meets. The rhythm that moves people.

By the end of that song, nearly eighty thousand Brits in the stadium and billions more around the world were standing, stomping and clapping to Queen's beat. *Forty percent of the world's population*, all listening, moving, dancing, and singing—connected. A 2005 music industry poll acknowledged it as "the greatest live rock and roll performance of all time." By the end of the night, the trickle of donations had turned into a flood. Nearly $150 million came in. On that day, at least, Queen ruled.

Such a simple beat. STOMP STOMP CLAP. Such an obvious thing to do. As May reflects, it's "one of those things that people think was always there!" But it nearly didn't happen at all.

The original 1977 recording of "We Will Rock You" was faster and had none of the audience engagement. It wasn't until a particularly rowdy night in Birmingham that May and Mercury realized something unusual was happening. "They were singing along with everything we did," he says. "And I said, 'Obviously, we can no longer fight this. This has to be part of our show.'"

But what seemed like a new level of interactivity to May and Mercury was actually ancient—as old as music itself. "Throughout most of the world and for most of human history, music making was as natural an activity as breathing and walking, and everyone participated," Daniel Levitin, professor of neuroscience at McGill University and author of *This Is Your Brain on Music*, explains. "Concert halls, dedicated to the performance of music, arose only in the last several centuries."

The morning after the Birmingham show, May woke up with the STOMP STOMP CLAP beat in his head. "I was thinking, 'What can you give an audience that they could do while they're standing there?'" May told NPR's Terry Gross. "They can stamp and they can clap and they can sing some kind of chant," he says. "To me, it was a united thing. It was an expression of strength."

"It has only been in the last hundred years or so that the ties between musical sound and human movement have been minimized," says John Blacking, the anthropologist and author of *How Musical Is Man?* "The embodied nature of music, the indivisibility of movement and sound, characterizes music across cultures and across times."

That's why May's insight to empower his audience with the simplest tools available—their hands and feet—to enact one of the simplest beats available was such genius. It worked. First time. Every time. For everyone.

"Our culture, and indeed our very language, makes a distinction between a class of expert performers," Daniel Levitin explains, "the Ella Fitzgeralds, Paul McCartneys [and Freddie Mercurys]—and the rest of us. The rest of us pay money to hear the experts entertain us." And not just a little bit of money, Levitin argues. "Americans spend more money on music than on sex or prescription drugs *combined*."

But Queen had the intuition to see that people would give even more to be part of the performance. The "two-way process" that they had first experienced in Birmingham wasn't an innovation after all—it was a restoration to the way music had always been.

So after that Birmingham show the band went to an abandoned church-turned-sound-studio to record a fresh cut of "We Will Rock You." They piled up a bunch of loose boards that were lying around and started stamping on them to simulate the clapping of a large crowd. It sounded great, but May, a physicist at Imperial College before becoming a guitar god, wanted more.

"When we recorded each track, we put a delay of a certain length on it," May explains. "And the distances were all prime numbers. None of the delays were harmonically related. So there's no echo on it whatsoever, but the clapped sound—they spread around the stereo, but they also kind of spread from a distance from you—so you just feel like you're in the middle of a large number of people stamping and clapping."

And with that physics-geek recording trick, Queen did something magical—they re-created the timeless experience of "feeling like you're in the middle of a large number of people stamping and clapping." By the time they walked onstage at Live Aid, everyone listening already knew their part by heart.

That feeling of connection to others through the power of rhythm and song is, according to ethnomusicologists, even older than language itself. "Musical instruments are among the oldest human-made artifacts we have found [and] predate agriculture in the history of our species," Levitin writes. "*We can say, conservatively, that there is no tangible evidence that language preceded music* [emphasis added]. In fact, the physical evidence suggests the contrary. Music is no doubt older than the fifty-thousand-year-old bone flute, because flutes were unlikely the first instruments."

Think about that. In most histories of civilization, we pin language right up there with tool-making and fire as the cornerstones of our leap from hairy ape to human. "For millions of years, mankind lived just like the animals," physicist Stephen Hawking wrote. "Then something happened which unleashed the power of our imagination. We learned to talk. We learned to listen. Speech has allowed the communication of ideas, enabling human beings to work together to build the impossible."

But if Levitin is right, learning to talk and listen happened even earlier than that. Quite possibly, while we were still grunting and pointing, and hadn't developed anything resembling the complex syntax we might associate with formal language, we were calling and responding, listening and speaking—connecting and coordinating—with the primal power of rhythm, melody, and voice.

"Humans are social animals," Levitin explains, "and music may have historically served to promote feelings of group togetherness and synchrony, and may have been an exercise for other social acts such as turn-taking behaviors. Singing around the ancient campfire might have been a way to stay awake, to ward off predators, and to develop social coordination and social cooperation within the group. Humans need social linkages to make society work, and music is one of them."

Robin Dunbar, a professor of evolutionary psychology at Oxford University, believes that a few hundred thousand years ago, when ancient humans began to make music, dance, and sing, they did it not just to connect with each other but to transcend themselves. When the synchronized breathing, chanting, drumming, and dancing reached a peak, individuals likely entered trance states.

In his book *Human Evolution*, Dunbar describes one of the oldest surviving cultures on the planet and how they make the most of music to enhance social cohesion. "Among the San Bushmen of southern Africa," Dunbar writes, "trance dances are particularly likely to take place when relationships within the extended community have started to unravel as people bicker among themselves. A trance dance restores the equilibrium, almost as though it wipes the slate clean of the toxic memories of the injustices and slights that poisoned relationships."

Think of it as an archaic Groove and Reconciliation Committee. Batch forgiveness. No talking stick or therapist required. As Alice Walker puts it in the title to one of her essay collections, *Hard Times Call for Furious Dancing*. In these times of hypersensitivity, micro-PTSD, and nonstop culture wars, we could heed this advice.

So when concerned mothers and fathers of the 1950s and '60s fretted about the destabilizing power of rock music on their impressionable children, when they lamented that Elvis, Beatlemania, and

Woodstock heralded the decline of civilization, they had it backward. Sex, drugs, and rock 'n' roll weren't the end of civilization, they were its beginning. For tens of thousands of years, they have served as the building blocks of culture—heightening group cohesion, honing our ability to communicate, and providing glimpses of the Sublime. Without them, we might still be pointing and grunting, cowering in caves.

STOMP STOMP CLAP. STOMP STOMP CLAP.

Ancient. Primal. Profound.

For twenty-one minutes at Live Aid, the world was united against hardship and suffering by doing what comes naturally. Celebration. If music really is the food of love, we'd do well to turn it up.

By Their Beats Ye Shall Know Them

You probably haven't heard *of* Will Henshall. But odds are good that you have heard him. Putting a spring in your step as you wander through that big-box hardware store. Inspiring you to tap your fingers as you cruise down the highway.

One of the founding members of the English '90s pop band Londonbeat, Henshall penned over six hundred tunes for his label, Warner Music. The soundtracks for the first Harry Potter and Lord of the Rings films were recorded on his tech, as were albums by U2, Eric Clapton, and Phil Collins.

"As a writer," Henshall says, "I discovered early on that I had an intuitive ability to fine tune the thing that makes a tune catchy. Songs are like these little tiny memory hooks and when they go into the earworm, into the collective consciousness as they do, they become woven into the infrastructure of our society."

Levitin, the McGill neuroscientist, explains exactly how this happens: "When we love a piece of music, it reminds us of other music we have heard, and it activates memory traces of emotional times in our lives. The story of your brain on music is the story of an exquisite orchestration of brain regions, involving both the oldest and newest parts of the human brain. . . . It involves a precision choreography of neurochemical release . . . and emotional reward systems."

Henshall's natural talent for hacking those emotional reward systems bore fruit. "I'm blessed that I've had a few of those breakout hits," Henshall says. "Some of my songs have been the most played songs ever in the world on the radio."

In 1992, he received the BMI Songwriter of the Year award and was seated as the guest of honor at the same table as Paul McCartney. More excited by his tablemate than his award, he asked the Beatles' master songwriter, "'So how do you write songs, Paul?' And he goes, 'I don't know. I can look over there and just fucking wait.'"

That awards show got Henshall interested in the balance between the art—the intuitive part of the process that McCartney had summed up so succinctly—and the science. Analyzing creativity has become the second half of his life's work.

Levitin confirms Henshall's hunch that there was more to the art of music than what McCartney had let on. "Music listening, performance, and composition engage nearly every area of the brain that we have so far identified, and involve . . . a network of regions—the mesolimbic system—involved in arousal, pleasure, and the transmission of opioids and the production of dopamine."

Neuroscientist Oliver Sacks expands on this notion. "Our auditory systems, our nervous systems, are indeed exquisitely tuned for music. How much this is due to . . . its complex sonic patterns woven in time . . . its insistent rhythms and repetitions . . . and how much to the immensely complex, multilevel neural circuitry that underlies musical perception and replay, we do not yet know."

But Henshall really wanted to know. So he didn't limit his research to twelve-bar blues and rock and roll. His curiosity led him to the booming world of electronic music too. "Really great DJs know the neurological element of music," Henshall explains. "They're managing the amount of bass on the dance floor. They're managing the speed in real time. Watching them spin, they're in real time managing the neuroscience part of people's brain."

"Recording engineers and musicians have learned to create special effects," neuroscientist Levitin agrees, "that tickle our brains by exploiting neural circuits that evolved to discern important features of our auditory environment."

"My aha moment was when I went to see [superstar DJ] Paul Oakenfold live a few times and just watched what he was doing," Henshall continued. "And I was like, 'What speed is this at?' Trance techno. Wait a minute. I've got a speed thing on my phone here. I'm like, '128 BPM [beats per minute]. Just a bit over.' And then the DJ does a big drop. Every two minutes there's a little drop where they pull the bass out and people are like 'Put your hands in the air!' Every two minutes they do that, they drop the bass, the dopamine hit comes in from the bass coming back."

But about every twenty minutes, the DJ plays a big one and they make you wait for it, Henshall noticed. "When they drop the bass, DJs speed the track up a little bit. When it comes back in, it comes at 132 beats per minute. What they're doing all night is constantly changing the entrainment of these notes to help to keep someone sustained in a focused state.

"Map the 'peak to peak transient timing' of the musical pulses happening and it is 8.2 Hertz," he continues. "And if you know anything about brain entrainment . . . 8 to 14 Hertz is how you can entrain someone to be in an alpha wave, which is a focused state. It's a trance state [and common in meditative states, flow states, and other nonordinary peak states].

"That was the aha moment when I was like, 'Wow. These guys are intuitively using science, proven and repeatable.' And then I did a list of the 50 most successful trance techno tracks. What speed are they at? 128 BPM. All of 'em."

Like Brian May tinkering with prime number ratios while recording Queen's anthem, Henshall had found another mathematical structure hiding under the dance floor. Trance DJs had intuited that "sonic driving," a technique used for hundreds of thousands of years to shift the state of hominids, works even better hooked up to high-tech sound systems and dazzling light shows.

From a few dozen Neanderthals gathered around a campfire banging on animal skin drums, to a few thousand congregants in awe of the giant pipe organs of cathedrals like Notre Dame, to a few hundred thousand ravers gathered at EDM festivals, we have always been chasing the unity and transcendence that music has provided. "You can think of music," Brunel University psychologist Costas Karageorghis explains, "as a type of legal performance-enhancing drug."

They weren't the first, and they certainly won't be the last, but today's DJs are some of the best acoustic chemists the planet has ever seen.

Jehovah's Favorite Choir

Fresh out of my sophomore year in college, I headed to the beach for a summer as a lifeguard. I had to wear the dorky red trunks, strap the big rescue buoy to my back, and climb up on the beach patrol stand at ten a.m. sharp every morning, no matter how hungover. This was the era of peak *Baywatch*, and David Hasselhoff and Pamela Anderson were on everyone's screens and minds. To this day, I have an allergic reaction to red clothing.

Less than a month into the summer I found myself torn between love and duty. The prior semester, I'd met Julie and we'd spent every minute together since. But now she was about to embark on a road trip out West with some of her girlfriends in a rusty old VW bus. We made a plan: There was a concert for a band that neither of us had seen before—the Grateful Dead, in Washington, D.C., the day before she was about to leave. We agreed to meet at the entrance to the stadium and catch the show together.

So I lied to my crew chief, told him I had a family wedding to attend and needed the days off. Then I did something I'm embarrassed to admit. I made Julie a care package and a mixed tape. I took my newly issued patrol pack and filled it with things that I thought she might need on her trip. A poncho. Chewing gum. Beef jerky. Coloring books. Some postcards to mail if she felt like talking (this was before cell phones or e-mail).

On the morning of the show I drove from the coast to D.C. with my roommate. We pulled into the parking lot at RFK Stadium. A gypsy carnival had rolled into town and mushroomed up overnight. A cute girl wearing a Holly Hobbie patchwork smock ambled up to us and sweetly asked, "Would you like to try a Humboldt Triangle?" Sure, we said, why not? We started nibbling on the oddly greenish, three-pointed brownie. It tasted like it was made of rancid butter and lawn clippings.

But I was on a mission: to meet Julie at the entrance to the concert. I started walking around the outside of the stadium and my heart sank. RFK Stadium is round. It's built like an old Roman coliseum. Every hundred yards or so, another, identical arched gateway leads in. There wasn't a single main entrance—there were *seven*.

I could hear the music rocking inside, could hear the roar of the crowd. I kept looking, but after an hour I gave up. Dejected, I went into the concert, light-headed and off-kilter. That Emerald Triangle was really packing a punch. Holly Hobbie had sandbagged us.

I shuffled to my seat, high up in the stands. Then I looked around. Tens of thousands of people dancing in their seats, mobbing the floor, singing along with every tune.

I wasn't feeling it. The music felt lumbering, atonal. It would gel for a moment into something, then splooge out again into undifferentiated noodling. I thought about leaving and going to sleep in my buddy's car until the show was over.

Then the fat gray-haired man playing lead guitar kicked off a riff. A Hammond B3 organ layered in, two drummers started driving a straight-ahead rock 'n' roll rhythm. The whole thing snapped to grid. The lights on the stage powered up, the volume jumped, and suddenly we were on a galloping, rollicking runaway freight train.

Going down the road feeling bad, Jerry Garcia warbled in his world-weary voice.

Don't wanna be treated this a way
Going where the climate suits my clothes
Don't wanna be treated this a way

Going where the water tastes like wine
I don't wanna be treated this a way

And somewhere in the midst of this, the first concert of my life, bushwhacked by an edible, rudderless from my missed meeting with my girlfriend, I heard someone next to me hoot and holler with pure, unrestrained joy.

It was such a raw sound, what Walt Whitman might have termed a "barbaric yawp," that it startled me. I opened my eyes to see who it could have been.

But there was no one for two seats beside me. I had met the Yawper, and he was me. I *had* been going down the road feeling bad after all. And I definitely didn't want to be treated that way. And who wouldn't want to go where the water tastes like wine and the climate suits their clothes? I couldn't help but shout out in joyful recognition. The main character in that tune was me. But not just me. Everyone there. Isolated in our despair, united in our defiance.

Reading this, the idea of a young kid cheering at a concert might seem pretty unremarkable. But for me, a locked-down English boy raised in a military household—that hoot was a *revelation.*

My whole life, that was the sort of thing that "one simply didn't do." As Monty Python's John Cleese once said, "It can be considered the singular goal of every Englishman to make it to his grave unembarrassed." And a spontaneous, totally unironic hoot of happiness— well, that was potentially deeply embarrassing. But there, with my head addled and my heart broken open, I had found a way past all of that repression, into something that felt alive and good.

* * *

A few years earlier, mythologist Joseph Campbell sat on a UC Berkeley panel at the Palace of Fine Arts in San Francisco. The evening was titled "Ritual and Rapture, from Dionysus to the Grateful Dead." The band loved Campbell's book, *The Hero with a Thousand Faces,* and recently the scholar had broken his normal aversion to pop culture and gone to one of their shows.

"Rock music has never seemed that interesting to me," Campbell admitted up front. "It's very simple and the beat is the same old thing. But when you see a room with young people for five hours going through it to the beat of these boys [the Grateful Dead] . . . The first thing I thought of was the Dionysian festivals, of course.

"This is more than music," he continued. "It turns something on in here, the heart? And what it turns on is life energy. This is Dionysus talking through these kids."

Campbell, ever the comparative mythologist, saw parallels to other gatherings too. "Down in New York we have a big Russian Cathedral. You go there on Russian Easter at midnight and you hear *Kristos anesti!* Christ is Risen! Christ is Risen! It's almost as good as a rock concert. It has the same kind of life feel."

For Campbell, once you could see the deep structures of that death/rebirth ritual, of that collective uncorking of vitality, you could spot it all over the place. "When I was in Mexico City at the Cathedral of the Virgin of Guadelupe, there it was again," he continued. "In India, in Puri, at the temple of the Jagannath—that means the 'Lord of the Moving World'—the same damn thing again. It doesn't matter what the name of the God is, or whether it's a rock group or a clergy. It's somehow hitting that chord of realization of the unity of God in you all, that's a terrific thing and it just blows the rest away."

Campbell had nailed it, and explained what I'd stumbled into at that D.C. stadium. A modern-day Dionysian ritual that "turns something on in the heart . . . life energy . . . that chord of realization of unity." And while many scholars have since critiqued Campbell's broad-brush universalism, the fact that he spotted something timeless in the Grateful Dead's postmodern bacchanal was spot-on.

The show ended and the stadium lights came up. Finally the bouncers herded us all out the gates. But this time, rather than being awash in a sea of freaks and misfits, I was awash in a sea of faith. Rather than feeling like a stranger in a very strange land, I felt at home among brothers and sisters. By the next morning, it had faded, but it was a new and not unwelcome feeling.

It was what Quakers would've called a "gathered meeting," where members could feel the spirit and "speak when spoken through." What Joseph Campbell called a modern-day rite of Dionysus. What others might call "Church." Not the place with the steeple. The space with the people.

Either that, or the Humboldt Triangle had really done a number on me.

That's why kids ran away from home to join the traveling circus touring with that band. That's what cynics listening to scratchy cassette tapes and claiming the music sucked could never understand. This wasn't a rock 'n' roll show after all. It was an electric-kinetic *liturgy*. The high priest just happened to have an electric guitar instead of a bishop's staff. What I'd stumbled into that day in D.C. was a gnostic initiation ceremony disguised as a concert.

I had to wait until the end of summer to finally give Julie that care package. She gave me a rubber-banded bundle of unsent postcards from the edge of the Grand Canyon, the coast of Big Sur, and the redwoods of Sequoia. Even though we missed each other at that show, we've been together ever since.

That fall, I went back home to visit my parents for a weekend, and I was listening to a Grateful Dead concert on the stereo. As the band jumped into "Going Down the Road Feeling Bad," my dad walked through the living room and started chiming in. He even added a few variations on the lyrics.

"Wait, how do you know this song?" I asked him. This was *my* newfound music, after all. It was countercultural, accessible only to those "in the know." How in the hell did my dad know anything about the Dead?

"'Going Down the Road'?" he asked. "That's an old Woody Guthrie and Pete Seeger tune. They called it 'Lonesome Road Blues.' Here, gimme a minute." He brought out his old mahogany banjo, fiddled with the tuning pegs, and jumped into a finger-picking rendition.

It turned out that back in the early sixties, between tours of duty as a test pilot on aircraft carriers, my dad had been a part of the London folk scene. That banjo he'd been playing for me had been given to him by Peggy Seeger, Pete's kid sister. (It's sitting next to me now as I write this, though I can't play it half as well.)

My dad got up, rummaged for a minute through his musty record collection, and pulled out an album called *Old and in the Way*. The cover was a goofy cartoon of a jug band—but there, dead center of the picture, was a bearded dude sitting on a stool holding a banjo. Black haired rather than gray. Not quite as chunky as the psychedelic Santa I'd seen back at RFK Stadium, but it was definitely him—Jerry Garcia.

In the mid-'70s, Garcia, mandolin virtuoso Dave Grisman, and fiddle legend Vassar Clements had come together to record that album. It's still the top-selling bluegrass record of all time—crossing over fans of gospel, bluegrass, country, and Deadheads (as fans of the Grateful Dead are often known). Through my whole childhood, it had been sitting there on our bookshelf, just waiting for me to connect the dots.

Arcana Americana

Once I started connecting them, those dots crisscrossed America from Nova Scotia to Appalachia to California to Africa before popping back up in the strangest of places—like full moon "polyethnic cajun slamgrass" tribal stomps in the mountains of Colorado and flashy headliners' sets at Coachella.

But no matter where those dots led—tracing the catalog of the Grateful Dead, the coffeehouse folk of Bob Dylan, or the blues-infused revival of the British rock invasion—they kept coming back to a mild-mannered guy named Alan Lomax.

Lomax was a music geek who'd grown up in the early 1900s in Austin, Texas, and bounced between Harvard and other schools before finding his vocation. He started out by helping his father, a folklorist, gather field recordings of cowboy tunes. But Alan really came into his own when he took over leadership of the Library of Congress's Archive of Folk Song in 1937.

He lugged clunky metal-and-wax recording equipment along with him all across the country. Lomax made over ten thousand field recordings and captured the voices and sounds of an America that most people never knew existed. He became fascinated by "the seemingly incoherent diversity of American folk song as an expression of its democratic, inter-racial, international character." He interviewed the famous folk singer Woody Guthrie, jazz legends Big Bill Broonzy and Jelly Roll Morton, Chicago blues icon Muddy Waters, and dozens of others.

While a meaningful number of Lomax's recordings captured the folkways of the African American South, the music of this country really emerged as a mishmash of traditions and influences. From the Scots-Irish Celtic tunes of hardscrabble Appalachia that grew into bluegrass and country music, to the French Catholic fiddle strains of Acadian music that then became the Cajun zydeco of Mardi Gras. Everywhere displaced people suffered and prevailed, these redemption songs became a way of giving point and purpose to their struggle.

"*Homo Americanus* is part Yankee ingenuity, part backwoodsman/ Indian or gamecock of the wilderness, and part Negro," Albert Murray, the founder of Jazz at Lincoln Center, said of the country's essential character.

"The blues tradition itself," he wrote in *The Hero and the Blues*, ". . . is the candid acknowledgment and sober acceptance of adversity as an inescapable condition of human existence—and, perhaps in consequence an affirmative disposition toward all obstacles . . . whether political or metaphysical."

When 1920s bluesman Furry Lewis lamented "I been down so goddamn long 'cause it seem like up to me," he was embodying Murray's "affirmative disposition" toward the obstacles of life. Naming it, claiming it, transcending it. Apparently his sentiment struck a chord—everyone from Nancy Sinatra to the Doors to the hip-hop superstar Drake have covered his song.

Murray's protégé Stanley Crouch gave a name to this balance of adversity and triumph—*swing*. "It's that combination of grace and intensity we know as swing. In jazz, *sorrow rhythmically transforms itself into joy*, which is perhaps the point of the music: joy earned or arrived at through performance, through creation" [emphasis added].

And that's the thing that we're really trying to tease apart here: that somehow, buried in this polyglot mishmash tradition of the American songbook, lies something potentially profound. A philosophy, a way of being, a secret scripture—an *arcanum*—that not only sheds light on where we've come from but hints at a way forward for all of us.

Because these redemption songs aren't just about looking on the bright side of lousy situations. They're powerful calls to radical transformation. "The question's not having hope," Cornel West insisted at a lecture at Harvard Divinity School, "the question is *being* a hope. Having hope is still too detached, too spectatorial. You got to be a participant. You gotta be an agent. 'You keep on pushing,' Curtis Mayfield says. 'Be a force for good,' Coltrane says. 'Mississippi god *damn*!' says Nina Simone. That ain't having hope. That's *being* a hope. Courageously bearing witness regardless of what the circumstances are because you're choosing to be a kind of person of integrity to the best of your ability before the worms get your body. Boom! that's it. That's blues. Beautiful tradition."

Courageously bearing witness before the worms get your body—and singing about it—is a uniquely American path to salvation. It's transformative to name the pain rather than minimize it. But to take it from broken lament into triumphal celebration? That's alchemy.

"Spiritual rebirth in the American Religion . . . is far closer to the patterns of Hermeticism than to doctrinal European Christianity," Yale historian Harold Bloom writes in *Omens of the Millennium*. Bloom's saying that American spirituality has always been more subversive, more mystical, and more experiential than either the Protestant or Catholic churches of Europe would have allowed. Drawing from the same impulse that prompted Quakers, Shakers, Puritans, Mormons, Adventists, and dozens of other sects to flee persecution and seek their own Promised Land in America—American spirituality is wilder, weirder, and ultimately more subversive than many of the traditions it sprang from.

"The American mode of self-knowledge is essentially Hermetic *not*

Christian," Bloom explains. "Initiation in American spiritual rebirth commences a process in which we become 'healed original and pure' *Anthropos*. Rebirth is emphatically not a repetition of physical birth, but a bursting into a new plane of existence previously unattained."

It's this death/rebirth sacred mystical initiation—this move from suffering to salvation, from mortal human to twice-born "Anthropos" that is so central to the American experience. It's what Joseph Campbell was getting at when he connected the rock concerts of the Grateful Dead to the Dionysian rituals of ancient Greece.

As Zora Neale Hurston once said, "You've gotta *go* there to *know* there!" This is the secret scripture, the alchemical instruction manual, hiding in plain sight in the American song tradition. *Hermetically* sealed. Secretive. But accessible if you have the key (often little more than a record album or concert ticket). Think of it as the *Arcana Americana*. We don't need to pen new verses or gin up new stories to guide our way forward. They've been with us all along.

Bloom's assertion, that scratch the surface of American Christianity and you'll find a magical mystical body of initiatory knowledge, isn't widely shared. That's in large part because religion in America is either embraced by true believers who take it entirely at face value or dismissed by nonbelievers who deny there's anything there to notice.

"Gnosis [or direct experience of reality]," Bloom asserts, "has been domesticated in America for two centuries now, so *we have the paradox of a Gnostic Nation that does not know it knows!*" [emphasis added].

A Gnostic nation that does not know it knows. We have literally forgotten the tools we forged to help ourselves remember. A bitter irony, but also a chance to redeem it.

* * *

If all of this seems dryly historical, academic even, look around today and you can see signs of this Gnostic Revivalism everywhere. You can hear it in Dolly Parton's Grammy/Oscar/Golden Globe–nominated performance of her song "Travelin' Thru." The lead single for the soundtrack to the film *Transamerica*, it connected the contemporary struggle for LGBTQ rights to the longer-standing American folk tradition of the rambling seeker. The Academy Awards gave her top billing to perform, and when she did, she brought the house down (younger stars like Amy Adams and Jake Gyllenhaal can be seen politely clapping along in the video, but an older, wiser Jack Nicholson is on the edge of his Cheshire Cat seat).

Questions I have many, answers but a few, Parton sang.

But we're here to learn, the spirit burns, to know the greater truth
We've all been crucified and they nailed Jesus to the tree
And when I'm born again, you're gonna see a change in me

What starts out as vintage Grand Ole Opry Dolly Parton becomes something else by the end. Standing on the Academy Awards stage, all alone in a form-fitting white pantsuit, Dolly brings it. The tune begins as a typically plaintive country ballad, a catalog of woes. Then it drops down to an a cappella *Graceland*-style call and response with the gospel choir backing her. Slowly out of the mud of that suffering and confusion her voice picks up, the band comes with her, and she starts belting out the refrain. Strutting up and down the stage, raising her hands in praise and testimony, encouraging the black-tie crowd to "sing it with me now." Nothing less than Soul Church.

"This ability to articulate this tragic-comic attitude toward life explains much of the mysterious power and attractiveness of that quality . . . known as 'soul,'" Ralph Ellison explained. He could just as easily have been writing about Dolly Parton's Oscar performance or Jerry Garcia's plaintive ballads. "An expression of American diversity within unity, of blackness with whiteness, soul announces the presence of a creative struggle against the realities of existence . . . of ordeals, initiation ceremonies, of rebirth."

While Parton's stint at the Academy Awards might have smuggled a little bit of the hillbilly sacred into the Hollywood secular, lately it's been going back in the other direction. New-school secular has been reinvigorating old school sacred.

* * *

In April 2018, at Grace Cathedral in San Francisco, the fifty or so regulars for the midweek service had to make some room for newcomers. A lot of room. Eight hundred and fifty fresh faces were crowding into the pews. All colors, all shapes, some flamboyant, some quiet. But everyone had come to attend the inaugural Beyoncé Mass—a Christian worship service inspired by the life and music of Beyoncé Knowles.

"Black artists have always been central to the struggle for black freedom, whether we're talking about Nina Simone or Harry Belafonte or . . . Sweet Honey in the Rock," Rev. Dr. Kelly Brown Douglas, dean of the Episcopal Divinity School at Union Theological Seminary, told *The New York Times*. "Beyoncé is a part of this legacy. There is this natural correspondence between the kinds of things she does in her music and the black church."

The Mass, which was inspired by the Reverend Yolanda Norton, chair of Black Church Studies at San Francisco Theological Seminary, treats Beyoncé's story and songs as a springboard to explore and celebrate black women and LGBTQ people through the lens of the Christian Gospels. And of course, lots of banging Beyoncé singalongs to drive the point home.

Video recordings of that first service went viral and soon communities from Los Angeles to Lisbon were clamoring to repeat the experience. "I haven't been involved in the church for years," one participant in the first L.A. service said, "but stepping back into that space felt amazing. It felt warm and inviting, and I left feeling healed. By the end of the service, people were weeping, people were joyous, people were hugging each other."

Which isn't too surprising really. Compared to reedy renditions of "Ave Maria," or stilted recitations of the Nicene Creed, cutting a congregation loose with Beyoncé's anthem "I'm a Survivor" is asymmetrical warfare. Many of her songs contain the same blueprint we've been exploring so far—soul, blues, swing, jazz. Being hope, not having hope. Seeking rebirth and redemption.

"This isn't about bringing pop music into the church," one of the

Mass organizers told the *Times*. "It's about giving people a new lens for Christianity, and showing them that it's not about a bunch of old stories in an old book."

"There's been pushback," Reverend Norton acknowledges. "There has been a misunderstanding about what we're doing and even from people in the church, but this is about bringing people together, not pulling them apart. . . . If you listen to the words [of Beyoncé's songs] in an ecclesiastical context, it's a very faithful, honest, raw acknowledgment of the imperfect relationship we have with God."

It's less an aberration to see a church featuring Beyoncé than it's a full-circle completion for the artist. Knowles grew up in Houston singing in her church choir. She was steeped in gospel and spirituals. Her father is African American, but her mother (from whom she takes her French-inflected name) is Louisiana Creole, Jewish, Spanish, Chinese, and Indian. By the time she had embarked on her professional career, she was drawing freely from that treasure chest of references, rhythms, and lineages, and bringing out something truly, deeply, and uniquely American.

But really, the Arcana Americana is even bigger than Beyoncé.

* * *

In 1996, the famous Iranian filmmaker Abbas Kiarostami premiered his film *Through the Olive Trees* at Lincoln Center in New York City. At the Q&A afterward an audience member asked why he had scored a film that was set in a remote village in northern Iran with classical music. Kiarostami responded, "Classical music has long ceased to belong to the West. It belongs to the world now."

The same can be said of gospel, blues, jazz, and folk music—the Arcana Americana. These redemption songs were forged in the fires of our collective hope and despair. Slavery, wars, exiles, homecomings. Racism. Intermarriage. Multiculturalism. Nationalism. The African Diaspora. European reformations. Chinese railroad workers. Japanese internment camps. Vietnamese boat people. The Irish potato famine. Trails of Tears, Ghost Dances, and reservations. Revivals and Awakenings—great and small. Marches. Protests. Assassinations. Tragedy. Triumph. Tribulation. Transformation.

The Arcana Americana, perhaps even more than classical music, doesn't belong to any country anymore. It belongs to the world now—an expression, forged in the fires of suffering and survival— that speaks to a deep and universal experience. Of being knocked down again and again, but each time, rising up singing. A soundtrack for the Infinite Game.

When Alan Lomax looked back over his more than ten thousand recordings archived in the Library of Congress, he marveled at "the seemingly incoherent diversity of American folksong as an expression of its democratic, interracial, international character, as a function of its . . . turbulent many-sided development."

Picking ourselves up, and doing it all again. Dancing to forget. Singing to remember. While much of this tradition is steeped in the idiom of the Judeo-Christian tradition, as Harold Bloom reminds us, there's a secret hidden within that secret too. The Arcana Americana is a living hermetical *and heretical* tradition. It rejects the doctrine of Original Sin—that we are forever cast out East of Eden to suffer and atone.

In the place of guilty prostration, the Arcana Americana defiantly claims a second act, a transfiguration based upon the innate perfectibility of humankind. *Anthropos*, Bloom calls it. HomeGrown Humans, if we prefer something more accessible.

As we try to mend our crisis in meaning, and the fractures that threaten to tear us apart, our redemption songs can bring us together. Giving us hope, *being a hope*. Shining the way, in our hymnals and our hoedowns.

Chapter 8

Sacraments

A Mic Drop Moment

In the 1870s and '80s, the Peyote Church spread rapidly from its origins in Northern Mexico to Indian reservations across the western United States. Its ceremonies included all-night rituals of song, dance, prayer, and repeated consumption of the psychoactive buttons of the peyote cactus. Anglo politicians grew deeply concerned by the rise of the "Peyote Cult" and, fearing Indian rebellions, outlawed its use.

A decade later, Comanche chief Quanah Parker stood up to testify in front of the Oklahoma legislature on whether that prohibition should be repealed or upheld. Parker assured the senators that his experience within the Peyote Church had provided him and countless others healing, had inspired them to make the transition from their traditional way of life, and that the eucharistic experience of consuming the sacred plant had rescued many from alcoholism and despair. "The White Man goes into his church house and talks *about* Jesus," Parker explained, "but the Indian goes into his tipi and talks *to* Jesus."

The spluttering congressmen had no ready reply. Parker's testimony was one of the first in a series of victories for indigenous use of sacramental plants that continued all the way to the Congress's passage of the Indian Religious Freedom Act of 1978. Today, the Native American Church, as the movement came to be known, has over a quarter of a million adherents, hailing from Mexico to Canada.

Parker's distinction—between arm's-length discussion of the sacred and full-body immersion in the sacred—is an important one. As Michael Pollan mentions in *How to Change Your Mind*, there's a profound difference between truly transformative entheogens—literally "a substance that engenders the sacred"—like peyote, and the "placebo sacraments of the Catholic eucharist."

That difference all boils down to pronouns.

Talking "about Jesus" or any other deity is a third-person he/she/it kind of conversation. There's Us (the subject) talking about Them (the object). Arm's length. Relatively abstract. The realm of academics and scholastics counting angels on pinheads.

Alternately, there's a second-person experience of the divine—what philosopher Martin Buber memorably called the I-Thou relationship. That's the talking *to* Jesus that Quanah Parker championed. This is most typically expressed in direct supplicative prayer: *"Dear God, please help me/give me/spare me/save me."* It's definitely more intimate than abstract third-person discussion.

Finally, if we enter the rarefied world of mystics like Saint Francis of Assisi in Christianity, Maimonides in Judaism, Rumi in Islam, Padmasambhava in Buddhism, and Ramakrishna in Hinduism (to name only a handful), we see the grammar collapse. It moves from I-Thou relationship into a straight *mystico-unio* I-I communion. First-person humanity recognizing its own first-person divinity.

Wade Davis, *National Geographic*'s Explorer in Residence, told me that when studying Vodou trance possession in Haiti, a *houngan* (priest) expanded Quanah Parker's original distinction: "When the white man goes to church you talk *about* god, when the Native American goes into his tipi he talks *to* god, when we conduct our Vodou ceremony, we *become* our gods." That's about as first-person as it gets.

You could make the case that while all three expressions—third-person, second-person, and first-person—are part of a healthy human relationship to the sacred, we've become imbalanced in our allocations. Most of our contemporary rites of passage, from senior proms and fraternity pledging on the secular side, to bar mitzvahs, Communion, and weddings on the religious side, are third-person pantomimes, no longer delivering the goods. Placebo sacraments in all but name. These days we're far longer on third-person discussion than first- and second-person immersion. And we're suffering because of it.

"Without somehow destroying me in the process," American theologian Frederick Buechner wondered, "how could God reveal himself in a way that would leave no room for doubt? If there were no room for doubt, there would be no room for me."

But there are experiences that deliver direct connection to the sublime and obliterate both self and doubt. We just need to expand our search parameters.

That's where sacraments like the Native American Church's come in.

"Every culture has found such chemical means of transcendence, and at some point the use of such intoxicants becomes institutionalized at a magical or sacramental level," NYU neuroscientist Oliver Sacks says. "The sacramental use of psychoactive plant substances has a long history and continues to the present day in various shamanic and religious rites around the world . . . some people can reach transcendent states through meditation or similar trance-inducing techniques, or through prayer and spiritual exercises. But drugs offer a shortcut; they promise transcendence on demand. These shortcuts are possible because certain chemicals can directly stimulate many complex brain functions." That neurological stimulation, that "transcendence on demand" kicks down the walls of third-person speculation and gets us into second- and first-person communion.

While Sacks rightly observes that psychoactive sacraments are as old as human culture, there's an increasingly urgent need for them these days. As we have demystified the world, both our selves and our doubts have grown heavier. To stand a chance of escaping the gravitational pull of the cynicism, neuroticism, and despair we're facing, we're going to need a bigger rocket. And much better guidance systems.

The Rolling Monks of Carmel

Sometimes it's not about pouring old communion wine into new bottles. Sometimes it's about dumping out the wine and filling up those bottles with an altogether stranger brew.

If you meet Rick Doblin, Harvard PhD and founder of the Multidisciplinary Association for Psychedelic Studies (MAPS) today, you might mistake him for a shape-shifter. One day, in a coat and tie, he'll be sincerely coordinating with DEA officials or testifying in Congress on the benefits of MDMA therapy for veterans. The next, he's dressed in a rainbow patchwork jacket, hosting psychedelic harm-reduction workshops at a desert festival.

But if you wind the clock back thirty years, you'd find him in a different form again—a mischievous Johnny Appleseed, bringing the Fruit of the Tree of Knowledge to those who'd pledged their lives to tending it.

Back in 1984, MDMA was an entirely legal research chemical, and Doblin was still formulating his core thesis that it could help people heal and become more effective human beings. He met some monks from the Benedictine Immaculate Heart Hermitage in Big Sur and made a proposal: He wanted to offer them MDMA, or "ADAM" as it was known then, as a supplement to their normal daily prayer routine. The monks, skeptical but open, agreed. Doblin proceeded to hook some brothers up.

That day, they all went about their sitting meditation in customary silence. As they did the time-released capsules flooded their brains with serotonin, oxytocin, dopamine, and prolactin. Brother David Steindl-Rast, a psychologist before he entered the monastery, described his experience. "It's like climbing all day in the fog and then suddenly, briefly seeing the mountain peak for the first time. There are no shortcuts to the awakened attitude, and it takes daily work and effort. But the drug gives you a vision, a glimpse of what you are seeking."

Another monk commented that "in thirty years of meditating on the love of Christ, today I felt His presence more strongly in my heart than at any other time."

The next day the abbot called Doblin into his office, looking concerned. "What have my monks been doing with your drugs?" After a searching conversation Doblin said felt like a dissertation defense, he convinced the abbot. The monks could keep on rolling.

By swapping out the "placebo sacraments" of wafers and wine, Doblin had provided contemplatives who'd dedicated their lives to a third-person relationship to God with something more immediate. Through first- and second-person I-I and I-Thou communion, they experienced a chance to lift themselves above the fog of obedient practice, and to glimpse "the mountain peak for the first time."

Consuming the appropriately nicknamed "ADAM," in conjunction with decades of discipline and the natural beauty of their monastery, gave them the chance to live *as* Adam—firstborn, reborn, primordial Man. Bathed in the "peace that passeth all understanding" (if only for a dreamy afternoon), they could taste the fruit they'd dedicated their lives to tending.

After that moment of grace in 1984, things went south. Use of the substance broke out of its therapeutic and sacramental confines and exploded as a club drug in the rave scene. A few hospitals began seeing ER visits from users. Newspapers amplified the coverage, calling it an international epidemic. MDMA got reclassified as a Schedule I controlled substance. The next thirty years of Doblin's work began to take shape in front of him. With ADAM (rebranded as the far more marketable "ecstasy") cast out of Eden, it became Doblin's mission to get the forbidden fruit back past the gatekeepers.

Everything I Needed to Know about Drugs I Learned in Kindergarten

Not long after our son was born, my wife, Julie, and I went back East to see our families. After fawning over her new grandson, my mother asked Julie if she wanted to see some pictures of me when I was that age. She pulled out the most embarrassing family favorites. Me, aged eighteen months, in a white christening dress with long flowing hair down past my shoulders (she had really been hoping for a girl). Me, aged three, proudly standing up in my bath, wearing a bright yellow Sou'wester rain hat and nothing else. And then, something I hadn't seen in twenty-five years—my report card from kindergarten.

My mother and wife opened it up, looked down the page, and promptly got the giggles. My teacher, Mrs. Fisher, wrote the line that really got them going at the bottom of the form: "James might find that he would make a few more friends on the playground if he wasn't always correcting them on the proper way to play all the games!"

And that has pretty much been the story of my life. That's how I'm wired to think—in terms of logic and consistency—feelings be damned. Apparently, even way back then. But it's a questionable strategy for winning friends and influencing people.

Since then, I have experienced a number of meaningful encounters with psychedelic compounds. From picking Liberty Cap mushrooms off cow pies in college with a rogue biology professor, to taking ayahuasca with a Colombian shaman, to getting launched down the ketamine hole by an anesthesiologist during surgery (not recommended).

The most profound of those encounters left me feeling very much like "today is the first day of the rest of my life." Except, looking back over thirty years, I think I was wrong about that. All of those sunrise epiphanies were less first days of a new life than they were, unavoidably, the *next* days of my old one.

Which brings us back to that report card. My teacher's insight, that I was by and large an opinionated on-the-spectrum little sod, arose *before* all the "adverse childhood events" I could think of that might explain my character defects. And her description still fits *after* all the psychedelic insights I've experienced since. That's why my mother and wife were laughing so hard.

Despite my best efforts, I'm remarkably close to the little dude who came into this world, christening dress, yellow rain hat, report card, and all. As much as I've had my world turned inside out and backward, and felt utterly transformed by entheogenic experiences, a large percentage of my personality structure remains humblingly intact.

I don't think I'm alone in my efforts to sabotage my own growth. After all, if psychedelic benefits extended linearly from the studies we've been reading lately, then by all accounts, baby boomer hippies would be Galactic Time Lords by now. If three sessions of MDMA therapy can cure everything from depression to PTSD, why aren't thirty-three sessions turning that Cat in the Hat Raver into a Bodhisattva?

Because there's a dark underbelly to the groundbreaking research that's been pouring out of places like Johns Hopkins and Imperial College over the last decade. Beyond the truly astonishing statistics and accounts of complete remission of depression and PTSD symptoms in just a few sessions are the quieter, sometimes desperate queries from patients six months later. And six months after that. Once the all-too-real limitations of their flawed world and selves return. Back to the bottom of the slide, only this time, there's no going back to their old games.

Old-timey mystics used to call that the "Dark Night of the Soul"— the hair ball period after you've seen the light, and then had it unceremoniously whisked away. It's always darkest (and coldest) just before the dawn. Sometimes, that next sunrise takes a lot longer to arrive than we hoped.

Which begs the broader question: How transformative can entheogens, or "sacred substances," really be? And are we using them right?

This is a real issue. Arguably, it is *the* issue when it comes to appropriate use of psychedelic substances. Can we ever, as scholar Huston Smith once mused, "transform our passing illuminations into abiding light?"

As asymmetrically positive as initial experiences can be (especially in structured, therapeutic settings), there appears to be an equal and opposite asymmetrical drop-off in benefit to subsequent efforts.

Once we look beyond the neurochemistry of the experience, how much of the breakthrough healing is prompted by a new direct sense that there is, in fact, Capital M More to life? What at first is revelatory and uplifting—i.e., "I don't have to live a life of suburban conformity!" or "I am worthy of love!"—can quickly become existentially overwhelming. Once I've had my Eureka experience, I realize that all of that More still irreducibly contains the human condition within it.

Welcome to the Brotherhood of the Screaming Abyss. There's a good reason why most never peer over the Edge. Sometimes More isn't always Better. It's just More. A lot more.

Superegos

It's the Pareto principle gone wrong. If the first 20 percent of my experience of cathartic healing delivers 80 percent of the whizbang insights and breakthroughs, I am going to rationally conclude, "Holy shit! This is the most game-changing thing *ever*. I need to clear the decks and dedicate my life to this transformative practice—at this rate, I'll be enlightened in no time!"

Except that's rarely how it goes. Pareto twists on us, and we're now facing the disappointing reality that the remaining 80 percent of our time, money, and effort will be dedicated to gleaning only 20 percent more growth and integration. And that can take a lot of frustrated searching to figure out.

The principle applies to ecstatic techniques of any stripe—psychedelics, group work, breath work, body work, tantra, music: succumb to the irrational exuberance of your initial hits of healing, and you can lose yourself. We can become addicted to the states without ever raising our stage.

We're familiar with the overprescription of antibiotics and how it's creating superviruses. The same can be said of excessive and unstructured use of psychedelics. When they're used for everything from therapy to biohack to weekend fun, we can end up overprescribing them too. Only in this case, we don't get superbugs coming back to plague us, we get super*egos*. The very medicine intended to get rid of our selfish attachments can actually create even more virulent versions of the selves we were so desperate to transcend in the first place.

The technical term for this is what Tibetan Buddhist teacher

Chögyam Trungpa called "spiritual materialism"—often, our practices can become a source of pride that calcifies our egos even more. Instagram shamans. Venture capitalists "called in" to disrupt the psychedelic therapy space. Preening yogis who care more about how their butts look in leggings than their adherence to any eight-limbed path. Self-appointed mystics convinced their "downloads" hold the keys to unlocking Ancient Egypt or Atlantis.

This is the downside of Oliver Sacks's observation that "drugs offer a shortcut; they promise transcendence on demand." No need to practice Vipassana or pranayama for years. No prerequisite to cultivate ethics and right-livelihood ahead of time.

"Buy the ticket, take the ride," as Hunter Thompson said. Millions of people are heeding that advice. It's not surprising that with such inconsistent preparation and repeat visits to the cosmic carnival, some of those roller coasters go off the rails.

* * *

Our current relationships to "entheogens" or substances used with sacramental intent are erratic and without precedent. Today, you can order the strongest psychoactives ever discovered and have them delivered two-day priority to your front door. Ayahuasca tourists flock to the Amazon. Twentysomething kids puff DMT (one of the most powerful and disorienting drugs out there) at EDM shows, and Silicon Valley CEOs smoke Sonoran toad venom as one more merit badge for the "tech-titan who has experienced everything!"

This is not normal. It's like breaking the sticks off bottle rockets and still hoping they'll go where you point them. Never have we combined such unstructured and open access to such powerful tools in all of human history, anywhere, *ever*. The medical and recreational use models aren't up to the job of guiding us safely and ethically through this complex terrain.

Fortunately, there are examples of how to properly integrate sacramental use into a culture—we just need to poke around a bit in the anthropological literature to find them.

Open Source Revelation

The Mountain Ok people of Western New Guinea have an especially elegant approach to the role of substances in their culture. They have twelve levels of initiation involving three main plants—ginger, tobacco, and mushrooms. The first ten levels represent the standard stages of initiation, while the final two are steps toward senior eldership.

The sacred substances are ordered into a hierarchy that reflects the level of initiation and the social status of the initiates. The first three rituals involve ginger, the middle six involve tobacco, and the final three involve varying species of psychoactive mushrooms. All stages involve increasing degrees of privation—fasting, sleeplessness, dehydration, chanting, dancing, and drumming to intensify the experience.

Once you have been initiated, you are permitted to use the substance. But you are not allowed to sample one ahead of schedule or out of order. In that respect, it's very much like a Montessori classroom, where a child is allowed to work with whatever materials they want *provided they have already been instructed in the proper use by the guide.* Same concept—freedom within order. Different materials.

"The whole cycle is orchestrated by elders belonging to the highest degrees," writes Oxford anthropologist Richard Rudgley, "who, having passed through the lower ranks, attain a profound and detailed understanding of the entire system of ritual knowledge."

In the final two stages, things get interesting. The initiate retreats to the highest mountains, undergoes grueling days and nights of deprivation, then consumes large quantities of highly toxic (and psychoactive) mushrooms. Plants that, taken outside of this ritual context, would likely kill someone. But once they have accessed the sacred and earned their position as elders, their insights are added to the living tradition of the tribe. "They are invested with the authority and insight," Rudgley explains, "to add their own individual subjective perceptions to the existing bodies of knowledge."

Most religious traditions are inherently conservative. At some point in a distant past, a founder, and possibly an elect group of initiates, had access to revelation. After that, the veil closed, history turned, a priest class grew, and the rest of us had to settle for hand-me-downs and Just So stories.

Sure, there are third-person efforts to talk about the Divine, to add commentary like the Hebrew midrash, or the Church writings of Augustine. But direct second- or first-person I-Thou or I-I encounters with the Numinous? Generally frowned upon, or outright persecuted as heresy. Illumined certainty and orthodox authority have often been at odds. Few powerful priests have been willing to get upstaged by hair-on-fire mystics.

So for the New Guineans to include an open-ended update to their living scripture? That has a subtle and surprisingly contemporary genius to it. After all, even the most vibrant mountain stream goes stagnant if you dam it. Long before Linux, Wikipedia, or blockchain, the Mountain Ok people pioneered a way to open-source revelation and keep the currents of inspiration flowing freely.

Freedom within limits. Innovation building upon tradition. Those are lessons we might draw from as we explore open-source sacraments for Meaning 3.0.

Hedonic Calendaring

Now that we have considered the utility of sacramental use, we should address how often to use those sacraments. For starters, we might state the obvious. Not everyone should consume entheogens willy-nilly. It's entirely possible that 10 percent of the population should never touch them, especially those with adverse medical or family histories (as well as Dark Triad narcissists, Machiavellians, and psychopaths).

It's probable that only 10 percent of the population should try them more than a few times. This would be consistent with the distributions we saw in New Guinea, where initiation into elder status and the most intensive ceremonies occurred only for a select few. Not everyone wants to be—or should be—an elder. For the remaining 80 percent in the middle of the bell curve, what would a lifetime calendar of appropriate initiations look like? The three milestones of adolescence, marriage, and death are obvious candidates to consider.

In the opening chapter of Alex Haley's landmark account of the African diaspora, *Roots*, a Gambian father lifts his newborn son up to the dazzling Milky Way and exclaims, "Behold Kunta Kinte—the only thing in the universe greater than you!" How much less anxiety and depression might we endure, if every one of our children was welcomed into the scheme of things like that?

A rite-of-passage initiation into adulthood with 3 grams of psilocybin, surrounded by elders, mentors, and peers, could fit here. This is the "Goldilocks dosage" perfected by Johns Hopkins to prompt insight and healing without excessive destabilization. If the sorts of positive effects that the Hopkins teams have found in their studies were extended to these coming-of-age ceremonies, they could set an adolescent on the path toward an ethical and engaged life in society and on this earth.

While in the context of drug wars and teenage substance abuse this sort of initiation might seem reckless, keep in mind that we willingly ply our children with high-dosage amphetamines, antidepressants, and antipsychotics, often to catastrophic effect. Tightly structured, community-supported initiation into periodic use of sacred substances has been practiced around the world for millennia and is of an entirely different category of application.

The obvious next "placebo sacrament" we endure is the wedding. These days it's often reduced to little more than photo ops, virtue signaling, and status displays. Little in the way of initiating a couple into *hieros gamos*—divine union—ever happens. What if, as part of the nuptials and in the company of a therapist, minister, or cherished members of the wedding party, the couple were to take 150 milligrams of MDMA (the MAPS therapeutic dosage) and share their deepest heartfelt hopes, fears, and commitments to the life they are about to cocreate?

What if at each anniversary, they repeated the ritual? They could reconnect after twelve months of hope and heartache, and recommit to the year ahead. It might prevent the slow accretion of frustration, grief, and resentment that so often drive wedges between life partners. It would go a long way to keeping deep connections and intentions alive through the trials of life.

Finally, how could we create a culturally appropriate initiation to stepping off the mortal coil altogether? Many survivors of near-death experiences report that it has radically reshaped their experience of life, because they now know what's coming and they're not afraid anymore. Subjects in Johns Hopkins end-of-life psilocybin trials reported much of the same—a meaningful reduction in "existential dread."

Whether the physical death of an NDE, or the ego-death of a psychedelic therapy, it seems that getting a dry run at dying can meaningfully increase folks' equanimity and grace when they ultimately have to face the real thing. By all accounts, the compound 5-MeO-DMT provides the closest analogue to the white-light experience that many report in NDEs. One to three sessions of that for elders or those facing terminal conditions could help answer nagging existential questions, make the most of the time they have left, and prepare them to say goodbye on their own terms. It would be a definite step up from drawing our last breath surrounded by hourly workers, hooked up to monitors and IV drips, sedated to oblivion.

These three examples are obvious ones where we could augment existing third-person "placebo sacraments" with more immediate and transformative first- and second-person encounters with the Sublime. Experiences where we're not talking about the Mystery, or being talked at by others about what it supposedly means. Instead, we are talking *to* the Mystery, or we are partaking *of* the Mystery. Direct sacramental, culturally integrated, and celebrated occasions for communion. Supported by our loved ones. Affirmed by our own understandings. Steered by a living tradition. No middleman required.

Essential Substances

If we're sticking to our IDEO design guide, then we need to pay attention to the intersection of "open source" and "anti-fragile." Traditionally, sacred substances have been rare and closely guarded—the opposite of open source. We still don't know the true ingredients for Hindu soma, Greek kykeon, or dozens of other classical concoctions that were often guarded on pain of death. That's still true today for Schedule I and Schedule II compounds, especially classes like psychedelics, which carry potential life sentences for possession and use. While the lifetime calendar of rites of passage we just considered above might sound promising, or even profound, at this point it's not even allowed.

If ancient and recent history are any guide, even cautious moves toward legalizing these drugs could be reversed at the stroke of a pen. Prometheans run a distinct risk of getting their matches confiscated by the priests, all in the name of public safety. All it would take is an attorney general with a prosecutor's distrust of the Weird or Revolutionary, and decades of work could be frozen overnight.

Open source means we have to share recipes made with widely accessible ingredients so communities everywhere have access. We can't afford to chase mad chemists or exotic plants and animals for our raw matériel. Anti-fragile in this case means "resistant to persecution." Especially if people start taking these liberating experiences seriously, and get impatient for meaningful social change.

The game then becomes how to diversify from an overreliance on Schedule I and Schedule II substances that, however promising, are vulnerable to marginalization and interruptions in supply. When those rare or restricted compounds are available, therapists, scientists, and ministers can incorporate those more powerful tools into their ongoing work, like farm-to-table chefs featuring what's in season on their menus. In the meantime, we can pull together viable candidates from our unscheduled medicine cabinets and less restricted Schedule III and Schedule IV compounds (i.e., those available via prescription, like cannabinoids, nitrous and nitric oxides, carbogen, oxytocin, and ketamine).

In other words, we need to create a list of widely available "essential substances" that grant inspiration, healing, and connection. Experiences that deliver us to the Sublime with little more than a driver's license or a doctor's note.

Church, then, could become something else altogether. Self-organized synchronized consumption of prescription pharmaceuticals in a revelatory, celebratory environment. B.Y.O.*E*. Bring Your Own Entheogens. Brought to you by your local Groove and Reconciliation Committee.

CHAPTER 9

Sex, Part I

EVOLUTION IS AMORAL

In the summer of 1980, *The Blue Lagoon* premiered in American theaters. It starred a fourteen-year-old Brooke Shields, who would go on to become a famous actress, befriend Michael Jackson, and marry tennis star Andre Agassi. On its way to a Top 10 box-office gross, the film scandalized audiences.

The movie poster read:

The director of *Grease*, Randal Kleiser brings to the screen a sensual story of natural love. Two children, shipwrecked alone on a tropical island. Nature is kind. They thrive on the bounty of jungle and lagoon. The boy grows tall. The girl beautiful. When their love happens it is as natural as the sea, and as powerful.

The Blue Lagoon updated Rousseau's fantasy of the Noble Savage living in paradise. The film coyly asked, "In a *Swiss Family Robinson* idyll, what is our true nature? Are we hardwired for innocent love and passion, or are we doomed by our instincts?"

At first Emmeline and Richard live happily off the fat of the land. But as "the boy grows tall [and] the girl beautiful," things happen.

Emmeline gets her period and both worry that she's been somehow wounded. Richard notices her budding breasts and teases Emmeline that she looks like the "hoobly booblie" pinups the sailors had on the ship. Emmeline counters that she's been spying on Richard and "I've seen you playing with it . . . I've seen it all, and what happens when you've been playing with it for a long time."

Then, one day after skinny-dipping in the lagoon and sharing a messy mango, they kiss.

"I feel so funny in my stomach," says Richard. "Me too," admits Emmeline.

"My heart's beating so fast," Emmeline shares. "Mine too," Richard agrees.

With a gorgeous waterfall backdrop and a swelling orchestral soundtrack, they get it on.

A few soft-porny tropical montages follow. They make love in various photogenic spots around the island. But then Emmeline starts putting on weight, going off sex, and getting irritated with Richard. In other words, she's pregnant. Nine months after their initial bliss, they have a baby. Everything changes. Heaven's Gate clangs shut.

As predictable as the film was, and as hard as the critics slammed it (the site aggregator Rotten Tomatoes gave it an 8 percent Rotten score, while Shields won the first ever Razzie Award for Worst Actress), audiences ate it up. Only *The Empire Strikes Back*, *Airplane*, and *Smokey and the Bandit II* outgrossed the film that summer.

But in its own goofy way, it also highlights a simple fact of life: Humans always figure out how to reproduce, no matter how clueless or misinformed. For millions of years we pulled this off *with no instruction manual*. It's the single most effective biological impulse beyond breathing and eating. It must be, or nearly eight billion of us wouldn't be here. This overwhelming imperative underpins some of our deepest pain and our highest potential.

At some point, for reasons they can't fully explain, boys and girls get to exploring each other's bodies, just as Richard and Emmeline do at the lagoon. The funny feelings in their stomachs and their racing heartbeats? Norepinephrine, dopamine, and testosterone flooding their systems and rewarding them for their efforts. "Keep going, you're nearly there!" whispers Mother Nature.

The boy's alert member, packed with over seven thousand discrete nerve endings, the most anywhere on his body, bumps up against the girl's midsection. There, tucked between her thighs, is a secret spot, more inviting than any place he has ever been.

The girl's body also responds to the visual and olfactory cues of arousal. It releases vasoactive intestinal polypeptide (VIP), which increases blood flow to her vagina. Plasma seeps from the vaginal walls, making it wet. Two pea-sized glands on either side of the introitus and the cervix secrete mucus. The end result is a lubricant literally slicker than snot—even the synovial fluid that greases our creaky knees isn't as slippery. Nature saved her best chemistry for this high-stakes hot spot.

So when the two young lovers fumblingly figure out how to put their bits together, it feels amazing. But also, not fully satisfying. No sooner than he's figured out what goes where, some deep impulse prompts the boy to reverse course. Backing-and-forthing until a lightning bolt of sensation explodes up his brain stem and out his body. It feels like the best sneeze of his life backed with a pint of ice cream. Supersaturated contentment (and a drowsy desire to do it again).

But then nine months later, *seemingly unconnected in any way to those prior romps*, out pops a baby! That same fascinating nether region is now co-opted for an entirely different purpose—delivery. There's nothing thematically, aesthetically, or logistically that connects these two activities—sex and childbirth. One is passionate, pleasurable, and typically brief. The other takes nine months of sustained effort, is agonizing and scary at the crux—and the consequences last a lifetime. The joke's on us. And every generation falls for it, like, no one could have seen it coming.

It's one of Mother Nature's dirtiest tricks, but also some of her strongest juju—getting a bunch of distractible primates to fornicate often enough to ensure the survival of the species. The savage within us all may or may not be noble, as Rousseau wondered. But evolution is most certainly amoral. It's not that love is blind, we are. We barely acknowledge the driving force that shapes much of our lives.

In no small part, humans are puppets on the strings of evolution. Helen of Troy was the "face that launched a thousand ships." Tristan and Iseult. Romeo and Juliet. Richard Burton and Elizabeth Taylor. Brangelina. We like to think our epic tales of romance are testaments to the power of free will and the human spirit. But really, they're just as much a catalog of hormonal imperative. Evolution doesn't care at all for our preferences, promises, or taboos. All it cares about is creating the conditions for the most robust gene pool possible. 'Til death do we part be damned.

* * *

Think about the first mad rush of lust and love that sweeps every new couple off their feet. Our libidos skyrocket. We can't keep our hands off each other. Kissing, calling, sexting, shagging.

This! We think to ourselves, and spout off to any friends and family who will listen. This is true love! Except it's not. It's technically closer to true lust. The testes and ovaries secrete testosterone and estrogen and fill us with a powerful urge to couple. The hypothalamus pumps out oxytocin and vasopressin, creating potent feelings of trust, attachment, and connection. No one else matters as much or feels this good to be around.

That profound attachment has a dark side too—blind jealousy—the kind that prompts jilted lovers to dump furniture on the street or run a key down the side of a rival's car. But never mind all that—we're fully committed to the ride at this point.

Then the hypothalamus starts to secrete dopamine—an incredibly pleasurable reward chemical that peaks with orgasm. Throw a little norepinephrine into the mix and our hearts race. We can't eat or sleep. The caudate nucleus, one of the brain's major reward centers, lights up like fireworks when we see images of our lover. All we can do is scheme and long to reconnect with the object of our affection. Being apart for a day can feel like forever. We must be together.

But too much dopamine, like too much oxytocin, isn't all fun. It can lead to bingeing, addiction, and impulsivity. When Parkinson's patients are given too much L-Dopa, a synthetic substitute for dopamine, sweet-as-peaches Granny, once content to sit on the couch watching her "stories" on the TV, steals her kids' credit cards and racks up thousands of dollars in gambling debt. Lower the dosage of L-Dopa, or stop the meds altogether, and old relatives come back to themselves, as if they've been in a dream.

But turn the dopamine drip up to puppy-love highs, and all bets are off. The English playwright George Bernard Shaw called romantic love "the most violent, most insane, most delusive, and most transient of passions." We're crazy in love.

To make things worse, the neurotransmitter serotonin plummets during early courtship. It's the hormone connected to both mood and appetite (and the primary system affected by antidepressants like Prozac and psychedelics like psilocybin). When it's low, we become fixated on romantic and possessive thoughts and feel so lovesick we stop eating. Neurochemically, some researchers believe this infatuation closely mimics obsessive-compulsive disorder (OCD). While we're in the throes of low serotonin and decreased prefrontal cortical activity, we chalk up our punch-drunkenness to true love. But from a clinical perspective, we've quite literally lost our minds.

To a degree that our modern selves might find insulting, we're still driven by ancient programming. In a 2016 study in *Frontiers in Psychology*, the researchers concluded that "romantic love is a natural (and often positive) addiction that evolved from mammalian antecedents by 4 million years ago as a survival mechanism to encourage hominin pair-bonding and reproduction." Everyone knows you should never trust an addict. And yet, that deep coding is what animates some of the most profound and personal decisions in all of our lives.

As obvious as this derangement appears when it's happening to someone else, once afflicted, we're all a bit more obsessive, impulsive, and reckless. We leave perfectly good mates to chase new dates. We break leases and quit jobs to move across the country to pursue a flame. We have impulsive flings with milkmen and work wives. We abandon families to go and start new ones. We imagine that this love, this time, is going to be our everything and is going to fill all our deepest needs and longings.

And sometimes it does. Just long enough to fulfill our biological imperative to conceive, birth, and wean a small child. But four to seven years later all those lusty attraction hormones shut down, like Hot Slots Grandma weaning off her L-Dopa gambling binge. The infatuation and fornication peter out, and we see a major uptick in affairs and divorces. That "seven-year itch" made famous by the Marilyn Monroe film turns out to be real. Hardwired into our genes, and right on schedule.

We start to yearn for novelty, adventure, and passion. We'd do almost anything to get our groove back. Mother Nature's got us covered on that front too. As slyly as she coaxed us into these unions, she whispers in our ears to double down at another turn at the roulette wheel.

In a new study just published in 2020, scientists found that every month, many women grow especially dissatisfied with their long-term partners. Last week may have been fine, but this week, they can't stand the way their lover talks, the way he smells, the way he dresses and moves. Even though men can't always put their finger on it, they know something's up too. They bristle or cower, depending on their tolerance for risk.

Most people would guess that this irritation coincides with premenstrual syndrome (PMS). But it doesn't. It actually maps to the week of peak ovulation. Researchers speculate that female irritation coincides with peak fertility to boost the chance of one-night stands with more virile partners.

So let's just imagine that right around day fourteen of the ovulation cycle, the couple starts to fight. The woman, seething but secretly relieved, storms out the front door. Maybe she heads out to a local bar. In every sense, she's heated.

Scientists have found that when strippers are ovulating they earn up to 30 percent higher tips. They speculate it's pheromonal attraction—men don't even know what they're experiencing, but deep down their Spidey senses are tingling (and urging them to make it rain dollar bills). If our newly liberated woman shares that pheromonal boost with her go-go dancing sisters, she's that much more likely to attract a potential suitor herself.

Only now, she's searching for the exact opposite of her safe, reliable domestic partner. She's craving strong, dangerous testosterone-laden excitement. And she finds it. She knocks back her drink, throws caution out the window, and pursues what Erica Jong memorably called the Zipless Fuck. Hot, heavy, forbidden. *Fantastic.*

And here's where Nature throws one of her cruelest twists. When a woman climaxes, especially with a new, virile lover, her ability to conceive can slide up to three full days in either direction. Evolution wants that new genetic material, and it will go to incredible lengths to secure it. So even if by the next morning, the woman feels ready to go back to her old life and man, she might not get the chance. Odds are higher than average she's just conceived with her dangerous new baby daddy.

It's not just women who wander. For many men, as they crest the forty-year mark, they begin to sense their own mortality for the first time. "Why am I soft in the middle now?" sang a pensive Paul Simon. "The rest of my life is so hard." Fearing their best may be behind them, middle-aged men can grow restless for adventure and excitement. Some, against their better judgment, start shopping for convertible Porsches or wondering if it's too late to get an earring or a tribal tattoo.

Except what's really going on underneath this predictable malaise is a drop in testosterone. Around midlife, this central hormone tapers and the man can experience a sag in mental clarity and stamina. It takes longer to recover after hard workouts. His body begins to droop downward, pooling disconcertingly around his dad-bod middle. He begins to nurse a nagging suspicion that it's a slippery slope to the grave from here.

Researchers have found that one of the surest ways to reduce that existential crisis and boost testosterone production in middle-aged men is having sex with a new younger partner. It's the Coolidge effect busting out of the henhouse and into the suburbs. The ultimate arbiters of all things amorous, the French, have found this event so common, so utterly predictable, they've even given it a name, *l'affaire de la quarantaine*. Literally—the Affair of the Forties. Like clockwork, every generation. Almost as if it were planned.

Once past the intoxicating honeymoon romps, the man might realize he has less in common with his new lover than he thought. He's Nintendo. She's XBox. He's a vintage Cabernet. She's a Fireball shooter. Different music tastes. Different movies. Different friends. Just not. That. Compatible.

Shaking off the fog, he belatedly realizes what he's done. Only now it might be too late to go back. Too much heartache, too much scar tissue. Maybe even a new love child to really complicate things. When in reality, all of it could've been avoided if he'd just had the foresight to go to his family doctor and ask for a testosterone patch. And maybe settled for a Volvo instead of a Porsche.

Meanwhile Mother Nature laughs, all the way to the sperm bank.

If that were the last of it, we'd be right to shake our fists at the sky. But the practical jokes don't end there. Even the selfless and faithful get snookered by evolution. When a woman experiences menopause, estrogen, vasopressin, and oxytocin taper off with it. In the same way that lovers coming off the chemical high of early infatuation see things (and partners) more clearly, a woman leaving behind her child-bearing years can come to a fresh reckoning of her own. Namely, that she is absolutely *done* looking after everyone else in the home.

Freed from the mother-hen priming of hormones, which for so long made her feel connected to her brood and committed to making a nurturing home, now she dreams of Virginia Woolf and a room of her own. "Gray divorces" for fifty-something couples are the fastest-growing segment of separations, doubling in the past decade. A majority are initiated by women.

That's not to say that we are blind victims of our hormonal programming. We all have choice, and the culture we grow up in radically informs how we experience our urges, longings, and desires. To be a gay man in 2020 living in San Francisco, for example, is to have a fundamentally different experience than Oscar Wilde did in 1890s London when he saw his career ruined by accusations of sodomy. To be a politician caught with a lover fuels a very different news cycle in France or Italy than in the United States.

Culture matters. Psychology matters. But so does biology. And because we are so steeped in the psychological and social, we tend to ignore the biological underpinnings of much of our experience. We insist we are captains of our ship, never noticing the tides that sweep us out to sea.

* * *

So far, we've discussed largely consensual relationships, and how little of our choices are truly our own. But there's an even sadder side to the evolutionary impulse—where the sex is tragic, violent, and unwanted.

From an evolutionary perspective, once a girl begins menstruating, she is a fertile woman. Younger mothers tend to have healthier pregnancies than older ones. This is why so many traditional cultures betroth girls at that age.

But from a developmental perspective, she is still very much a child, with a heart and mind playing catch-up to her body. Babies having babies isn't great for either of them. Which is why there's a global movement to stop the practice of arranged marriages.

It's not until her early twenties that a woman's prefrontal cortex, and with it, executive function, situational awareness, and delay of gratification, fully comes online (boys take a bit longer). That gap between physical and psychological development turns out to be a gauntlet every young girl has to run. Nearly two out of three sexual assaults are perpetrated on children and young adults. Girls aged sixteen to nineteen are four times more likely to be victims of rape or sexual assault than at any other time in their lives.

When you think about what percentage of adverse childhood events (ACEs), domestic violence, and trauma has a sexual component forced upon victims, and you realize how much of that is driven by the cold dictates of biological impulse, it's enough to make you weep. Throw in the more common but no less painful elements of our romantic lives—jealousy, infidelity, divorce, betrayal, obsession, resentment, abortions, and miscarriages—and it's a wonder we manage at all.

To top it all off, add the mind-boggling fact that even today, in the so-called developed world, *half* of all pregnancies are accidental, no better than a coin toss deciding one of the most momentous decisions in life—whether or not to create another one. We can put men on the moon and split atoms, but we haven't come close to civilizing our most basic instinct.

We might think that we're in charge of our romantic destiny. We might insist that the "heart wants what it wants" and equate that with the fulfillment of our highest desire. But really, the "heart"—in the sense of our deepest bodily longings—wants what evolution wants. And in the space between our highest expressions and our deepest compulsions—is written the tragic comedy of our lives.

Forgive us, for we truly know not what we do.

*   *   *

The Stoned Ape (or the Horned Ape?)

In the mid-1990s, Terence McKenna, the infamous psychedelic philosopher and heir to Timothy Leary's throne, took a wild swing at the origins of consciousness. He believed he'd found the answer to the central paradox of human existence—namely, how'd we get so damned smart all of a sudden?

According to McKenna, about one hundred million years ago our ancient African grandparents climbed down from the trees and began to explore the savanna. As they hunted and foraged for food they came across grazing animals like impala, gazelle, and wildebeest. Those massive herds left piles of dung behind them. The droppings hosted millions of insects that were an easy-to-harvest protein source, and well worth picking through to find.

The dung hosted another plentiful food supply—fungi. Among the best-known varieties that sprout on cow pies are *Psilocybe cubensis*, a.k.a. "magic mushrooms." Entomologists speculate that these mushrooms first secreted psychedelic compounds as a natural insect repellent. Tripping dung beetles, they theorized, often wandered off and forgot to finish eating the rest of the mushroom. Problem solved.

McKenna, though, saw a much grander role for those humble toad-stools. He mused that complex linguistics sprang from the synaptic superconductivity of the psychedelic trip. It was, according to Mc-Kenna, the most likely candidate for how we went from grunting and pointing to poetry and song. And the truly heroic, blow-out-the-pipes shamanic adventure—or, as he so memorably put it, "Five grams in silent darkness"? The catalyst for nothing less than the prehistoric birth of awe and the origins of religion.

Serious anthropologists never gave the Stoned Ape theory much credence. Even sympathetic scholars found that McKenna was play-ing fast and loose with citations and ignoring counterfactual exam-ples in the literature (like bloody Aztec mushroom sacrifices, violent ayahuascan Amazonian tribes, or sociopathic CIA programs). But the theory never disappeared, either. If anything, it's enjoying a recent resurgence along with all things psychedelic these days. We might not have to stretch as far as McKenna's ramblings, though, to find what distinguishes us from our nearest primate cousins.

To refine our search for the causes of consciousness we need to ask what else could have provided the neurological boost to transform us from the ape who stands (*Homo erectus*) to the ape who *knows* (*Homo sapiens*)? A plausible alternate candidate to the Stoned Ape hypoth-esis would have to check three boxes: It would need to be strongly instinctive, feel powerfully rewarding, and enjoy widespread adop-tion. It would have to meaningfully shift physiology and psychology, and be able to do so repeatedly over time. In sum, the transforma-tive substance or practice would need to be what psychologists call *autotelic*—meaning it would have to have its own intrinsic reason and reward for doing.

It might not have been the Stoned Ape that tripped us awake, but it could have been his far more widespread cousin, the Horned Ape, the ape who differs from all his primate relatives in the way he en-gages love and sex. The Horned Ape is a more plausible missing link between *Homo erectus* and *Homo sapiens*. Or, to give him his proper Latin name, *Homo coitus*—the ape who gets it on.

* * *

Jared Diamond, the Pulitzer Prize–winning UCLA anthropologist, makes exactly this case. In *Why Is Sex Fun?: The Evolution of Human Sexuality*, he compares us to different primate and animal species and comes to a controversial conclusion: Growing bigger brains didn't create our sexual habits, as Freud would have insisted. Instead, our sexual habits created our bigger brains.

If true, this upends everything we've assumed about how human consciousness and culture developed. "While paleontologists usually attribute the evolution of [culture, speech, and complex tools] to our attainment of large brains and upright postures," Diamond argues, "our bizarre sexuality was equally essential for their evolution."

In the prior section we discussed how powerful lust and attraction are, and how little we understand of our romantic lives. What we experience as our deeply personal love stories turn out to be highly predictable, largely subconscious evolutionary scripts. That's not to say we don't ever consciously think about our sexuality. We do. All the time.

There's a cottage industry of books, from *Sex at Dawn* to *Bonk* to *Mating in Captivity*, that attempt to contextualize how we behave in terms of our most elemental drivers and impulses. Even these recent books are too close to the problem to see how unusual our sexual behavior really is. They encourage us to embrace our innate drive for pleasure and break free from social conditioning, but they do so from a wholly anthropocentric stance. These authors try to normalize a wider range of behaviors, like promiscuity, polyamory, and infidelity. But they don't question how atypical our sexual nature is in the first place.

In 1999, the Bloodhound Gang released a novelty song, "Bad Touch," that went where anthropologists and psychologists were afraid to go. Their catchy lyrics put human courtship back within the broader context of love in the animal kingdom. The tune struck a chord, rocketing to the Top 10 charts worldwide and getting sampled by the rapper Eminem.

You and me baby ain't nothin' but mammals
So let's do it like they do on the Discovery Channel
(Gettin' horny now)

But really, the Bloodhound Gang should've watched a little more Discovery Channel before they penned their pickup lines. After all, have you seen how animals have sex?

It's brutal.

Ducks practically drown each other in their efforts. The male mounts the female, wings beating, crushing her underwater until the deed is done. Leave the cooing to the turtledoves. Ducks fuck.

Dogs hump frantically but can get tied up and twisted on the dismount. Stuck facing backward for hours, they have to wait sheepishly until the swelling goes down and they can both be on their way.

But the big cats—the cats have it maybe worst of all. Lions, for instance, only mate every couple of years in the wild. When they do, they make up for lost time, copulating up to fifty times in a twenty-four-hour window. And it's not because they like it. The male's penis has over a hundred tiny barbs on it, which gouge the vaginal walls of the lioness. The spikes serve two purposes: to scrape out any competing semen from prior males and to stimulate ovulation in the female. Fun comes in a distant third.

When Thomas Hobbes wrote in *Leviathan* that the life of man was nasty, brutish, and short, he could just as easily have been thinking of love in the animal kingdom. Sex, for the overwhelming majority of animals, is violent, dangerous, and brief. There's barely a lick of enjoyment for anyone involved.

And that's what's so fascinating about our own sexual habits—how thoroughly different they are from those mammals on the Discovery Channel. "All these features of human sexuality—long-term sexual partnerships . . . private sex, concealed ovulation, extended female receptivity, sex for fun . . . constitute what we humans assume is normal sexuality," Diamond explains. "But that proves to be a species-ist interpretation. By the standards of the world's 4,300 other species of mammals, and even by the standards of our own closest relatives the great apes . . . we are the ones who are bizarre."

We're among only a handful of animals on the entire planet who have sex outside of a narrowly defined window of fertility. Sure, dolphins and bonobos do sometimes, but they're two of the most intelligent species on the planet. Their friskiness only strengthens the linkage between elective sexuality and complex cognition. But even they lack many of the other factors that render human sexuality so distinctive, like concealed ovulation and frequent female orgasm.

Animals ignore their sex drives until they are briefly consumed by them. But humans think and act on their impulse anytime, all the time. Most women, unless they're on the Pill or using a fertility app, do not know for certain when they are in estrus—a simple fact of life that cows and baboons readily understand. Men definitely can't tell when their potential mates are ovulating, and experience high sex drive and a desire to copulate year-round. Women mostly humor them.

* * *

Over the past ten million years, human natural selection has unmistakably diverged from our cousins. And those differences show up in both sexes of our species. We can see how different we are by how far we've branched from our family tree.

Let's start with the most obvious and visible.

"Men possess penises that are much longer, thicker, and more flexible than those of other primates," writes evolutionary psychologist Geoffrey Miller. "These are more likely to reflect female choice than male competition," he adds.

In 2015, Miller and a team of researchers at UCLA wanted to answer the perennial question asked in men's and women's magazines alike: does size really matter? They went about it in a novel way. Rather than showing women pictures of penises, they 3D printed actual ones made of silicone. Then they conducted a survey using "improved shape identification based on haptic information from 3D objects"—which is apparently peer-reviewed journal speak for "we let them rummage around in a bag of dicks and pick the one they liked best."

As it turns out, for women, size does matter, just not as much as porn stars hope or most men fear. In general, women in the study chose an ideal penis size of 6.3 inches (compared to an average size of 5.0 inches). When invited to select for a one-night stand, they preferred slightly larger, girthier implements. "Women's penis preferences may vary with their relationship expectations," the paper explains primly. "Women prefer more masculine partners for shorter-term sexual relationships. . . . More masculine traits, such as lower voice pitch and (to some extent) larger penis size are correlated with testosterone levels, which also may influence men's mating goals and attractiveness. Since a larger penis size is perceived as more masculine, we predict women will prefer a larger penis for shorter-term sexual relationships."

This preference for penis size does not exist in our primate cousins. It is a unique feature of *Homo sapiens'* sexual selection, and it developed quite suddenly. Our family tree branched from our nearest relatives, the chimps and bonobos, about seven million years ago, from gorillas about nine million years ago, and from orangutans fourteen million years ago.

That may seem like ages to us, but in evolutionary terms, it's not long at all. Gorillas' erect penises, for comparison, measure about 1.25 inches in length, despite mature males weighing up to five hundred pounds—three times larger than most men. So much for the Big Hands theory.

One might then reasonably wonder if human penises grew longer to support the more adventuresome sex positions we seem to prefer. But orangutans, whose units clock in at only 1.5 inches, engage in gymnastic couplings that would humble a circus performer. And they pull out all the stops while hanging one-armed from tree branches.

"Starting from a ¼-inch ancestral ape penis . . . the human penis increased in length by a runaway process," Jared Diamond explains, "conveying an advantage to its owner as an increasingly conspicuous signal of virility . . . in effect . . . boasting 'I'm already so smart and superior that I don't need to devote more ounces of protoplasm to my brain, but I can instead afford the handicap of packing the ounces uselessly onto my penis.'"

*   *   *

Females have optimized for mate selection as well. Women maintain visible and shapely breasts throughout their sexually reproductive lives, even when they're not lactating. Virtually no other species does this. It impedes mobility and other survival functions but helps in mate selection. Primatologists call this a "false signal" because milk is produced by the underlying glandular tissue and not from breast fat. So bigger boobs don't make for better mammas.

But that isn't how men assess it. "Women . . . evolved to incarnate male sexual preferences," explains Miller in his book *The Mating Mind: How Sexual Choice Shaped the Evolution of Human Nature.* "Women have enlarged breasts and buttocks, narrower waists, *and a greater orgasmic capacity* than other apes" [emphasis added].

Over millennia of selection, those desired genetics have inspired a matching aesthetic—the curvy curves of prehistoric Venus goddess figures. Some of the earliest figurines found in archaeological dig sites across Europe showcase this idealized female form. Forty thousand years ago, tits and ass were venerated.

And they still are today. A quarter century ago, noted gender theorist (and rapper) Sir Mix-a-Lot lobbied for a return to that timeless Venusian ideal.

> *I like big butts and I cannot lie*
> *You other brothers can't deny*
> *That when a girl walks in with an itty-bitty waist*
> *And a round thing in your face*
> *You get sprung, want to pull up tough*
> *'Cause you notice that butt was stuffed!*

In 2014, Kim Kardashian famously "broke the internet" with a nude portrait for *Paper* magazine showcasing her improbable proportions by balancing a champagne glass on her rump. Heroin chic was definitely out. VaVaVoom was back.

Instagram Face

If you really want to see how powerfully these primitive mating signals shape our desires, consider how ingeniously we modify what we're given. More now than at any other time in the past, we've hacked the mating game. In today's sexual marketplace, sellers have so thoroughly blurred the lines between honest and deceptive signaling that buyers literally have no idea what they're getting into.

What used to get doled out by the dumb luck of natural selection can now be worked into an outpatient procedure. The linkage between healthy genetics and desired aesthetics has broken down entirely.

We're approaching a cosmetic singularity where all looks are converging into one uniform appearance. "What seems likely to be one of the oddest legacies of our rapidly expiring decade," Jia Tolentino recently acknowledged in *The New Yorker*, [is] the gradual emergence, among professionally beautiful women, of a single, cyborgian face."

Her assessment of how radically beauty standards are mutating and converging is worth quoting in full: "It's a young face, of course, with poreless skin and plump, high cheekbones. It has catlike eyes and long, cartoonish lashes; it has a small, neat nose and full, lush lips. It looks at you coyly but blankly, as if its owner has taken half a Klonopin and is considering asking you for a private-jet ride to Coachella. The face is distinctly white but ambiguously ethnic—it suggests a *National Geographic* composite illustrating what Americans will look like in 2050."

Tolentino concedes that impossible beauty standards for women have always been around, from foot-binding in China to tiny-waisted corsets in Europe. But she then points out how pervasive and pernicious the role of "self as selfie" digital presentation has made things.

"Social media has supercharged the propensity to regard one's personal identity as a potential source of profit—and, especially for young women, to regard one's body this way, too," she says. "For those born with assets—natural assets, capital assets, or both—it can seem sensible, even automatic, to think of your body the way that a McKinsey consultant would think about a corporation: identify underperforming sectors and remake them."

It's not only women. In an increasingly competitive workplace, male tech executives in particular take great pains to maintain youthful appearances, so as not to seem over the hill to their twentysomething coworkers. The end result is that faking young, hip "alpha male" status, which was damn near impossible in the era of hunter-warrior societies, is now only a TAG Heuer watch and a Tesla away. For any aspiring beta male looking to fudge his reproductive bona fides, chest implants, a tummy tuck, and some Botox are increasingly welcomed.

That's not all. Guys are constantly tempted to tinker with their junk. Ads for nonsurgical penis enhancement fool up to half of all men into believing that kind of change is possible. Creams, pills, and pumps abound.

There are even some field studies we can review to understand the signaling power of a large package. Specifically, what happens when men have the chance to design their own? In Papua New Guinea, the men of the Ketengban tribe collect an array of penis sheaths the same way a businessman might manage his tie rack. Ranging in size up to two feet, these "phallocarps" vary in decoration and even angle of erection. Without them, the otherwise stark-naked men report feeling undressed. For the Ketengban, penis sheaths are essential clothing.

It's not just exotic islanders that have augmented their jocks. In Renaissance Europe, the codpiece—a padded cup covering the penis and testicles—became mandatory fashion. One two-and-a-half-pound steel version featured prominently on Henry VIII's royal armor. Rabelais, the French satirist, took the piss out of the whole trend, working a sly reference to *On the Dignity of Codpieces* into the foreword to *Gargantua and Pantagruel*.

Even though codpieces fell out of fashion, they've always hung around. Within the past few years, they've made a return to haute couture, gracing runway exhibitions for Gucci. Between the Marvel and DC Comic universes, there are plenty of superhero bulges to go around as well. Batman sports an especially daunting one. Rock stars do too. Both Guns N' Roses front man, Axl Rose, and the lead singer of Jethro Tull wore them. Derek Smalls, the fictional bass player for the British spoof band Spinal Tap, took matters into his own hands with a DIY "trouser helper." He crammed a zucchini into his pants to "put the expand back in his Spandex." "Certainly less painful than collagen," he conceded.

* * *

All this adjusting and manipulating our bodies to boost our desirability—from fillers to dyes to surgeries—highlights how motivated we are to optimize our reproductive fitness. We've nurtured the hell out of our natures, just to boost the chance of getting laid. And while we can't help trying to increase our chances of standing out, the fact is that as a species, we are already far more sexualized than any of our nearest relatives.

Concealed fertility, abundant recreational sex, permanent female breasts, frequent female orgasm, and larger penises occur nowhere else in the animal kingdom. We are so different, in fact, that any accounting of our rapid acceleration into *Homo sapiens* has to consider our divergent sexuality as a prime candidate fueling that change.

"Within the relatively short period during which our ancestors and the ancestors of our great ape relatives have been evolving separately," Diamond explains, "along with posture and brain size, sexuality completes the trinity of the decisive respects in which the ancestors of humans and great apes diverged. . . . *Recreational sex . . . was as important for our development of fire, language, art, and writing as were our upright posture and large brains*" [emphasis added].

The reward circuitry that prompted romance at the Blue Lagoon encourages us to go back to those waters, again and again. Over time, those altered, more expansive and connected experiences became a permanent part of our thinking and being. Norepinephrine energizing us and sharpening our focus. Dopamine rewarding our explorations and new discoveries. Endorphins easing our aches and providing brief relief from the grind of life. Oxytocin bonding us to our lovers and offspring. Slower brain waves allowing subconscious thinking and inspiration. Our altered states became altered traits, one orgasm at a time.

* * *

So Stoned Ape or Horned Ape? Terence McKenna argued that our ancestors must have eaten magic mushrooms to wake ourselves up. But that's a tenuous theory, impossible to prove from here. Based on the anthropological record, the Horned Ape—the primate that sexed itself into higher consciousness—seems a more likely candidate.

If we agree with Diamond and other anthropologists who argue that sexuality accelerated human consciousness and culture, we also have to reckon with all of the pain and suffering that those unconscious drives continue to cause. Sure, we can bowl strikes all day long, aiming precisely for the romantic path we desire. But on either side of that narrow path, gravity and biology beckon. A lapse in attention, or a slip of the wrist, and the gutter ball waits for us all.

That realization offers us a shot at redemption. We can transform the suffering and confusion that our sexuality has often caused. All of that imprinting, all of that relentless drive to procreate can be repurposed. Rather than dancing like puppets on the strings of indifferent evolution, we can untie those strings and begin to stand on our own two feet.

We can hot-wire evolution.

Sexuality doesn't have to lead to misery. It helped transform us from *Homo erectus* to *Homo sapiens* after all. Informed by these recent findings in neurobiology and anthropology, we can repurpose sex from something impulsive and constraining to something intentional and liberating. We can complete the move from *Homo sapiens* (the ape who knows) to *Homo ludens* (the ape who plays).

In the next chapter, we will move from the realm of sexual anthropology into neurophysiology—to look under the hood of all of these biological drivers and map out what hedonic engineering—a pleasurable path of healing, inspiration, and connection—might look like.

CHAPTER 10

Sex, Part II

HIGHER LOVE

One summer right after grad school, my wife, Julie, and I signed on to an expedition guiding in the Himalayas. It was a great program—taking college students trekking to monasteries and mountain communities in Nepal and Tibet, capped off with a climb on the North Face of Mount Everest. While we were acclimating, we hiked up to a remote monastery high up in the Tibetan mountains. So high, in fact, that the Chinese had never made it up there to shut it all down.

Before we got to the hobbit-like door to the temple, I pulled aside our students and told them how lucky we were to get to glimpse "untouched" Tibetan culture. We approached the gate in reverential silence, only to have it opened by a young monk in a yak-butter- and soot-stained Chicago Bulls letterman's jacket. To his credit, the burgundy sleeves matched his robes perfectly.

We dropped our packs and set up camp on the flat rooftops of the monastery, right beside a roaring river and hot spring. A huge cloud of vultures circled the ridge above the compound. Then we noticed a Buddhist priest in full garb with a scythe-like curved blade, cutting chunks of something and feeding it to the waiting birds. We asked our Tibetan guide what was going on—he replied it was a Sky Burial, where a monk who had recently died was being offered up to the carrion eaters as a direct route back to Source. Gruesome. *Awesome.* The Circle of Life—not just a metaphor in those parts.

Exhausted after our long climb, and excited to watch the sun set in such a spectacular spot, we grabbed our trunks and climbed down to the steaming riverbank hot spring. After a few minutes of soaking, one of our students looked down at her leg and screamed, "There's a snake coiled around my ankle!" We were sure she was altitude sick and hallucinating. But then, in the fading light, the walls of the pool began to ripple and shimmer. I blinked hard and dozens of snakes came into focus, like something out of an Indiana Jones movie. Turns out this little colony of serpents had survived up there at over fifteen thousand feet by cozying up to the thermal springs. They were harmless, but their impact on the vibe was fatal. Our soaking session was done.

Just below the springs, the whitewater punched a hole straight through a granite wall and gushed out the other side. It's worth noting, that's not how rivers usually get around. Typically, they erode a water course over millions of years, etching a path of least resistance from high up in the mountains down to the sea.

When we asked that young monk how on earth this river had bucked that trend, he told us it was Padmasambhava, one of the patron saints of Tibetan Buddhism. Took the river, he said, and magicked it straight through a mountain. Then he pointed to the cliff a thousand feet above us.

Way up on that face sat the tiny shadow of a cave entrance. It was in the middle of a sheer drop that dwarfed the big walls of Yosemite, with no possible way up, down, or in. "That's Padmasambhava and his consort Yeshe Tsogyal's cave," our guide explained. "They retreated to practice their hidden teachings of Vajrayana Buddhism, Bon shamanism, and sacred sex." We craned our necks to spot it—but how on earth did they get up there?

"Oh, they flew on a magic carpet!" he said.

I couldn't stop staring up at that cave. What a strange overlay of geology and mythology this remote valley had. Padmasambhava is like Tibet's King Arthur—a loose mix of the historical woven in with the legendary. Also known as Guru Rinpoche, he is venerated as one of the main transmitters of the Dharma to Tibet and a second coming of the Buddha. Even casual students of Tibetan Buddhism know all about Padmasambhava. He's kind of a big deal.

But Yeshe Tsogyal? She's a slightly deeper cut, revered only by those who have slowed down enough to learn her story. She was born into a royal family in Kharchen, Tibet, toward the end of the eighth century. A headstrong princess from an early age, she ran away from home to avoid an arranged marriage. She risked everything to become an adept and survived a list of trials fit for Hercules. She even fought and beheaded a tiger.

Once initiated as a Tantrika—a carrier of psychosexual initiation—she made her way back to her family's province. But before she could get home she was robbed and raped by seven bandits. Rather than being traumatized by the assault, Yeshe used the experience to demonstrate her power. Afterward the seven men were so humbled by her transmission that they all dropped to their knees weeping and vowed to become her bodyguards for life.

Padmasambhava himself acknowledged the power of Yeshe's attainment. "The basis for realizing enlightenment is in a human body, male or female. . . . But if she develops the mind bent on enlightenment *the woman's body is better*." Yeshe became Padmasambhava's consort and teacher, bringing him to god consciousness and teaching him how to fly on her magic carpet (which was crucial, because the elevator to their love cave never worked).

The legend of Yeshe Tsogyal embodies the relationship between sex, suffering, and consciousness. On the one hand, she, like many women before and after her, was a victim of sexual violence. But on the other, she was able to master her body and mind to such a degree that she could not only withstand assault but could transform her assailants.

She was a *dakini*—a woman who mastered the erotic and the divine. "It is implicit that if [yoginis] were able to help others fully realize the nature of their minds," Harvard-trained scholar Miranda Shaw writes in *Passionate Enlightenment: Women in Tantric Buddhism*, "these women had fully realized the nature of their own minds." It's that alchemical power that allowed her to wake up Padmasambhava too—giving birth to some of the deepest teachings of Tibetan Buddhism, including the practice of Tonglen we learned about in Chapter 6.

In the last chapter we explored the simple truth that our sexual impulses often pull the strings of our lives. Like the castaways of the Blue Lagoon, hormonal imprinting drives many of the triumphs and tragedies of our romantic experience. But it doesn't end there. Human sexuality might, as anthropologist Jared Diamond has argued, also hold the key for the development of complex consciousness. Prolonged exposure to the shifted states that come from sexual arousal may well have nudged us toward expanded awareness. And as Yeshe's story suggests, that expanded awareness might even hold the key to healing trauma and full awakening.

All of the neurochemical priming that makes babies inevitable—our animal nature—can also give us access to higher states of awareness—our angel nature. That is the terrain that tantra in the East and sex magick in the West have always explored—the notion that peak states don't need to be focused on transcending the body through denial and asceticism. In fact, the path to transcendence can begin in the most immanent place of all—our bodies.

If you scratch beneath the surface of most mystical traditions around the world, sooner or later you'll find some form of sexual yoga. Closely guarded. Often persecuted. Slandered and distorted beyond recognition by those on the outside peeking in. But there, nonetheless. "The ghostly imprint of sacred sex can still be discerned in every mainstream religion today," psychologist Jenny Wade writes in *Transcendent Sex*. "It can't be eradicated from the pool of human experience, and it keeps popping up randomly and irrepressibly."

Ranging from Shaiva Tantra in India, to Vajrayana Buddhism in Tibet, all the way to the mystic celibacy of the Cathars and the scandalous rites of the Templars and the Masons, these practices hold some of the most powerful techniques of ecstasy ever discovered. But, as with most religious traditions, they came bundled with mythologies, superstitions, and arcane terminology. Which you might expect from secret sects practicing secret sex.

Until fairly recently, no one had tried to separate the functional protocols—the actual, evidence-based mechanism of action—from the hand-me-down explanations of eroto-mystic practice. But that has changed in the past half century and has given rise to an entirely new field. Combining neuroscience and optimal psychology, it seeks to strip out the shame, guilt, and taboo that surround so much of our sexuality, and revisit this central driver of life with fresh eyes, open minds, and evidence.

Welcome to the era of Hedonic Engineering.

The Hedonic Engineers

Hedonic Engineering—The human nervous system studying and improving itself: intelligence studying and improving intelligence. Why be depressed, dumb, and agitated when you can be happy, smart, and tranquil?

—Robert Anton Wilson

Way back in 1953, University of Pennsylvania neuroscientist John Lilly began researching pleasure in primates. He wanted to see what lit up our brains and minds. To explore these previously hidden realms, he tapped specially designed steel sleeves into the skulls of rhesus monkeys. Once those guides were located over certain regions of the brain, Lilly would then push in thin wires to stimulate different parts of the nervous system. While he found that primates are hardwired to seek out pleasure, their overwhelming favorite was the experience of orgasm. Given the choice, male monkeys would self-stimulate orgasm until exhaustion. Pass out. Wake up. Do it all over again. Predictable. But now proven.

With all that careful probing, Lilly noticed something else: Orgasm, erection, and ejaculation—almost always thought of as a bundled hat trick of responses—were each actually discrete neurological

processes. You could have any one of them without the other two involved. The more Lilly explored the primate nervous system, the more
he came to an overarching conclusion: Our ecstatic reward circuitry
maps one to one with our sexual arousal network. "Sexual urges," a
Kinsey Institute researcher explained recently, "are built on the basic
brain architecture that underlies all emotions and motivated behaviors, from anger to joy."

All of those feel-good neurochemicals that we've been discussing,
from dopamine and endorphins, to endocannabinoids and oxytocin,
are directly triggered by sexual stimulation. And while a finding like
that might have seemed scandalous in the buttoned-down '50s when
Lilly first floated it, it's little more than common sense today.

After all, nature is efficient. Our mouths let us chew food and
breathe. Our noses filter air and decode smells. Even our genitals let
us both pee and procreate. So it makes sense that, as evolution wired
us up to make babies, it would lay that reward circuitry into the foundational level of our nervous system. Since Job #1 was getting it on,
everything else we find enjoyable got built on top of that bedrock.

The same year that Lilly published his findings, Albert Kinsey
of the University of Indiana released the second of what came to be
known as "the Kinsey Reports"—exhaustive observational studies on
human sexuality. By actually watching people while they had solo or
partner sex, Kinsey and his colleagues established a six-point "Kinsey
Scale" for sexual orientation. It dismantled the obvious binaries of
hetero- and homosexuality into a more nuanced (and realistic) gradi-
ent. He debunked Freud's theory that clitoral orgasms were immature
compared to "real" vaginal orgasms, and a host of other misconceptions. Those reports helped spark the sexual revolution of the 1960s,
drawing praise and blame in equal measure.

Hot on Kinsey's heels, Virginia Masters and William Johnson
set up their own sexuality study at Washington University in Saint
Louis. There, they observed prostitutes and couples engaging in sexual acts and mapped an enduring framework—their four-stage model
of sexual arousal—excitement, plateau, orgasm, and resolution. They
also studied a range of sexual dysfunctions, shedding new light on

issues from premature ejaculation to women's anorgasmia to geriatric sex.

Along with Kinsey's, their work came under fire for projecting social morals onto homosexuality and women's pleasure, and over-relying on sex workers as study subjects. But between them, their curious, courageous observational studies did more to advance our understanding of the human sexual response than anything in the modern era.

Kinsey, Masters, and Johnson all found their research methods and personal lives scrutinized. Like the first wave of psychedelic studies in the early 1960s, sex research experienced a fierce backlash. Their provocative findings filtered out into the mainstream and started shaping sexual behavior. Not everyone cheered.

Despite the controversy and pushback, those were the briefest of glory days for sex ed in the United States. There have been a couple of spikes of interest since—the AIDS/HIV epidemic grudgingly forced money and attention to sexuality as a public health issue. The blockbuster drug Viagra so thoroughly reshaped the sexual landscape that many pharmacology studies found funding, just to discover the next billion-dollar pill.

But since then, an increasingly focused and sophisticated alliance of religious conservatives and anti-porn activists have targeted federal funding, pressured universities and research institutions, and put a withering spotlight on the study of human sexual response. "That's one area where there's been a big influence on what can be studied and what data can be disseminated," says Beverly Whipple, PhD, a Rutgers University psychobiologist and a legend in the field. "That's been somewhat of a stymie to people doing sexuality education research."

Researchers can't even put the word "sex" or "orgasm" in their funding proposals, or an overzealous politician finds them via key word searches and gets their grants blocked. "Program officers at the National Institutes of Health instruct you not to include the word 'sexual' in any of your grant applications," one Kinsey researcher admits. "Apparently, congressional aides run regular searches of funding databases to look for studies they can make examples of, and 'sexual' is one of the words they search."

"On every ground, it's a triumph of ideology over reality," leading social psychologist Elaine Hatfield told the American Psychological Association. "It's like a throwback to the fifteenth century."

Despite a near-constant barrage of hypersexualized imagery in movies, media, and marketing, actual sex research in America is a dying profession. In 2014, the last of the Kinsey Institute's psycho-physiologists resigned to take a position in Belgium, where they are free to study what they want. Other leading scientists have decamped for Canada and Australia. As it stands, only two U.S. labs are still federally funded to study sexual arousal. Research on the most central human experience—one responsible for our very existence—has been marginalized almost out of existence.

The Sisters Kinsey

This lockout of institutional funding and support has pushed the next generation of Kinsey Institute researchers out of academia. They've had to take their study of people's privates private. And for at least two Kinsey alums, Drs. Helen Fisher and Nicole Prause, their passion projects have offered new insight into the relationship between biology, psychology, and healing.

Helen Fisher, a Kinsey Institute senior research fellow and professor at Rutgers, took a position with the dating service Match.com as their chief scientist. With their ample funding and massive database, she pioneered a new personality profile to compete with the standard Big Five trait test.

Close to twenty million people have now taken the Fisher Temperament Inventory (FTI), making it one of the largest statistically validated tests of its kind. It's also the only widespread personality test with a neuroscientific foundation. The well-known Myers-Briggs Type Indicator personality test (MBTI), in comparison, was invented in the 1940s from whole cloth by a homemaker who happened to be really into Carl Jung. Despite its mass adoption and popularity, the MBTI and most other personality quizzes have little science to back them up.

The Fisher Temperament Inventory breaks down personality types into four categories based on which neurochemicals drive a person's sexual and romantic attachments. The **Explorer**: the novelty-seeking adventurer who primarily expresses the traits linked with the dopamine system. The **Builder**: the cautious, socially compliant rule follower who primarily expresses the traits linked with the serotonin system. The **Director**: the analytical and rigorous thinker who primarily expresses the traits linked with the testosterone system. And the **Negotiator**: the pro-social empath who primarily expresses the traits linked with the estrogen system. Our most intimate and personal of experiences—falling in love—might have as much to do with our neurochemistry and neuroanatomy as Cupid's skills with a bow.

There are reasonable criticisms of Fisher's test. Psychologists question the reductionist hypothesis that personality expression can be explained by singular neurochemicals. "There is no 'sex' center in the brain," a colleague of Fisher's notes, "so we will never be able to really 'control' your sexuality." People, they insist, aren't automatons and any explanation of how and why we do what we do cannot be reduced to a mechanistic explanation.

But other studies are finding positive corroboration with the FTI's neurochemical model, "ranging from religiosity, political orientation, and attitudes about sex in a relationship." It seems that the way we fall in love informs the way we live the rest of our lives too.

While this kind of integrated neuropsychology is still in its infancy, the premise that how we feel is strongly informed by the hormones and chemicals surrounding our sexuality is unlikely to go away. It's the Horned Ape hypothesis of consciousness, compressed from thousands of generations into our own lifetimes. From Jared Diamond to Helen Fisher in a hop, skip, and a hump.

If Fisher's work seems overly deterministic—giving an outsize role to neurochemicals in the formation of love and attachment—we can reverse the inquiry and see if pharmaceuticals can actually generate love itself. If both natural and chemical methods work similarly, then their shared mechanism of action seems more valid. "The time to think through such questions is now," write Julian Savulescu and Brian Earp, ethicists at Oxford and Yale Universities, in *Love Drugs: The Chemical Future of Relationships*. "Biochemical interventions into love and relationships are not some far-off speculation."

Fortunately there is some parallel research exploring how pharmacology can shape our psychology that can serve as a helpful test case. For thirty years, the Multidisciplinary Association for Psychedelic Studies (MAPS) has been advancing clinical studies using the chemical MDMA in conjunction with therapy for sufferers of PTSD. Their results have been so significant that the FDA has fast-tracked the Phase III trials, earmarking this approach as an essential therapy for people suffering from trauma. Interestingly, what makes MDMA work so well for therapy are the same neurochemicals that Fisher tracked for romance.

Within an hour of onset of MDMA, serotonin levels rise considerably, boosting mood and heightening perception. Oxytocin follows, reducing fear and stress and increasing trust and connectivity. Therapists suggest that the calming effect of these neurochemicals allows them to bond with patients and encourage them to revisit and rewrite traumatic memories from a more resilient state.

Soon after, MAPS researchers explain, prolactin is released in the patient's brain, "contributing to a post-orgasmic sense of relaxation and receptivity." The neurocircuitry of PTSD is shut down. Hypervigilant amygdalas and ventromedial prefrontal cortices reset and patients who have been tormented for months or years by traumatic memories get to rewrite their pasts from a safer and more expansive present.

"One man who had been sexually abused as a child," clinicians wrote, "told us that he had spent his adult life observing that other people were having an experience that he presumed must be what they called 'happiness'—something he had not experienced and had always assumed he was incapable of experiencing. By shifting his neurochemistry he gained access to a range of feeling that had been inaccessible since his abuse."

A female subject said: "I feel like I'm walking in a place [of safety and happiness] I've needed to go for so long and just didn't know how to get there. . . . I've been through some bad stuff, but . . . those are things that happened to me, not who I am."

She was more right than she knew. MDMA prompted the specific blend of serotonin, oxytocin, and prolactin in her brain that allowed her to emotionally get to the place she "needed to go for so long and just didn't know how to get there." But she also intuited, "This is me . . . this is *in* me."

It's not just her. "The medicine" is in all of us. We don't even need external compounds to experience these feelings. We just need to re-learn how to make love to experience more of it.

Last year Rick Doblin, the founder of MAPS, and I were speaking on a panel and I asked him about this dynamic—about how their research into trauma could be extended to other interventions. "You know," he said, "from our research mapping patients' state in MDMA therapy, the closest analogue we can find, with those high serotonin, oxytocin, and prolactin levels, along with the feelings of safety, connection, and openness, is the postorgasmic state."

I was surprised by what he'd just said.

Option 1: Take thirty years and tens of millions of dollars to navigate a Byzantine federal process to decriminalize a Schedule I drug. Powerful and important work, but slow, costly, and subject to marginalization.

Or

Option 2: Pioneer some utterly novel, groundbreaking way to get people to that exalted state known only to scientists as "postorgasmic," and do the work from there.

* * *

Another Kinsey Institute alum, Dr. Nicole Prause, has taken up that exact question—how to boost health and well-being by replacing prescription drugs with orgasm. Prause was an early prodigy, earning her doctorate at the University of Indiana and Kinsey Institute and doing her postdoc work at Harvard. She worked at the Veterans

Administration and then landed a research position at UCLA. There, her unapologetic interest in bringing data-driven science to the most taboo of topics ran into political and social reality.

"I had been an academic for nearly ten years and just promoted to an Associate Scientist at the University of California, Los Angeles," she told an interviewer. "In one year, I was unable to get a simple orgasm protocol through the ethics review process (the same protocol passed through another university easily), then the university refused to accept a grant that I had received to study sexual partners in the laboratory. It became clear that I was either going to have to move to Canada, as most of my colleagues had, or get the research done under a completely new model. I chose the latter."

So she founded Liberos, a private research and biotech company funded by foundation and federal grants. There she and other researchers are free to focus on studying orgasmic response and the role smart technologies like magnetic and electrical brain stimulation can play in sexual health.

But it hasn't been a seamless transition from the public university to the private laboratory. With every new project Prause has faced resistance to clearheaded inquiry into the subject matter, and not just from politicians and activists (although there's been plenty of both). Sometimes it's from colleagues in the field.

"The biggest misconception about sex is that using sex to feel better is unhealthy," Prause explains. "This view is widely promoted even by therapists. They are quick to shame patients who, for example, masturbate after a tough day at work, as having 'poor coping.' Relatedly, partners often shame one another for seeking sexual activity for a health purpose like managing stress. . . . *Shaming the use of sex for coping is an extremely harmful and regressive attitude not different than religious 'sex only for procreation' wrapped in a new banner of 'health'*" [emphasis added].

In one study, Prause is looking to measure the health benefits of orgasm. Ultimately, her goal is to validate orgasm-as-prescription like a pharmaceutical, for a spectrum of conditions ranging from sleeplessness to anxiety and depression. Her approach looks to mimic MAPS's

efforts with MDMA. But rather than taking a drug to prompt healing, she's figuring out how to trigger our own natural chemistry to
provide similar benefit.

"We have strong evidence that sex (whether masturbation, watching adult films, or having sex with your partner) is an excellent
method of improving mood, can be a primary method of coping,
and can be engaged in on a regular basis," she says. "If we understand
direct manual genital stimulation makes this happen in your brain,
maybe we can find out it works in some way to help depression. It
might not have the same effect as antidepressant medication, it might
not be as strong, but maybe we've found that it's been able to sustain
people who had to come off of meds because [insurance stops and]
they can't pay for them anymore."

It's not just helpful for emotional disorders. Orgasm also eases
physical suffering. The combination of natural opioids in our system,
plus endocannabinoids (responsible for the famous "runner's high"
where pain and exhaustion give way to energized euphoria), all serve
to alleviate persistent discomfort. "One of the best things for chronic
pain disorders is regular exercise," Prause notes. "But that's a very
hard sell for someone who's hurting. What if I could tell them to try
regular masturbation?"

A recurring theme in our exploration of human sexuality is that the
same experiences that can lift us out of our lowest lows can also provide
glimpses of our highest highs. Catharsis—or the deep alleviation of
suffering, often goes hand in hand with ecstasis—the peak experience.
Anything that can provide the former quite often does so via the latter.

In another study run by colleagues of Prause, researchers specifically wanted to know if orgasm not only could lessen mental and
physical pain but could deliver glimpses of the ineffable—of mystical
experience. And they wanted to see how it compared to the current
leading candidate for epiphany-on-tap, psilocybin (the active ingredient in the "magic mushrooms" that Terence McKenna was so bullish
about).

Because these researchers wanted to make the comparison as close to
"apples to apples" as possible, they turned to Johns Hopkins University

psychedelic pioneer Roland Griffiths. Griffiths's lab had developed a thirty-question survey known as the Mystical Experience Question-naire (MEQ30) to deploy for test subjects undergoing psilocybin ther-apies. This is the scale he used to validate the famous Good Friday Experiment, confirming that mystical religious experience was indis-tinguishable from psychedelic states.

When subjects at Hopkins were given moderate dosages of psi-locybin it successfully treated nicotine addiction, treatment-resistant depression, and end-of-life anxiety. All three of these conditions are notoriously hard to address using mainstream methods. Across a num-ber of groups, subjects also reported their sessions as "the most mean-ingful experience of my life" (20 percent of respondents) and for a whopping 60 percent of patients as "one of the top five most mean-ingful experiences" of their lives.

In ways that the researchers are still trying to tease apart, those mystical experiences appeared to play a direct role in the healing ef-fects of the sessions. Address the underlying issues, and chronic symp-toms often resolve on their own. That's the interlocking relationship between ecstasis and catharsis.

The study of women's orgasm looked to see if fifteen minutes of manual clitoral stimulation could deliver a similar boost in mood, shifts in time perception, ineffability, and sacredness as the psilocybin stud-ies. They took eight hundred participants of varying ages, ethnici-ties, and gender conducting the fifteen-minute practice, and surveyed them afterward with the MEQ30.

The study revealed three interesting results:

First, "These findings suggest that [clitoral stimulation] can trigger a substantial mystical experience, *comparable in strength to a moderate dose of psilocybin*," the researchers wrote in their findings.

Second, "The proportion of participants who reported a complete mystical experience *was slightly higher than that found by the maximum dose of psilocybin* administered in Griffiths and colleagues' 2011 study (62 percent vs. 56 percent)."

And third, "While both partners reported moderate to strong mys-tical experiences, *women reported a stronger response than men*."

Psychedelics have alternately been praised, then villainized, and most recently rehabilitated as a powerful tool for psychological growth and healing. Compared to other classes of medicine, they stand out by leaps and bounds for their efficacy. But they're tricky to manage, still tightly restricted, and have unpredictable side effects.

Simple, "no frills" stimulation of a woman's clitoris—no candles and incense, no chanting, no Enya or John Legend on the stereo—is potent enough to deliver "substantial mystical experience" comparable to those substances. In fact, in a head-to-head matchup between the maximum dose of psilocybin that the Hopkins team administered and the orgasm protocol, simple sexual stimulation prompted more mystical states by over 6 percent.

This has meaningful implications for the rest of us. Mystical states, arguably one of the essential yearnings of humans throughout history, and now proven to have a strong correlation with well-being, healing, and existential equanimity, are attainable through one of the most accessible, inexpensive, low-tech methodologies available. No tracking the deserts of Sonora to find a toad to lick, no traipsing through the Himalayas looking for a sadhu to follow, just the simple act that brought us all here in the first place. Practiced purposefully, with an intent not to procreate but to integrate.

And it doesn't even require special skills or esoteric practices to get there. In *Transcendent Sex: When Lovemaking Opens the Veil*, a study of nearly one hundred subjects who had self-reported powerful mystical experiences during sexual encounters, Jenny Wade explicitly sought out "naive practitioners." That means regular folks who weren't deploying some tantric techniques to intensify their experience. She found that "probably one in twenty people have had a spontaneous transcendent episode during sex." If those numbers hold up across geographies and cultures, that would amount to nearly *half a billion people worldwide* having had a breakthrough experience of awe, ineffability, and oneness through the accidental and intuitive exploration of their own bodies.

Finally, this study delivered proof of what Yeshe Tsogyal so fearlessly demonstrated over a thousand years ago in the mountains of Tibet.

That women *are* smarter. And possibly more enlightened. Women appear to be even better suited to experience transcendence through sex than men. Padmasambhava said that "*if [a tantrika] develops the mind bent on enlightenment the woman's body is better.*"

It's taken a while, but the science has finally caught up.

Garden of Earthly Delights

A few years ago, I was invited to brief the U.S. Naval Special Warfare Development Group (officially known as DEVGRU, but since 2011, when famously loose-lipped then Vice President Joe Biden outed them—SEAL Team 6). I was conflicted about what to share. On the one hand, I'd grown up around the naval community and had a ton of respect for the caliber and competence of these Tier One special operators.

And on the other hand, these guys' lethality was decoupled from their morality. The mandate to disobey "unlawful orders" is insufficient compared to the juggernaut that is U.S. military capacity. They were at the whim of a commander in chief who told them who the "terrorists" were that needed to be taken out.

So after briefing the team on the neuroscience of group flow states and peak performance, I turned to the final part of the presentation: *The Ethics of Weaponizing Consciousness*. It felt like important grounding for the use of these powerful tools.

Unsure how far back these Gen Y super soldiers' memories went, I recapped a little of the United States' questionable involvement in clandestine psyops projects like MK-ULTRA and COINTELPRO in the 1960s and '70s. Then I briefed them on a different, lesser-known operation.

High up in a mountain hideout in the Qazvin Province of Iran, a Shia Muslim warlord was training fighters for suicide missions. He was using highly effective methods of indoctrination and brainwashing to create utterly loyal, fanatical soldiers who could penetrate almost any defense and target key officials for assassination. With no regard for their own survival, their reach was almost unlimited—they had successfully inserted operatives in power centers of the region and taken out dozens of key officials. And in the battle for "hearts and minds," they had seized the psychological edge that all terrorists strive for—they instilled irrational fear in their enemies.

As I opened this description, I could see the room tighten. These twentysomething special operators, who'd been casually lounging like young lions after a kill, sat up, eyes trained on me. If this was bin Laden's successor, or a new ISIS commander, they wanted to know everything about him.

But Hassan-i Sabbah, the warlord of the Shia Nizari Isma'ili sect we were discussing, wasn't going to be in their crosshairs anytime soon, no matter how hard they searched for him. He was a ghost. A cipher. Untouchable. Inscrutable. Plus, he'd been dead for a thousand years.

Hassan, or the Old Man of the Mountain, as he was known, was one of the first historically documented masters of Hedonic Engineering. Marco Polo wrote about him, as did Dante, and Nietzsche, who called his warrior clan "free spirits, par excellence." The Beat writer William Burroughs offered lines of reflection on these infamous operatives. The film *The Manchurian Candidate* immortalized the idea of a "sleeper agent" programmed for assassination inspired by this legend. The blockbuster video game series *Assassin's Creed* situates its origin story there too, at the Castle of Alamut—Hassan's mountain stronghold.

In short, there's far more imagined about the Assassins (as they came to be called) than is known for certain. Even the origin of their name is disputed—some believe it sprang straight from "Hassan" while others insist it's a nod to the *Hashashin*—those smokers of hashish who became his soldiers. But his methods remain a fascinating case study in the power of manipulating bodies and brains to control hearts and minds.

Candidates for the Order were brought in pairs to the castle and invited to dine with Hassan himself. Hassan would tell them that he had the power to deliver them to Paradise, but only if they pledged undying loyalty to him. Slipped into their meal was a time-release capsule containing opium, which sent them into a dreamy half-slumber. Servants would then carry the initiates into a beautiful walled Garden of Earthly Delights filled with exotic animals from far-flung corners of the world, and flowers and fruit trees like oranges, called "paradise apples." It would have seemed utterly fantastical to rural Persian boys.

Then the capsule would release ephedra (a prolific bush throughout the Middle East that is the raw ingredient for amphetamine) and hashish, reviving the candidates and adding a shimmering glow to everything they saw. They looked around and reasonably concluded that they had been delivered to Heaven. Beautiful houris, divine virgins accompanying martyrs to paradise in Muslim legend—in reality, courtesans gleaned from the finest brothels of Cairo—would then surround the initiates, playing flutes, dancing, and playfully disrobing until they were naked.

Eventually, as Robert Anton Wilson recounts, "some fell at the candidate's feet and kissed his ankles; some kissed knees or thighs, one sucked raptly at his penis, others kissed the chest and arms and belly, a few kissed eyes and mouth and ears. And as he was smothered in this hashish-intensified avalanche of love, the lady working on his penis sucked and sucked and he climaxed in her mouth as softly and slowly and blissfully as a single snowflake falling."

Around that time, a second slug of opium would release into their bloodstream. They would drift back to sleep, until they were returned to Hassan's chambers. There they would be revived.

In one telling, Hassan buried one of his existing operatives up to his neck in the dirt floor in front of this throne, tricking the candidates into believing that he had the power to communicate with the dead. He sealed the illusion by beheading the unlucky volunteer and leaving his head on a pike for the initiates to see on their way out.

In another account, he would carefully interrogate the two initiates after their initiation to determine what they had learned and what was to be done next.

"Truly," the first exclaimed, "I have seen the glories of Heaven, as foretold in the Koran. I have no more doubts. I will trust Hassan-i Sabbah and love him and serve him."

"You are accepted for the Order of Assassin," said Hassan solemnly. "Go at once to the Green Room to meet your superior in the order."

When this candidate had left, Hassan turned to the second, asking, "And you?" "I have discovered the First Matter, the Medicine of Metals, the Elixir of Life, the Stone of the Philosophers, True Wisdom and Perfect Happiness," said he, quoting the alchemical formula. "And it is inside my own head!" Hassan-i Sabbah grinned broadly. "Welcome to the Order of the Illuminati!" he said, laughing.

And that bifurcation—between the candidate who pledged blind loyalty to Hassan in the hopes of being returned one day to Paradise, and the other, who recognized that "perfect happiness" resided in his own head and that he was the master of his own realization—is the difference between a brainwashed assassin and an illumined adept.

Because when it comes down to it, the psychotechnologies of mind control and alchemy are nearly identical. The only difference is that one erases sovereignty while the other enhances it. That's how dark psyops projects like MK-ULTRA coincided with the hippie Aquarian ideal of Turning On, Tuning In, and Dropping Out. It's how the infamous "Rolls-Royce guru" Osho managed to harness thousands of blissed-out sannyasins to build a city from scratch in the sagebrush of Oregon. It's how dopamine-looped social media algorithms, originally touted as tools to connect the world, have enslaved us, like silicon-chip slot-machined monkeys.

"Hassan-i Sabbah was not the first or last student of the ways in which sexuality can be transmuted into . . . rapture," Wilson acknowledges. "Further to the East, there were Tantric schools within Hinduism, Buddhism and Taoism, which taught techniques by which prolongation of the genital embrace could explode into dramatic brain change. In the West, underground cults of Gnostics, Illuminati, alchemists and witches kept similar techniques as closely guarded secrets, for if the Holy Inquisition ever learned of such practices the participants would be denounced as devil-worshippers and burned at the stake. . . . In our own time, there has been a revolutionary up-surge of these ancient neurological secrets, with an admixture of more modern techniques."

Hassan was one of the founding fathers of Hedonic Engineering (or at least, a Crazy Uncle you can still pick out in the old family photos), and his life and legacy are substantial. The simple idea that you can use sexuality, substances, music, dance, and awe to reformat consciousness is radical.

But as Robert Anton Wilson notes, it is also ubiquitous. Whether to liberate or enslave, Hedonic Engineering is arguably one of the most potent and least understood technologies ever developed. "Remember . . . remember," the Old Man of the Mountain whispered on his deathbed, *nothing is true, everything is permitted!*"

CHAPTER 11

An Immodest Proposal

I am not so violently bent upon my own opinion as to reject any offer, proposed by wise men, which shall be found equally innocent, cheap, easy, and effectual.

—Jonathan Swift, *A Modest Proposal*

The Celebrated Jumping Frog of Double Blind County

There's an old joke among biologists that goes something like this:

A researcher is experimenting on frogs to learn more about their athletic abilities.

He gives the frog on his lab bench the verbal command "Jump!"

The frog leaps ten inches across the table. The scientist whips out his tape measure and jots down the measurement in his notebook.

He then takes a scalpel and cuts off one of the frog's legs and repeats the command "Jump!"

The frog, a little worse for wear but still game, leaps 7.5 inches.

The scientist repeats his grim surgery three more times, lopping off a leg every round. Each time he gives the command to "Jump!" the frog's distance scores dwindle understandably.

Finally, the poor legless frog is just sitting there on the workbench. The researcher gives the command "Jump!" for the fifth and final time.

The frog doesn't move.

He repeats the command to "Jump!" twice more, to be sure. Finally, he opens his notebook and writes in careful pencil, "The four-legged frog displayed substantial jumping abilities, which was observed to decrease by approximately twenty-five percent with the loss of each limb. However, the most exciting finding to report is something totally unexpected—I have discovered that a frog with no legs . . . is deaf!"

And that's kind of where we are these days in the realm of experimental science: bending and distorting reality and common sense because our methods are often too clumsy to disclose the insights we're seeking. Time and again, we think we've come to a revolutionary new discovery, only to realize that how we conceived and ran our experiment has already shaped any outcomes we might find.

The Kitchen Sink Method

It's not that the double-blind method is broken, it's just that it's limited and not always the right tool for the job. Like the biologist and the jumping frog, it's best for tracking linear incremental change, but it breaks down when asked to make leaps of faith or logic.

But there is another method that does a much better job of tracking multivariable equations like the recipes from the Alchemist Cookbook. We'll call it the Kitchen Sink Method, or KSM for short. In the KSM, we don't isolate single factors at first. Instead, we do the exact opposite. We literally throw "everything but the kitchen sink" at the problem. We combine anything that has an evidence-based rationale for impact until we absolutely, positively get the result we're looking for. Blow yourself sky high, in other words, then go back to the lab to figure out what put the might in your dynamite.

With the desired outcome established and repeatable, we can work backward to figure out which elements were "nice to have" vs. which ones are "have to have." We can back off a variable at a time until we observe an undesired drop-off in results. Then we can tune the sweet spot for an optimally shareable protocol, confident that we're including the full spectrum of treatment options without adding unnecessary bells and whistles, or cost and complexity.

This is especially helpful when we move from seeking single-pointed solutions like a pill or piece of technology to combined therapies that rely on a bunch of smaller effects to add up to big change. Any one of them in isolation wouldn't poke their heads above the waterline of the placebo effect, but together they do something almost magical—they work.

That's the Kitchen Sink Method in a nutshell. It won't replace double-blind placebo-controlled studies, but it might be a more helpful method for figuring out the nuances of how we heal and grow, in all of our baffling contradictions and complexity.

Hedonic Engineering Matrix

If you threw everything from the Alchemist Cookbook together willy-nilly, you'd get some pretty hairball combinations. We need some guidelines to understand what pairs with what for safest and greatest effect.

For the past ten years, in consultation with many of the academics and experts we've met in this book (and others profiled in its prequel, *Stealing Fire*), the organization I help lead studied the research on peak states. At first, we wanted to catalog the biggest levers in our bodies and brains that affect our experience—from the neurological to the endocrine, cardiac, pulmonary, kinetic, and psychological. If we could learn to tune each, from its simplest expression to its most complex, we hoped to learn how to shift our experiences along with them.

In other words, rather than waiting to accidentally become "enlightened" or a Six Sigma Blackbelt or whatever superlative we're shooting for, why not adjust the settings of our bodies and brains first, and then see how life looks and feels like from there?

Instead of spending years trying to imitate wise old Tibetan monks, for example, never sure what was true mysticism versus mere mannerism, we could actually learn what makes them tick from the inside out. If we did, we might notice that these contemplatives consistently display lower respiratory rates, more relaxed alpha-wave EEGs, and higher vagal nerve tone than your average citizen (among a host of other biological and psychological markers). You could then take a regular person, put them into that same physical state, and see if they feel a little more resilient and compassionate. It's a pretty straightforward approach to human development that swaps out psychological rumination for physiological recalibration.

It also spares us the endless and largely frustrating search for accidental peak experiences. If we don't know what got us there the last time, it's much harder to re-create it the next time. People waste years of their lives rolling and re-rolling those dice. Rather than waiting for lightning to strike, we can build our own Tesla coil. We can tune the knobs and levers of our bodies and brains to trigger flashes of illumination. That's what reverse-engineering offers.

Unavoidably, the chart below isn't quite right. There's no way to compress the interwoven complexities of the human experience into a

Flow Genome Matrix	PRE-CONVENTIONAL	CONVENTIONAL	POST-CONVENTIONAL	INTEGRATED
Neuro-Electrical	Delta	Beta	Alpha	Theta/Gamma/Elective
Neuro-Anotomical	Amygdala	Prefrontal Cortex	Transient Hypofrontal	Global/Elective
Cardiac	Catabolic ◄——————————————————► Anabolic			
Endocrine	Cortisol/Epinepherine	Testosterone/Estrogen	Endorphins/Dopamine	Anandamide/Tryptamines
Postural	Frontal	Saggital	Transverse	Poly-axial
Respiratory	Parasympathetic	Thoracic	Abdominal	Dynamic
Psychological	N/A	Fixed	Growth	Self-Authoring
Temporal	Achronic (No time)	Diachronic (Linear)	Synchronic (Present)	Polychronic (Deep Now)
Vagal	Low ◄——————————————————► High			

21st Century Normal   HomeGrown Human

two-dimensional grid. But hopefully, it is *helpfully* wrong, and directionally accurate.

We can draw a few general conclusions, though. "Twenty-first-century normal" lives on the left-hand side of this graph, where we spend much of our time tired, wired, and stressed. That's the always-on of agitated beta-wave thinking with the steady drip of stress chemicals like norepinephrine and cortisol, poor air exchange in our lungs, low vagal nerve tone, and a fixed psychological mindset that tries to defend our safety and identity in an uncertain world. Things get consistently healthier, happier, and more interesting on the right-hand side, where many of the capacities we've explored in Part Two of this book start coming online.

The game to play, then, if we find ourselves stuck on the left, is how to tune our dials more to the right. There's no singular sweet spot to be in all the time, just like "balance" on a surfboard is an ever-shifting target. But an ability to fluidly adjust our state to match our task is invaluable. Range, rebound, and resilience are the name of this game.

As helpful as mapping our lives this way can be, there's a limitation to this model: No instruction on how to actually shift our states from less to more resourceful. It's informational but not all that practical.

We need to build a map that takes those academic insights and converts them to protocols people can actually use—like ones based on the Alchemist Cookbook. Every time we read a study or learn of a new technology or practice that reliably impacts neurochemistry, physiology, or psychology for the better, we can add it to this new chart. What results is a matrix mapping how to harness our deepest survival circuits in our bodies and brains for reproducible state-shifting transformation. Think of it like Build-a-Buzz Bingo.

Once we step back from all the research, we're in for a bit of a come-to-Jesus moment. Any way you slice it, this map has implications. If you're open-minded and sincere in your pursuit of the most effective protocols for healing humans, you end up in one of two places: sexy biohacking or nerdy kink. Neither of which is exactly our wheelhouse.

Hedonic Engineering	MILD	MEDIUM	SPICY
Nitric Oxide	Dietary (Beets, Pumpkin Seeds, etc.)	Supplements	ED Drugs
Vagal Nerve Tone	Throat Massage/Vocalization	Oral/Anal Stim/Plugs	Medical Device Stim
Endorphins/Dopamine	Sensation Play	Clamps	BDSM
Oxytocin	Kissing/Cuddling/Eye Gazing	Nipple Suction	Nasal Spray
Testosterone	Ice Bathing, Weight Lifting	DHEA	Gel/Intramuscular Supplementation
Psychoactives	CBD, THC	Nitroxygen, Ketamine, Carbogen	GHB, MDMA, 2CB*
Trauma Therapy	Biographical	Gender/Archetypal	Transpersonal
Respiration	Synchronized	Hyper-Ventilatory	Gas-Assisted Apnea

*Schedule I - Currently under no clinical studies "but" its inventor Alexander Shulgin ranked it as his favorite erotic psychedelic

Beyond the few pioneers of hedonic engineering that we've already mentioned, like John Lilly, Helen Fisher, and Nicole Prause, this is largely uncharted ground, littered with land mines. If you dig a bit deeper, you can decode signs of similar practices in the ethnographic literature, from Hindu tantrikas to Western sex magick.

But if you look to contemporary culture for examples of this kind of combinatory experimentation, you mostly find unreconstructed hedonism—bachelor and bachelorette parties in Vegas, underground dungeons in San Francisco, club scenes in Ibiza and Miami.

A couple of the most relevant examples to address: there can be powerful therapeutic value to intense physical sensation and pleasurable pain, as we explored with the 9/11 firefighters and their connection to the BDSM community. That's often been coupled to story lines that may seem off-putting to some. Leather and latex. Endless shades of gray. It's understandably not everyone's jam. But cultivating a full range of sensory integration can be.

If you survey catalogs for occupational therapists who work with sensory integration disorders, you'll see implements ranging from feathers to pinwheels, compression blankets, restraints, and blindfolds— the same assortment you might find in a sex-positive store. It's just different communities of practice surrounding it.

Now more than ever we need effective ways to discharge our

trauma and counterbalance our disembodied lives. We can leverage therapeutic sensation to help rewire our nervous systems and provide profound shifts in state. It's possible to provide these experiences for each other without resorting to demeaning or debasing narratives that have often come bundled with them. We can take the kink out of kinky (you can always put it back in later).

Another powerful taboo to negotiate is the notion of combining substances and sexuality. While that might bring up tawdry notions of "chemsex" (typically amphetamines, cocaine, and GHB popularized by the gay sex-party scene), the reality is we're all practicing chemsex already. We're just doing it badly.

Take three of the most common substances we consume—alcohol, hormonal birth control, and antidepressants. They are impacting our sex lives every day, rarely for the better. Despite its disinhibiting effects, alcohol is a dehydrating, disorienting depressant that dulls a woman's orgasmic response, and as Dr. Ruth loved to warn, "hangs right off the end of a man's penis!" Women on the Pill "scored lower on measures of sexual satisfaction and partner attraction," Yale's Brian Earp notes, "and were more likely to initiate separation. SSRIs can directly suppress activity in pathways for dopamine and norepinephrine, neurotransmitters that are involved in . . . romantic love." We take all of these distortions as normal and rarely think we could change them, despite their crippling effects on our experience and relationships.

It's not the chemsex that's the problem. It's which chems, and what sex. We need better options for both. As Earp and his coauthor, Julian Savulescu, write in *Love Drugs: The Chemical Future of Relationships,* "society should seriously consider the prospect of complementing psychosocial interventions [like marriage counseling] with interventions into love's biological side. To ignore this latter dimension is to obscure a crucial aspect of the ties that bind, and we ignore it at our peril."

So what to do about the implication of this research? Share it, and you run the risk of enabling hedonists, shocking conformists, and outraging purists. Don't share it, and you run the risk of sitting on information that might ease suffering and boost meaning in a world that needs both. This chapter is an attempt to snip all of the wires to that bomb. If it blows up in our face, it's not because we didn't try.

Cooking with Gas

We already know that any one of the interventions we've explored in Part Two are sufficient to prompt state shifts, healing, and connection. Breath work works. So does body work. Music. Substances. Sex. Pick any one of these paths, and they can lead to insight, integration, and bonding. "Enlightenment," the old Buddhist saying goes, "is *any path* pursued to its completion!"

We don't have to use them all. With enough time, money, and cutting-edge equipment, you can pretty much get to wherever you want to go—but cost and access become real issues. Not everyone has a biohacking researcher on speed-dial or access to six- and seven-figure medical devices. As hundreds of studies have proven, the longest levers to shift our neurophysiology, and with it our psychology, lie at the intersection of our ecstatic and erotic neural circuitry, and they are freely available to all of us. That's critical if we want to develop tools that are widely available around the world, regardless of privilege and access.

Here's what else we know: Once we've assembled all the ingredients, we can cook up whatever we want. If any particular intervention goes against moral, legal, or cultural norms that are important to you, *just skip that option.* All you will need to do to compensate is increase the intensity or duration of the remaining methods you do choose.

We're in charge of how we approach the body of knowledge in the Alchemist Cookbook. There are hundreds of recipes we can create. And we can break them down into three buckets:

Solo practices that can be done by anyone anywhere. Think breath work combined with body work and music.

Partner practices that either require a spotter for safety and comfort, or need another set of arms and legs to accomplish. Think partner yoga or massage.

Couple practices that may build on any solo or partner practice but include some component of emotional or physical intimacy/vulnerability best explored within a dedicated relational commitment. Think deep psychosexual work. Friends with (medical) benefits.

In sum, there are lots of newfangled ways to make more love in our lives, but if we want the least expensive, most effective, and most reliable methods, the oldest and simplest methods are often the best. Hedonic engineering. A deliberate set of neurophysiological practices designed to combine peak experiences in service of healing, integration, and connection.

* * *

To test these findings, we used the Kitchen Sink Method to design a twelve-week study. That means we opted to try a full combination of all Big Five disciplines together. There's ample research on each of these levers, but there's virtually none on how they work together. That's the biggest blank spot on the experimental map, and what we wanted to explore. So we came up with a flexible menu of activities for study subjects to choose from the Hedonic Engineering Matrix above.

Because roughly half of the interventions in the Hedonic Engineering Matrix have to do with physical intimacy and because there are so many issues surrounding the safety and ethics of that kind of practice (therapeutic sexual surrogacy, for example, remains in the legal gray zone in the United States), for this study we opted to select for consenting adult partners who were already in intimate relationships.

We accepted twelve couples who'd expressed interest in this research and who had enough stability and focus to successfully complete a three-month longitudinal study. Length of relationship ranged from two to thirty years. While we attempted to represent a variety of experiences and backgrounds, our first criterion was relational and emotional stability. Gender, religion, relational format, and ethnicity are better represented in this cohort than economic background, which tended to skew toward the WEIRD (western, educated, industrial, rich, and democratic).

Couples who elected to pursue more intensive use of pharmaceutical compounds did so under the guidance of their own overseeing physicians who were able to make off-label prescriptions of the relevant substances. (See the appendix for description of C³ physician oversight—Curious, Courageous, and Connected.) While we outlined the baseline protocols that subjects could follow, we left room for self-directed experimentation.

Partners were encouraged to explore and experiment within the Hedonic Engineering Matrix, selecting from Mild, Medium, and Spicy options, with an encouragement to "start low and go slow." They were then free to add additional intensity and complexity only after comfortably integrating prior practices. This approach is the opposite of a conventional study, which seeks to rigidly control for variables. By imposing minimal scaffolding, we were trying to support individual and collective exploration and innovation within boundaries.

An unexpectedly interesting finding was the self-organizing innovation that arose within the study cohort. Instead of sharing specific instructions, we dumped out a bunch of Lego blocks (in the form of the Hedonic Engineering Matrix and default practice schedule), showed how they can snap together in different configurations, and left a few potential recipes around to inspire creativity. That was the "liberating structure" of this experiment.

Over the course of those three months, couples continued to modify and innovate the beginnings of what can perhaps best be described as a Sexual Yoga of Becoming.

The Sexual Yoga of Becoming: An Experiment

While specific details vary tremendously, based on which levers you choose to throw and which tools you're comfortable deploying, the recipe for a Sexual Yoga of Becoming practice boils down to this:

Supersaturate your body and brain with endorphins, dopamine, nitric oxide, oxytocin, and serotonin.

Optimize your endocannabinoid system and boost vagal nerve tone.

Entrain your brain out of beta-wave executive functioning and into alpha and theta activity, with intentional spikes into gamma or deep dives into delta waves.

Reset your brain stem with cranial-nerve stimulation and/or selective exposure to molecules like nitrous oxide or ketamine.

Pulse energy, in the form of direct or alternating current, magnetism, light, sound waves, pain, or orgasm through your nervous system.

Engage and align spine, pelvis, limbs, and soft tissues for a full range of motion and proprioceptive integration and embodiment.

Breathe in deliberate patterns to upregulate or downregulate your nervous system by altering the ratios of oxygen, carbon dioxide, and nitrogen.

Play powerful music that syncopates and discombobulates your conscious thinking, and ideally inspires with lyrics that can serve as poetry/living scripture.

Take that ride. Don't flinch (or give in to astonishment). Remember what you forgot. Come home. Do your homework.

This set of basic protocols isn't set in stone. It doesn't come with taboos, superstitions, and prohibitions. It's the predictable assemblage of a lot of well-established neurophysiology. It amounts to experiential, experimental revelation.

* * *

Precisely because these experiences can be so discombobulating, we also wanted to track what we were doing. If this protocol wasn't helping people experience more peak states, healing, and connection—it probably wasn't worth the time or risks. So we identified a pair of objective metrics for each of those three categories–six in all. To better facilitate comparative analysis, we chose measurement tools that cross-reference to other studies in the field. This is no small point. If the nascent discipline of Hedonic Engineering stands a chance of addressing the Meaning crisis, we need objective, open-source research that can build on itself. Otherwise we'll remain stuck in the realm of unverifiable truth claims. Hopefully other academic and citizen scientists can use these initial baselines to advance their work.

We also included subjective self-reporting in the study, which while technically "anecdotal" would likely capture the experiences of the participants and provide context and color for the objective measures.

(For further detail, see the appendix for a summary of the study, metrics, profiles, and accounts of participants. For those interested in continuing this research, there's a solid framework to follow. And for anyone looking for the Easter eggs hidden in this book, there's a whole basket of them stashed in the back).

Insights and Reflections

After assessing the six metrics tracking ecstasis, catharsis, and communitas, over the three months of the study, it was clear that Hedonic Engineering can be a potentially effective tool for healing, peak experience, and relational connection. In the domain of communitas, or relational satisfaction, subjects experienced a meaningful uptick in their overall happiness and relational closeness. In the realm of catharsis or healing, people experienced a reduction in physical stress and residual psychological trauma. In the arena of ecstasis, or peak experience, couples reported an increase in daily peak states and meaningfully stronger mystical experiences than they had ever had.

Under the right conditions, Hedonic Engineering can outperform many more intensive or expensive interventions—including talk therapy and clinical psychedelic therapy. That in itself is a meaningful finding, and hopefully one that can help larger numbers of people mend trauma, reclaim purpose, and connect to those closest to them. More research needs to be done, but there is now at least a rubric to help focus and coordinate those efforts.

* * *

What is equally clear is that these methods don't work for everyone or all the time. As evidenced by non-completion, subsequent divorce, and self-reported struggles during the study, combining these methods into accelerated practice can make things worse before they get better.

Or, they can just make things worse. Calibrating the frequency and intensity of these protocols to match the psychology of participants, the cultural context of their experience, and their "constellation of care," i.e., the medical, psychological, and pastoral professionals in their orbit, is essential. Hedonic Engineering is deceptively strong medicine.

One couple documented their concern when dynamics around dependency showed up in their life. "Actually, we've kind of run into an issue that's pretty scary for us," one woman wrote. "I'm concerned this is becoming an addiction? . . . Once we started . . . combining with substances, it became something we started doing all the time—like our Sunday practice every day. We'd joke that I was like Charlotte in *Sex and the City* [where she gets a Rabbit vibrator and her friends have to stage an intervention]. But now I'm seriously having to question priorities and whether this is 'too much of a good thing'?"

There can definitely be too much of a good thing. Most of us are familiar with the concepts of physical and psychological addiction. In the former, you need to increase the dosage of a given substance or behavior to get similar results, and when you remove the high, you have physical withdrawal symptoms, ranging from nausea to organ failure. In the latter, you might develop an emotional dependence or

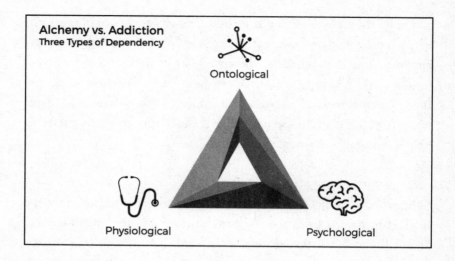

habituation, and when you remove the high you experience irritability, distractedness, or insomnia. Pushing all the buttons of our reward circuitry works better than most people imagine and can create reinforcement loops that can quickly become habitual.

But there is a third variation we should also consider in the field of Hedonic Engineering—ontological addiction. That is where the information or insights gleaned from a given set of practices prove so compelling that they override normal checks and balances. As some of the participants in the study noted, *"It was like looking at our life through a crystal ball"* and *"I was looking down on . . . this whole human experience from another dimension."* That's novel, potent, and potentially all-consuming.

In *Harry Potter and the Philosopher's Stone*, the young boy finds a magic mirror of Erised ("desire" spelled backward) that only reflects what someone yearns for most in the world. But the wizard Dumbledore cautions him: *"Men have wasted away before it, not knowing if what they have seen is real, or even possible. . . . It does not do to dwell on dreams and forget to live, remember that."* Hedonic Engineering polishes that magic mirror. If you're not careful, you can get blinded by the light.

When you intentionally hot-wire the full suite of evolutionary drivers, you may trigger stronger results than you intended. The only difference between a delightful flow state and a destructive compulsion is its positive or negative impact on one's life. Put bluntly, the only difference between an alchemist and an addict is the scoreboard.

If we're serious about providing ecstasis without the crave, and catharsis without the cringe, the final element of Hedonic Calendaring becomes essential—periodic abstinence. In the same way that mountaineers combat the pull of summit fever by agreeing on an ironclad turnaround time beforehand, we need to build into our annual hedonic calendars times where we go cold turkey, just to ensure we still can (go to www.recapturetherapture.com/tools for a full description of Hedonic Calendaring).

Lent, Ramadan, and Yom Kippur are traditional examples of ritualized abstinence. New Year/New You commitments and Sober October are more contemporary ones. For most practices, it's enough to have one month of each year serve as a period of abstention, where you can calibrate how sticky your habits have become. For the sort of full-spectrum sexual yoga explored in this study, we'd recommend adding one week per month to allow for quicker gut checks and course corrections.

It's helpful to think of Hedonic Engineering as NC-17 fifth-class rock climbing—definitely not for kids, and the falls can kill you. You wouldn't go wandering up a dangerous mountain without ropes, anchors, and harnesses. If you did, and you hurt yourself, you'd have no one to blame.

On the other hand, equip and train yourself, and venture humbly into consequential terrain with trustworthy guides and partners, and you'll be rewarded by the satisfaction of the ascent and the view from the top. It's precisely because it has risks that this experience is rewarding.

Once we understand the implications of the Alchemist Cookbook, we can tune our consciousness however we choose. We can access the numinous, discharge our trauma, and forge bonds that last a lifetime. To realize that the keys to our cage are also the keys to the Kingdom is a thrilling, if fearsome responsibility. But the gates swing wide open now. Our prison is unlocked. And so is the Garden.

PART III

Ethical Cult Building

But ye shall destroy their altars, break their
images, and cut down their groves.

—Book of Exodus (by way of Gary Snyder)

Mankind has *always* crucified and burned.

—Goethe

The only difference between a cult and a
religion is the amount of real estate they own.

—Frank Zappa

Part One, "Choose Your Own Apocalypse," surveyed the state of the world and the collapse in both Meaning 1.0 and Meaning 2.0. We established how critical it is for us to expand our perspectives, process our pain, and connect to each other to manage the road ahead.

Part Two, "The Alchemist Cookbook," explored five key drivers that give us the tools to wake up, grow up, and show up for ourselves—Meaning 3.0. In the last chapter we discussed a test case for what happens when we put all of these insights together, applying the tools of Hedonic Engineering to real lives and relationships.

But we're not done. The only reason we focused on intimate relationships in that study was the simple fact that evolution threw the kitchen sink at pair-bonding. There's no other relationship that we're more neurochemically incented to pull off. If we can't foster healing, inspiration, and connection at that level of relatedness, it only gets harder in larger numbers or under more challenging conditions. As Metcalfe's law reminds us, the complexity of a network goes up with the square of the number of nodes in it. Managing tight bonds across large numbers of people is exponentially harder—literally.

Regardless of our relational formats, it's essential for us to start small, go slowly, and forge intimate, deeply trusting connections with others as we find our way forward. Like climbers who commit to belay each other to the peak, we need to know that our travel partners have our backs, even and especially when we might be losing our grip.

Aristotle laid it out succinctly when he described the three most common forms of friendship—the transactional, the hedonistic, and the virtuous. The transactional bond is unapologetically mercenary—a quid pro quo where at least one member is only in it to get something they desire. The hedonistic relationship persists for as long as it's fun. When the party moves on, so do these friends. This kind of connection has become especially abundant as more people start playing with ecstatic technologies. The Party at the End of Time is attracting more than its fair share of gate crashers. Both angels and moths are drawn to the light.

In and of themselves, there is nothing inherently wrong with either transactional or hedonistic relationships. They only become problematic when it's not clear what kind of connection we have with each other and we start mixing and matching the euphoria of peak states and the vulnerability of deep healing.

The virtuous relationship is a much rarer and more valuable commitment. That's the hell or high water, in sickness and health, no one left behind kind of bond that is required to safely support each other through rough weather and challenging terrain. That's what it means to truly have each other "on belay."

"The first step in connectedness," Tyson Yunkaporta explains in his book *Sand Talk: How Indigenous Thinking Can Save the World*, "is forming pairs (like kinship pairs) with multiple other agents who also pair with others. The next step is creating or expanding networks of these connections. The final step is making sure these networks are interacting with the networks of other agents, both within your system and in others."

We need to take our duos and turn them into dozens, and take our dozens, and turn them into dozens of dozens. A flexible meshwork of HomeGrown Humans radiating across the world, doing the real work that needs to be done.

Combining peak experiences and deep healing into powerful connections has a chequered history, though. In fact, we're pretty bad at it. It's a rare community centered on these ideals that doesn't end up in one of three places: hedonization (the endless pursuit of pleasure), commodification (the selling of the sacred), or weaponization (the manipulation of these tools for personal or institutional gain).

So in Part Three, "Ethical Cult Building," we're going to tackle the final and possibly hardest problem of all—creating communitas without the cults. If we can pull that off in a way that is truly opensource, scalable, and anti-fragile, then we have a chance to bring these broader ideas to the world.

CHAPTER 12

Everybody Worships

You Ain't Frum Around Here, Are You?

Every year, on February 15, they do it again. The flag bearer carefully folds Old Glory so the stars are showing, and carries it toward the parade ground. GIs fall into line marching in step with their bayoneted rifles on their shoulders. The general, in his formal dress and sash, gives the order, and they raise the flag up the pole. The crowd cheers.

Then they wait.

But the guest of honor doesn't come. He never comes. They don't seem to mind.

They've been doing this for the better part of half a century, in the hopes that John Frum, a mythical U.S. infantryman, will return to their island of Vanuatu (an archipelago of islands in Melanesia in the South Pacific, recently made famous by the reality TV show *Survivor*).

No one is really sure who John was, but many think that during World War II, when the United States used the island nation as a staging base for Guadalcanal and other battles, so many soldiers introduced themselves as "John, from . . . Nebraska, or California, or Iowa" that eventually the name sort of made itself. John From. John *Frum*.

And that John, boy did he have a lot of cool stuff. A lot of it literally fell from the sky, pushed out the back of cargo planes, floating to earth by parachute. Canned goods, chewing gum, radios, medicine, washing machines, and motorbikes.

But in 1945, when the war ended, John picked up sticks and disappeared. And all of that magical cargo went with him. The locals were skilled in sympathetic magic and figured that if they could re-create the conditions that brought him in the first place, perhaps that would hasten his return. So they assembled bamboo rifles, painted uniforms on T-shirts, built full-size planes out of straw, lit tiki torches, cleared the jungle for a landing strip, and waited.

"John promised he'll bring planeloads and shiploads of cargo to us from America if we pray to him," a village elder recently told a journalist. "Radios, TVs, trucks, boats, watches, iceboxes, medicine, Coca-Cola, and many other wonderful things."

"Of course the cargo never comes," British anthropologist Peter Worsley noted. "The cults nonetheless live on. If the millennium does not arrive on schedule, then perhaps there is some failure in the magic, some error in the ritual. New breakaway groups organize around 'purer' faith and ritual. *The cult rarely disappears, so long as the social situation which brings it into being persists.*"

And the social situation that brings it into being is a group of people, torn between worlds, trying to make sense of life and a future worth hoping for. That intersection of the material world of cargo and the millenarian longing for redemption is a powerful one. While it's easy to dismiss John Frum's cargo cult as a goofy *Gilligan's Island* anachronism, the reality is, we're all cargo culters now. Waiting desperately for salvation, hopefully hoarding our talismans of transformation.

How many of us buy a fancy car, dreaming that it will attract a sexy mate or earn the admiration of our friends? Or wear a red shirt with a Swoosh so that we might take on the vitality of a Tiger, or slip on red-bottomed shoes so we might claim the swagger of a Cardi B?

And the Vanuatuans have a distinct advantage over the rest of us— the bamboo rifles and coconut tiki torches they need to work their magic literally grow on trees. The money we need to feed our cargo cults does not.

It's not just our fetish for magical material we share with those islanders. It's our urge to find and follow saviors, no matter how unlikely. "Everybody worships," David Foster Wallace acknowledged in his well-known essay "This Is Water." "The only choice we get is what to worship. And an outstanding reason for choosing some sort of God or spiritual-type thing to worship . . . is that pretty much anything else you worship will eat you alive."

Worship by Any Other Name

That's where we find ourselves in this conversation—figuring out what to worship, learning how to worship, and doing our level best not to get eaten alive. Because anytime you dip into the Alchemist Cookbook, anytime you uncork powerful experiences of ecstasis and catharsis, you tend to get boundary-dissolving, inhibition-lowering communitas hot on their heels.

If you don't watch out, that combination can get culty quickly. We succumb to magical thinking and give away our centers. We find ourselves led down the garden path by demagogues. We can't pretend those tendencies don't exist, either. It's time to reclaim our relationship to worship.

* * *

The original Latin word for "worship" is *cultus*. A traditional cult, as scholars of religion would term it, means a sect of practitioners oriented around shared beliefs and rituals. The Hindu goddess Kali had her cult, as did the Greek god Dionysus. The Eleusinian Mysteries were a cult. The Native American Church was a cult. For over three centuries before Emperor Constantine made it the state religion of Rome, Christianity was also a cult.

These historic cults asked members to submit to tradition, and to the lineage of hierophants (literally, "ministers of the sacred"). The vulnerability of an initiate was grounded and bounded by those who had come before them.

For thousands of years, these sorts of mystery cults flourished all around the world. Due to their intensive initiatory nature, they rarely grew to the kinds of numbers that more mainstream doctrines could. But they continued to pass on direct revelatory experience across generations of practitioners.

Then, in the nineteenth and twentieth centuries, travel shrank the world. As the power of Meaning 1.0 declined, some of those long-standing mystery cults jumped the tracks. Transplanted to a modernizing Western world thirsty for spiritual experiences, some leaders broke with tradition. Rather than situating themselves in a lineage, these gurus claimed "new covenants" that insisted theirs was an entirely original transmission, without precedent or deference to anyone or anything that had come before. Unfalsifiable. Unassailable.

Now the initiate was still expected to submit to the cult, only this time, it wasn't buffered or grounded in a lineage. It was submission of self to another, supposedly unimpeachable Self—the guru.

Orientalism, Columbia University professor Edward Said's term for Western romanticization of all things Eastern, only made things worse. Throw in a Sanskrit, Sufi, or Zen honorific title, insist on strict hierarchies developed centuries ago in monasteries, claim mystical abilities as the sole domain of the Realizer in Chief, and it's not hard to see how things could go sideways.

And sideways they went.

Bhagwan Shree Rajneesh (later renamed as Osho) broke with Hindu tradition and blazed a wilder path, filled with breath work, sensuality, and lots of Rolls-Royces. Adi Da, born Franklin Jones in Queens, began his spiritual career with some penetrating insights into the human condition. He ended it in exile in Fiji, hounded by allegations of abuse, baffled that the world had not recognized him as the World Savior. Timothy Leary abandoned his academic lineage at Harvard to become a Lysergic Trickster Priest in and out of federal prison.

Throw in the "mad, bad and dangerous to know" sex-magician Aleister Crowley, who burned through the Western mystery schools of Europe and left chaos, destruction, and addiction in his wake. L. Ron Hubbard, a sometime protégé of Crowley's teachings, spun his dabblings into Dianetics and then Scientology. "You don't get rich writing science fiction," Hubbard supposedly said to a convention of writers hoping to do exactly that. "If you want to get rich, you start a religion." On that point, at least, he was true to his word.

There are hundreds of others.

But the absolute corkers—the ones who put the capital C in Culty Cults—were Charlie Manson and Jim Jones. They bookended the 1970s with gory tragedies, immortalizing Helter Skelter and "drinking the Kool-Aid" as shorthand for people losing their minds (and even their lives) to gurus with feet of clay and hearts of stone. "Absolute power corrupts absolutely," Lord Acton once observed. "Great men are almost always bad men."

For a few decades, that seemed to dampen enthusiasm and heighten skepticism for culty cults. What had once been a simple academic term describing a community of believers had become an unqualified pejorative—a warning of the dangers of losing yourself when trying to find yourself.

But lately, that tide has turned. We seem to be backsliding down the slippery slope. We're freshly vulnerable to cultic tendencies. There are a host of reasons for this, which could easily be the subject of an entire book. But here are four that seem to be reinforcing each other these days:

Generational Amnesia: We always forget. If we didn't we'd likely go mad with grief. Whether the pains of childbirth or the horrors of war, sometimes it's better not to remember. "Fluidity of memory and a capacity to forget," anthropologist Wade Davis notes, "is perhaps the most haunting trait of our species." But this current rise of culty-cult dynamics all around us seems so much a chapter-and-verse repeat of the cautionary tales of the '60s and '70s, it's hard to understand why we can't seem to recognize what's staring us in the face.

Part of that might be exacerbated by the fact that the generation rising to power and prominence right now—the millennials—are the children of the baby boomers. And like all children individuating from their parents, they tend to assume two things—the first, that nothing their parents did could be cool, relevant, or revelatory, and the second, that anything the kids have discovered is new and has never been done before. That's leaving us with a wisdom gap, and we have an entire generation of echo-boomers putting it right in the same ditch, on the same hairpin turns that their parents did. Never mind the skid marks.

Instagrammers at Burning Man might not even know about Ken Kesey, the Merry Pranksters, and their original 1962 art car and Acid Tests. Ayahuasceros who first heard about the potion on a podcast might not even recognize the names of Harvard ethnobotanist Richard Evans Schultes or the Beat writer William Burroughs. Advocates of polyamory might never have heard of *Stranger in a Strange Land* or the Church of All Worlds that it spawned. "He who knows only his own generation," Churchill lamented, "remains forever a child." As we head into uncertain times, it's feeling increasingly like a Children's Crusade.

Techniques of Ecstasy: We've mentioned this before, but it bears repeating in this inventory. Never at any time in human history *anywhere* have so many had access to so much, with so few guidelines. The Age of Aquarius gets all the hype for being the era of Sex, Drugs, and Rock 'n' Roll experimentation, but really, that was a relatively small fringe population. It only looms so large in our collective imagination because the media loved to cover it.

Today, industrial-strength marijuana is legally available in most states, tens of millions of users are participating in the psychedelic "renaissance" (an order of magnitude more than dabbled in the '60s), polyamory and other forms of nontraditional sexual relationships are at an all-time high, breath work, sensory deprivation, ice and sauna bathing, intensive yoga, EDM concerts, immersive digital worlds—pretty much the entire Alchemist Cookbook—are available on demand. And there's quite a bit of demand. These are potent and destabilizing tools, especially when yanked out of context. Addiction is as likely an outcome as illumination.

Digital Influencer Culture: In the past, if you wanted to become an authority in a given field, you had to apprentice to a lineage. If you were a scholar you had to devote yourself to earning a PhD.

If you were a writer, you had to work your way up to the journals of record.

True also for martial arts, yoga, or meditation. Pick your tradition, find your teacher, submit to the practice, and maybe, just maybe, if you proved yourself out, year after year, at some point you'd get the nod and be given permission to assume the mantle of teacher yourself.

All that changed with the advent of the internet. The gatekeepers got disintermediated. Content got democratized. If you had the will, now there were a thousand ways. While there was a flourishing of creativity and greater inclusion of voices, quality control went out the window.

That kicked off a race to the bottom. The spiritual marketplace got thoroughly commoditized and its incentives flipped. In the past, traditions served an imperfect but vital function of boosting the signal of wise teachers and suppressing the signal of charlatans.

Today, pretenders to the throne can spin up a slick website, push out some digital ads, and start grooming their very own fleeceable flock. The naive seekers they target cannot tell the difference between the diamond sutra and a rhinestone knockoff. The money changers have sneaked back in the temple, only now they take Venmo.

Rapture Ideologies: On top of all that—things have been getting super weird lately. For all the reasons we've discussed so far—the collapse in authority, global systemic crises, and tangled mythologies—it's increasingly difficult to tell what's around the bend.

The seductive pull of Rapture ideologies beckons.

The more uncomfortable and the less certain we are, the more tempting it becomes to find comfort in community. And the most tempting community to latch on to? The one that confidently proclaims to know exactly what's going on and is certain it's going to be standing on the right side of history (just as soon as whatever Big-TimeCrazyThing that's gonna happen happens).

Rapture ideologies are like a giant ontological vacuum, devouring everything in their path. That slow sucking sound as you watch friends and family slip down the conspiratorial rabbit hole? It's not a rabbit hole. It's the black hole of the Intertwingularity as all of our

End Times End Games blend together. And no one, except the chosen few, gets out alive.

We should expect conditions to worsen on the road ahead. The year 2020 saw an exponential uptick in all four of these dynamics—Generational Amnesia, Ecstatic Technologies, Digital Influencers, and Rapture Ideologies—overlapping and amplifying each other.

As plagues, fires, famine, and floods (to say nothing of global cabals secretly running the world, or imminent alien disclosure) ricochet around us, it's hard not to read into things. Signs and portents abound. Omens of Millennium are everywhere.

Meanwhile the echo chamber of social media is taking our shadows and turning them into monsters. By the clicking of our thumbs, something wicked this way comes . . .

Fear, Fight, Follow, F*ck

It's a standard trope of cult-busting exposés. The narrator always asks the question, "But how could such a group of successful, intelligent, accomplished people fall for such a scam?" It was true for the varsity quarterbacks and homecoming queens of the Manson family, it was true for the heiresses and movie stars of the recent sex-slave group NXIVM.

There are countless justifications, many of them unique to each person, for trying to fill that "god-shaped hole in their hearts" or the mommy- or daddy-shaped hole, or whichever hole they're trying to fill. But there's also a more fundamental reason. We're tribal primates wired to seek the silverback among us.

And when an alpha monkey steps up who is truly extraordinary, someone who breaks the mold of convention and appears to embody a degree of attainment that we only dream of, something predictable happens. The cathartic release of profound healing, the social relief of "having found our people," and the neurochemical cascade of peak experience leaves us imprinting on the One Who Opened Our Eyes.

Like freshly hatched ducklings mistaking a barnyard pig for their mother, a "born again" human is susceptible to getting their wires crossed and following the wrong leader. We can't think straight or see straight when we feel all funny inside.

In her recent book, *How Emotions Are Made*, Lisa Feldman Barrett, a professor of psychology at Harvard Medical School, gives us a clue to what might be happening in these situations. Beneath the surface of our emotions, Barrett argues, we have a second layer, known as interoception. It's literally what we sense in our guts. Rather than having dozens of different emotions, at the interoceptive level things are simple. There are two core axes our experience maps to: positive to negative and active to passive. All of our interoception ends up in one of four boxes.

You can feel actively positive—like joy and excitement. You can feel actively negative—like anger or flight. You can feel passively positive—like calm or contentment. And you can feel passively negative—like melancholy or depression. On top of these visceral states, we assign words and thoughts, plots and characters, conjuring more elaborate explanations of what's going on for us and who's to praise or blame for the way we feel. But at our root level, it's always one of those four states.

The same four responses arise when faced with a charismatic leader—but in these emotionally heightened experiences, our interoception is off the charts. That's part of what makes culty cults so volatile.

If we fall head over heels for the whole project, the simplest interoceptive response is "positive passive." We feel really good in this person's company and want to follow them wherever they're going. The contact high leaves us blissed out of our trees. We happily accept our beta status to *follow* our new leader.

If things get more serious, peak states and deep healing create a charge of "active positivity." For many of us, we haven't experienced that surge of feelings outside of a romantic relationship. Even if the leader is impeccable with their sexuality (and many aren't), we can confuse Agape (spiritual love) for Eros (erotic love). At that point, following the leader isn't enough. We yearn for communion with them.

We want to love them, and mistake our existential yearning for romance. We want to *fuck* them.

But that's only half the interoception equation. We might not feel positive about this guru at all. We might feel unmoored by the deeper waters they're dragging us into. Whether right away, or slowly over time, we begin to doubt their sincerity or attainment. We might second-guess their truths, or get pulled back to Snug Harbor by friends and family who aren't onboard.

If you feel negative but passive in this situation, you come to *fear* the teacher, and then possibly flee. They are bigger than you and more powerful and you're not 100 percent sure—but the best bet seems to be to run. Get as far away from their reality distortion field as you possibly can.

In rarer situations, if you feel sufficiently threatened, or emboldened by a crowd, you might decide to challenge the leader, to *fight* them. Pitchforks, torches, crosses (or canceling) ensue. The only thing to do in this case is eradicate the one who makes you feel this uncomfortable.

So those are four foundational interoceptive responses to being in the presence of an avatar—real or imagined. We want to follow them, fuck them, fear them, or fight them. These patterns are so deeply entrenched that they account for nearly every outcome of transformational movements across history.

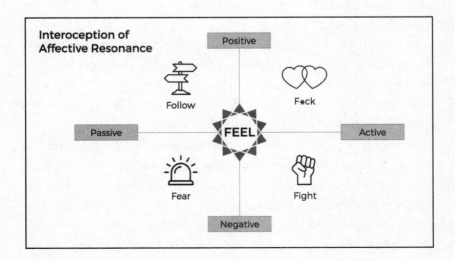

And it doesn't matter if the leader is a false front or the Real Deal. Our primate wiring calls the shots. From Jesus to Joan of Arc. From Manson to the Moonies. From Malcolm X to Martin Luther King. We've seen every permutation of this passion play. From the pedestal to the pit. None of them pencil out.

But there is a fifth option, a middle path that is less common but essential for building a scalable Meaning 3.0. When an exceptional person, a true Promethean, switches on powerfully enough to pass that spark to others, what if, instead of following, fucking, fearing, or fighting them, we stayed dead center at the intersection of our interoception—*feeling* all of it ourselves? Instead of dumping our own authority and agency, instead of projecting for good or bad onto the Other, what if we stepped up and actually owned our own power and potential?

"If you get to heaven before I do," the old spiritual "Swing Low, Sweet Chariot" asks, "open up the window and pull me on through!" In this version, it's less about who gets there first and takes the claim than it is about getting as many across that threshold as possible. As we step into our collective possibility together, the extraordinary should become simply ordinary.

While that sounds pleasant enough, it's actually harder than it looks. The concept of our psychological "shadow," i.e., those disowned or repressed parts of ourselves that are too dark to admit, is a well-known working concept in psychology. But the eminent twentieth-century Jungian Robert Johnson coined the term "golden shadow" to describe something else. Our golden shadow refers not to the dark parts we have a hard time owning up to but to the bright parts we are afraid to own. "The gold is related to our higher calling," Johnson writes, "and this can be hard to accept."

When we can't accept our own power, Johnson cautions that we "give away our gold." We hang it on the neck of our guru. They are wise, strong, and compassionate. We're not. They have solved the human condition and liberated themselves; we never could. No matter how strong and worthy they appear at first, the weight of all that projection brings these leaders and their communities to their knees eventually.

Abraham Maslow called this denial of our own power the Jonah complex. He named it after the Old Testament Jonah who tried to duck his God-given calling and ended up in the belly of the whale. In Maslow's reading, we fear our own greatness as much as our failure for two reasons—the first is "How on earth will I keep this up?" and the second is "What will the neighbors think?"

Which brings us to the third and least common version of cults in our survey. The *ethical* cult. Where traditional cults demanded subjugation of the self to the lineage, and culty cults demanded subjugation of the self to the guru, an ethical cult does neither. Instead, it seeks to enhance the sovereignty of the individual while increasing the intelligence of the collective.

That's a delicate balance, rarely achieved. Following, fucking, fearing, and fighting are easy and predictable responses. Feeling it all is much harder. Owning our own power while deferring to a higher power requires timing, humility, and skill.

If traditional cults were like taking your seat in an orchestra, and culty cults were like being in a marching band, ethical cults feel more like playing jazz. No sheet music or drum major to guide off. Just us, in the moment, listening for the pulse together.

But before we get to explore how ethical cults might function, we should clarify how culty cults have *dys*functioned. It's not enough to insist that our group is better, smarter, or more principled than all the others that have gone off the rails before us—that's what they've all said. Playing around with the high arousal of ecstasis, the profound vulnerability of catharsis, and the hive-mind buzz of communitas puts us right in a danger zone that's millions of years in the making. Everybody *cults*, as David Foster Wallace reminds us. The only question is what kind of cult.

Culty-Cult Checklist

What follows is a short checklist to spot cultic tendencies. It is based on an extensive survey of visionary and utopian communities, ranging from groups like the Oneidans, Millerites, and Mormons in the eighteenth and nineteenth centuries, to the standouts of the '60s and '70s mentioned above, to contemporary case studies in the spiritual marketplace. In the same way that Dr. Atul Gawande, author of *The Checklist Manifesto*, helped revolutionize standards of care in hospitals, by adopting preflight routines from pilots, this checklist helps ensure that critical errors aren't made in transformational community building. If it works for brain surgeons, it can work for ethical cult leaders and followers as well.

As we explore open-sourcing Meaning 3.0, we're going to see lots of experiments and variations. That "let a thousand fires burn" pluralism is essential. It's what we need to honor all of our collective diversity and to provide ample room for local innovation. But it's also going to lead to lots of misuse and even abuse of powerful psychosocial technologies.

These guidelines are intended as an open-source charter agreement by which different groups might voluntarily agree to play in the domains of ecstasis, catharsis, and communitas. They identify best practices for ethical culture building and can serve as a checklist for seekers as they enter the spiritual marketplace. It can provide faster pattern recognition and improved reaction time for where the slopes get slippery. It can help reclaim how we worship.

While there are nearly infinite ways to screw up ecstatic community-building, there are three common pitfalls to culty cults that have shown up over the ages: Grabbing the Ring, creating In/Out groups, and weaponizing Ecstasis and Catharsis.

Culty-Cult Checklist: What Not to Do

I. **GRABBING THE ONE RING OF POWER**— Absolute power corrupts absolutely. Like in *Lord of the Rings*, don't be the misguided warrior Boromir or the corrupt wizard Saruman, thinking you will bend the Ring, not that it will bend you. Be like Gandalf and the elven queen Galadriel—wise enough to know better. This one is nonnegotiable. Here are the top three ways leaders get seduced into claiming more than they've earned.

i.   **Mythologized Origin Story of the Founder**—Carefully curated, often repeated tales of exceptional conditions surrounding birth, childhood, or early signs of prodigious talent/insight. Or a Dark Night of the Soul/ Road to Damascus conversion experience that uniquely positions this person to lead. In extreme cases, these are confirmed with self-appointed name change. (In the age of info marketers, this has morphed to include the "I had it all, the big house, fast cars, sexy life, and then . . . I woke up one day in a hospital bed and realized [fill in the blank product or service] that I'm now here to share with you!")

ii. **Absolutist Claims of Attainment**—In the spiritual, intellectual, sexual, entrepreneurial, or artistic realms— typically reserved for the founder, occasionally extended to their inner circle. Once infallibility is claimed, all dissonance in relation to the founder must be either signs of supplicants' blind spots and projections or deliberate "crazy wisdom" being offered to liberate the subject—never signs of the founder's fallibility or humanity. This often extends beyond the blamelessness of the founder to the completeness and totality of their worldview, which is presumed to be comprehensive and supersedes all other modes of knowing. Two of the most prevalent expressions (often appearing together) are the one-two punch of absolute Enlightenment (with the leader implicitly or explicitly claiming such status) and a dismissal of objective reality as illusory in favor of the power of the mind, visualization, or positive thinking.

iii. **Ritualized Separation**—Keeping the leader distinct from operational tasks, duties, and common mingling. Most often done by adoption of Eastern monastic traditions and terminology (like *satsang*, which means "sitting in the presence of an awakened guru") but can also be accomplished by simple celebrity handling such as use of bouncers, greenrooms, and stage settings (which often include ornate seating, lily/lotus flower arrangements, altars, dressing in white or robes, or vestments rather than street clothes) that keep the leader apart from the community except in controlled and/or stylized encounters.

II. **CREATING IN/OUT GROUPS**—The dynamic of creating an Us and a Them is central for dysfunctional cults to take root. It is how otherwise well-intentioned seekers can get pulled into a reality distortion field where they lose track of their bearings. Any practice, experience, or community that lifts people "up and away"—from their traditions, connections, and culture—rather than bringing them "down and among" their fellow humanity, can be problematic. Here are three common viruses that prompt exceptionalism.

i. **Messianic Purpose**—The micro (of the community) is the macro (of the world) and the value of the work being done within the cloister has significance far beyond the lives of those directly practicing it. This sets up both the potential grandiosity of a world-saving mission and also can be used to suppress members' personal needs and concerns as petty, selfish, or small-minded in comparison (such as compensation vs. volunteer labor). In extreme cases, it may also invoke a "crypto-Puritanism" where those inside the group are considered pure, saved, or gifted, while those beyond the group are tainted, compromised, or in need of redemption.

ii. **Specialized Language**—Often culty cults use novel terms to describe or redefine everyday concepts or introduce pseudo-spiritual or pseudoscientific terms to convey legitimacy on otherwise unprovable truth claims. Over time this increasing lack of interoperability with everyday language or the concepts of mainstream discourse isolates the faithful from friends, family members, and healthy debate. "Quantum" used by non-physicists is a frequent catchall in the New Age scene.

iii. **Break with Past Precedent**—Very rarely do cultic leaders situate themselves within a lineage that would subject them to accountability or critique larger than themselves by others older or wiser than themselves (living or dead). Instead, they tend to declare a "clean slate" even if their own development began within a school or tradition. That immunity against precedent extends to charges of cultic behavior, as these leaders will often volunteer extended critiques of past gurus with feet of clay, holding their own transmission up as a corrective exemplar. They may even declare a complete break with the aggregate Human Condition, i.e., that they represent an end to suffering, ego, conditioning, fear, or trauma that has never been accomplished before (or has only been accomplished by Axial Age greats—Buddha, Jesus, Muhammad, Lao-tzu, etc.).

III. **WEAPONIZING PEAK EXPERIENCE AND HEALING**—Ecstasis and Catharsis create highly impressionable and susceptible states. While they can be used to enhance sovereignty, they can also rapidly erode it. Unscrupulous leaders make the most of this fact to control their followers in three consistent ways.

i. **Tightly Controlled Access** to techniques of ecstasy— drugs, sex, breath work, music/dance, prayer, charismatic transmission, or sensory deprivation, as well as to methods of catharsis—body work, encounter-type group therapy sessions, personal inquiry, specialized diets, cleanses, etc. Unsanctioned access and insights that contradict the leader's framing or group norms are often discouraged or suppressed. New or competing interpretations of peak states, healing, or broader philosophy by members are often treated as subversive or heretical.

ii. **An Emphasis on Regressive Practices That Value Feeling over Thinking** and an inoculation against thinking/discernment as signs of ego, projection, or resistance that is to be trusted less than either the "truths" of catharsis/trauma release or the insights and framing of the leader. Because the very methods of personal discernment (a.k.a. "trusting my gut") and logical critique are already discounted by the leader, even the most thoughtful and accurate concerns can be *ipso facto* dismissed as proof of a member's resistance to transformation—there is no way to crack the facade from within it.

iii. **Key Decisions and Commitments Encouraged or Forced While in Non-ordinary States**—Whether testaments of love, allegiance, atonement, or payment, these groups use the softened boundaries and impaired judgment of euphoric peak states or cathartic release as times to secure emotional, social, or financial commitments. Suitably primed members are encouraged to equate the visceral "truths" of the state they are in with the validity of all the prior truth claims of the guru. That is, if I am blissed out of my mind, or shuddering in trauma release, and that is an undeniable reality for me, then I am often compelled by the group to sign off on their entire mythology. Key decisions and commitments are encouraged or forced while in non-ordinary states, rather than deferring until a person returns to clearheaded sobriety and can offer full consent.

* * *

If it were as easy to spot culty cults as rolling down a checklist like this one, most of them would never get off the ground. Here are three additional edge cases that can dull our discernment and make it harder to know what we're looking at until it's too late.

False Negatives: Many healthy communities of practice will check several of these boxes (especially those regarding strong in-group identity and ritualized access to peak states). Religions, martial arts lineages, fraternal/sororal organizations, and start-ups can display positive versions of these dynamics, without devolving into cultic behavior. These "deep structures" of belonging have a tendency to emerge as natural parts of the collective meaning-making of tribal primates. We rally together around an inspiring shared purpose and we feel better/have more fun together. To differentiate between a healthy or pathological expression of these kinds of behaviors, an observer will need to exercise careful discernment and triangulate between all factors.

False Positives: Many cultlike communities will initially present with palpable energy, enthusiasm, and growth, *precisely because* they are harnessing many of the ecstatic and cathartic techniques described above. This can create cognitive dissonance for anyone applying the "by their fruits ye shall know them" filter to see if a community is legitimate. While the fruits appear to be abundant, it is tempting to conclude that the roots must be healthy. Using charismatic transmission, encouraging regressive catharsis, controlling ecstatic rituals of bonding, and advocating for magical thinking consistently produce potent effects. It is not that they don't work, it's that they work only too well (until they inevitably don't).

Talented but Tainted: Often, especially after a scandal or community collapse, pundits will label the leader as a fraud. In this judgment, the guru was only pretending to be spiritual and really only wanted money, sex, fame, or power. Everyone who followed them was duped. While those kinds of low-level hucksters are abundant, as NXIVM's Keith Ranière recently illustrates, at the higher levels of attainment, like Osho or Adi Da, it's rarely that cut-and-dried. As often, the leader had some remarkable skills and insights that fueled their own teaching and community in the first place. It was only over time that things visibly degraded/imploded. This is almost always due to Grabbing the One Ring of Power, which disconnects the leader from their humanity. When a gifted teacher accepts their followers' golden shadow, and allows themselves and others to believe that they are exceptional and even infallible, the rot invariably sets in.

The frequent use of altered states and regressive emotionality further disconnects followers from their common sense and discernment, making it harder to notice the decline.

These are all red flags and deal breakers. It is exceptionally rare for a leader to endorse any of those three behaviors—claims of infallibility, state-priming, and anti-intellectualism—and not have significant blind spots/ulterior motives. Even if not immediately apparent, they corrode the community over time.

CHAPTER 13

The Ethical Cult(ure) Toolbox

I must create a system, or be enslaved by another man's.

—William Blake

In the middle section of the book, we built on IDEO's human-centered design thinking in an attempt to revitalize the three functions filled by Meaning 1.0—inspiration, healing, and connection. We then grafted them onto three values of Meaning 2.0—open-source, scalability, and anti-fragility. Because a viable Meaning 3.0 needs to work across cultures, we have deliberately stayed away from prescribing any specific doctrine.

Which version of belief and belonging a given community chooses and what value systems they assign to their collective experience has to be figured out together at the local level. Not all are going to work out, but some are. They all need room to experiment and find the balance between tradition and innovation that works for them.

The tools that we have considered—respiration, embodiment, sexuality, music, and substances—intentionally used, just help us do the human thing a little better. They give us more reliable and effective access to ecstasis, catharsis, and communitas. That said, leaving everyone to their own devices, with no instruction manual, will likely result in a lot of wasted time and missed opportunities. It would be akin to everyone building rocket ships in their driveway rather than joining the team at NASA or SpaceX to put a man on the moon. It might work out, but there's likely to be a lot of flameouts and scrubbed launches.

Now that we have sketched the basic practices for individuals and small groups to wake up, grow up, and show up, we need to extend our design thinking to architecting culture more broadly. What are the essential ingredients for Meaning 3.0? What, in other words, is the tool kit for building ethical culture?

If we return to the field of comparative religion, we can find some clues scattered around the world and through the ages. While there are nearly infinite variations and permutations of how we worship, Meaning 1.0—organized religion—has tended to share five core elements.

First, you need a **Metaphysics**. Since the business of religion has always been as a mediator of the sacred, we're going to need reliable ways to make sense of the Ineffable. Otherwise we will get lost in the realm of the uncharted sublime. When we leave behind familiar signposts and landmarks and enter terrain that is fantastical or overwhelming, it's easy to get disoriented. Whether Hansel and Gretel leaving breadcrumbs to find their way out of the forest, or Theseus using his ball of string to retrace his steps out of the Minotaur's labyrinth, it's critical that when we venture beyond the pale, we have a way to keep our bearings. A solid metaphysics lets us make sense of paradoxes and epiphanies. It functions like a Cosmic Positioning System and helps us find our way back home.

Next, you need an **Ethics**. If there aren't guardrails to this experiment, no higher purpose or service, then it will be captured by Bliss Junkies endlessly chasing states, Epiphany Whores craving catharsis, or Gutless Groupies following gurus. Ethics are like the tail rotor on a helicopter—without them, we just spin in circles.

Then, you need **Sacraments**. If you don't have reliable techniques of ecstasy to deliver the sacred (however you define it) to your congregants, you will lack both the revelatory insights and potent bonding that fuel a spiritual community. "There can be no society," wrote Émile Durkheim, the founder of sociology, "which does not feel the need of upholding and reaffirming at regular intervals the collective sentiments and ideas which make its unity and personality."

Without reliably transformative initiatory rituals, you'll also end up with voltage drop, as the immediate gnosis of a founder dwindles as it gets handed down. Christ made more Christians than he did additional Christs. Buddha made more Buddhists than fellow buddhas. Bruce Lee inspired more copycats than true martial artists. Effective sacraments prevent this and anchor living traditions.

Over the long haul, you'll also need **Scriptures**. We live through our tradition's stories. We make sense of our lives through those who have come before us. We benefit from examples and exemplars to manage the human condition. We require narrative pegs to hang the events of our lives upon, so they don't end up in a pile on the floor.

Last, but certainly not least, you need **Deities**. They're the long pole in the Big Tent. If there isn't some higher power to aspire to, we're literally left to our own self-interest. That typically hasn't worked out too well. As Nietzsche warned, kill your gods and you tear the social fabric they came wrapped in. To be fair, a lot of suffering has been inflicted in deities' names too, so this whole category deserves a careful rethink.

In a survey of successful Utopian communities, almost all of those who persisted beyond the lifetime of a charismatic founder had a shared spirituality they considered bigger than their own personal needs. Harnessing our better angels (and better gods) will be important as we try to grow resilient social movements.

So that's it—the Ethical Culture Tool Kit for creating coherent communities. Metaphysics, Ethics, Sacraments, Scriptures, and Deities. "We are as gods," Stewart Brand wrote on the first page of the *Whole Earth Catalog*, "and might as well get good at it."

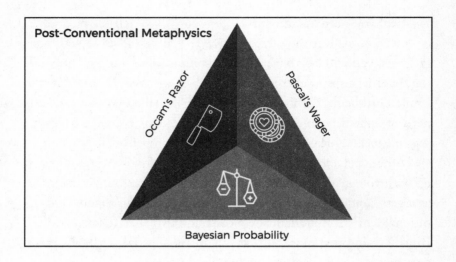

Metaphysics: Effing the Ineffable

Tradition has it that Plato had a sign over the door of his academy that said, LET NO ONE IGNORANT OF GEOMETRY ENTER HERE. That wasn't because the philosopher was a big fan of Common Core educational standards. He was warning students, on the brink of contemplating the Mysteries, to make sure they were bringing logic and reason to the table.

So what essential tools for sense-making do we need to consider? The long answer is a rigorous education in logic, rhetoric, and hermeneutics, as Plato would have insisted. But these are different times, and that sort of classical learning has fallen out of fashion. The shorter answer is a sturdy triangle made up of Pascal's wager, Occam's razor, and Bayesian probability. Between them, they should map most of the ground we need to cover.

Let's start with Pascal's wager. Blaise Pascal, a seventeenth-century French mathematician, famously figured that it was better to believe in God, on the off chance he was real, than to deny his existence and burn in hell for his doubts. Moral: *At least conceive of the inconceivable, just in case it turns out to be true.* As we enter the age of the Intertwingularity, everything from religious prophecies to global plots to existential collapse is on the table. We'd do well to consider them all, as Pascal did, just in case one or more of them end up happening.

The second guideline comes from William of Ockham, the medieval Franciscan who gave us the maxim known as Occam's razor. It boils down to "the simplest solution is usually the best." Moral: *Before galloping off into labyrinthine interpretations of our favorite conspiracy theory, late-night bender, or spiritual epiphany, consider the less exciting but more likely explanations first.* "Extraordinary claims," Carl Sagan cautioned, "require extraordinary proof!" Or, as Sigmund Freud drily observed, "Sometimes a cigar is just a cigar."

The third pillar comes from Thomas Bayes, a sixteenth-century statistician who gave us Bayesian analysis. The world is chaotic, complex, and confusing, Bayes suggested, and the best you can do is track all the variables and update them as you get new information. Rather than gunning for false certainty, he encouraged provisional uncertainty. Moral: *Don't get out too far over your skis.* Track everything that might be true but isn't yet certain, and update dynamically as you learn more. Fools rush in, in other words, where statisticians fear to tread.

More than ever, we are cut loose from our traditional moorings. We're both blessed and burdened with having to wrap our heads around a vast multiverse of confusing, confounding, and conflicting possibilities. Whether it's the staggering complexity of the human mind revealed by psychedelic research, or the disorienting weirdness of our increasingly digitized and simulated *Black Mirror* lives, we're in need of an upgrade to our Aristotelian/Cartesian epistemics. Just because I can't touch, taste, feel, or see something no longer means it isn't real. We've moved from the skeptic's stance of "I'll believe it when I see it" to the artist's, or adept's acknowledgment of "I'll see it when I believe it."

For the truly brave, willing to push off from the shore and voyage into the vastness of the unknown, there's a final set of guidelines for navigating the metaphysical deep end. This takes the trio of Pascal, Occam, and Bayes, cross references it with the Infinite Game, and throws the whole thing into warp drive.

These cautions and reminders draw on the collected experiences of Philip K. Dick, John Lilly, Robert Anton Wilson, Ken Kesey, and other modern psychonauts. What is important to notice about these provisional guidelines is what they *don't* say. Unlike religious epiphanies from times past, these postmodern adventurers trade false certainty for playful humility in the face of the Infinite. This open-endedness is an essential element to ensure that Meaning 3.0 remains experimental and nondogmatic.

After encountering the vastness of the mysterium tremendum, the "Great Mystery," Robert Anton Wilson maintains there are only two outcomes—you either go insane or become an agnostic. Think of this list that follows as a meta-metaphysics. It suggests an agnostic gnosticism—one that allows that a direct initiation into the nature of reality is not only possible but potentially desirable (that's the gnostic part), but holds back from asserting any fixed or definitive statement of What It All Means (the agnostic part).

If this isn't terrain you're already exploring, it will likely sound pointless or inscrutable (and feel free to turn the page to the next section on Ethics). But if you have been dipping your toe into the Mysto, these guidelines can serve as a trail of bread crumbs to get you (or someone you love) safely back home.

Cheat Codes for the Infinite Game

> *In the finite game the player plays within the rules. In the Infinite Game the player plays* with *the rules.*
>
> —James Carse

- The Game has an infinite number of levels in an infinite number of dimensions.

- The purpose of the Game is to remember you are playing it (anamnesis).

- The more levels of the Game you remember you're playing, the more fun (*and consequential*) the Game becomes.

- Higher levels of the Game bleed through into 3D: They often show up as coincidences, synchronicities, or absurdity. This is a "known issue" best taken as a reminder that the Game is afoot (and held loosely).

- The 3D level is the access point to all the other levels of the Game. If you die at the 3D level of the Game, it is Game Over (unless or until proven otherwise). So no matter what, don't die in 3D!

- Don't say anything, or think anything, that you don't want to become more true.

- Once you've figured out the Game, help turn as many NPCs (nonplayer characters) into Players and Players into Architects as you can.

- Stay awake. Build stuff. Help out.

Ethics: The Ten Suggestions

Those metaphysical filters can go a long way to helping us parse the Impossible. They give us some guidelines to steer by, but they are inherently value-neutral. They only help us consider all the paths that are possible. They cannot help us choose which path to go down. But we can't only pick the fun or self-serving explanations on the grounds that they're all make-believe. We shouldn't just choose our illusion.

So how do we deal with the partial truths of a nearly limitless number of perspectives? We have to bring our own logic and discernment along for the ride. If we're architecting ethical culture, we need a way to make effective value judgments. Otherwise we risk slipping into a moral relativism that could rationalize almost anything.

In trying to figure out how we should build healthy transformative cultures there's a stumbling block we have to acknowledge from the start: Ecstatic experiences are inherently Antinomian. Literally in the Greek *anti*, "against"; *nomos*, "law." That makes it tricky to establish rules for an inherently lawless domain. "There is such a sense of authority that comes out of the primary mystical experience," Johns Hopkins' Roland Griffiths writes, "that it can be threatening to existing hierarchical structures." The tagline of peak experiences could be summed up as "You're not the boss of me."

The U.S. Army learned this the hard way in the 1950s when they were testing LSD on troops to see if it could be used to disorient enemy combatants. Many pie-eyed soldiers had a bit of a rethink, put down their weapons, and walked away from the whole circus. This is why techniques of ecstasy haven't been widely distributed outside of tightly held lineages and traditions—they tend to blow apart systematic organizations.

But taking out guardrails altogether can be problematic, or even fatal to a healthy community. The comforting solidity of "thou shalts" and "thou shalt nots" doesn't pair that well with the Antinomian certainty of direct experience or the Bayesian uncertainty of *nothing is true, everything is permitted*. Our current times have grown too complex for the black-and-white binaries of the Old Testament traditions.

So can we come up with an alternative to the Ten Commandments, one that gives enough flexibility that people of varied beliefs and backgrounds find them helpful, while still providing enough steer to keep us on the tracks? To do that, we'll need what developmental psychologists call "liberating structures"—rules that help but don't constrain.

And that means replacing the certainty of morals—clear, unambiguous, and binary—with the situational relevance of ethics, where it's no longer the act that's right or wrong, but it's the relationship to the act that determines its value. As anthropologists joke, "It's only wrong to eat people if you're not a cannibal."

What follows is a working list of countermeasures to persistent issues that arise in today's transformative culture. They're not strict commandments. They're more like considered *suggestions*. As with everything we're discussing, these aren't intended to be the last word on anything for anyone. They are only examples of what can be built using the tools we're playing with in an open-source system. Some we cover in more detail elsewhere in the book; others are mentioned here in brief. Take what's helpful, leave the rest.

The Ten ~~Commandments~~ Suggestions

I.   **DO THE OBVIOUS.** There are entire industries devoted to personal growth, biohacking, and self-help. Most of them distract from the broader human project. Rather than getting overwhelmed by all of the options for optimization, just Do the Obvious: Sleep deeply; move frequently; eat real food; get outside; bathe often, play music, breathe deeply, grieve fully, make love; give thanks. You can put all that extra time and money left over toward living a vitalized and engaged life.

II. **DON'T DO STUPID SHIT.** We've never had more access to such powerful, transformative technologies free of guidance or restrictions. In this Brave New World, we're all operating on our own recognizance. So, no matter what, when playing with the Alchemist Cookbook, don't accidentally end up in: a cult, a body bag, a jail cell, divorce court, rehab, or a mental institution. You'll ruin it for the rest of us and provide an excuse for the Puritans itching to shut it all down. (Sometimes those setbacks happen for other reasons in life and deserve full support for anyone undergoing them—that's not what we're talking about here. Like mountaineers and big wave surfers, would-be Alchemists should know what they're getting into before they go, or they'll create accidents others have to clean up.)

III. **LET THE MYSTERY STAY THE MYSTERY.** The more you plumb the depths of the Mysto, the more you realize that it isn't something to be mastered or mapped. It really is turtles all the way

up, down and sideways. If you compare the accounts of the car-
tographers of the sacred through the ages, you quickly realize
they're wildly different. Their experiences were mediated by biology, the filters of selfhood, culture, and the prison house of language. "The answer is never the answer," Ken Kesey once said.
"What's really interesting is the mystery. If you seek the mystery
instead of the answer, you'll always be seeking. I've never seen
anybody find the answer, but they think they have. So they stop
thinking. But the job is to seek mystery, evoke mystery, plant a
garden in which strange plants grow and mysteries bloom. The
need for mystery is greater than the need for an answer."

IV. **80/20 AWOKEN TO BROKEN.** Because those early hits of ecstasis are so powerful, we are tempted to burn the remaining
80 percent of our energy chasing the long tail of our imagined
perfectibility. The reality is, we're human, and being human
contains an irreducible amount of grief and pain. So rather than
waste all that time trying to get our heads above the clouds, let's
look behind us and help some less fortunate people get their
heads above water. Go to the intersection of our trauma and our
talent—where we most acutely feel the wound of the world and
have the skills to do something about it. All we need is that 80
percent initial hit to remember what we forgot and what we're
here to do—and then GO DO IT!

V.   **F*CK YOUR JOURNEY.** Or as Saint Paul put it more encourag-
ingly: "Love keeps no record of wrong." Whatever chain of events
got us to the Deep Now is redeemed as an essential part of our
path and utterly irrelevant compared to the exquisite quality of
the moment we're blessed to share. We're all here, Now (or we're
not, and no amount of talking will change that fact). So, stop
being a carpetbagger of catharsis, rehashing your breakdowns
and breakthroughs. Show us how much you've grown. But, dear
God, please stop telling us.

VI. **DO THE HARD THING.** If you're focusing on peak states, which
often feel easy and effortless, you may get tricked into thinking

that's how it should be all the time. But that's not how it works. "Fortune," Louis Pasteur observed, "favors the prepared." Or as Mark Twain said, "If it's your job to eat two frogs, eat the biggest one first." If you want more flow, bliss, or grace in your life, tackle the gnarliest shit head-on. The Stoics were right about this one, the Obstacle is the Way.

VII. **NEVER LOSE THE ONE.** When musicians solo, they can improvise freely, *provided they can come back to the chorus on the beat (the beginning of the measure or the "One").* In fact, the farther from it they roam, the funkier the jam. But lose the One and it all falls apart. Same goes for athletes in action sports, where the One is their center of gravity (or *hara* or *dantian* in martial arts). They can flip, spin, and twist through the air, and as long as they remain centered, they can stomp the landing. It's the same for the far reaches of metaphysical exploration. You can go anywhere you want and think anything you want as long as you can make it back to the last known point of consensus reality—the One. So get funky, tweak it out, riff freely, *but be sure to stick the landing.*

VIII. **AND IT'S NOT THAT EITHER!** Whenever we think we've found It, we get a huge dopamine hit of pattern recognition and a sense of certainty that it's all overwhelmingly true—for us, in that moment. But whenever you take a lowercase truth and presume it's the capital "T" Truth, it becomes false, just by overstating the claim. You can no more become fully enlightened than you can become fully educated. Take your insights for what they are, integrate them, and keep going.

IX. **PRACTICE RESURRECTION.** Tibetan monks spend their entire lives meditating so at the moment of dying they can stay awake in the Bardos and step off the wheel of reincarnation for good. But what if we were to practice that every day? What if we practiced dying to our stories, our pain, and our pleasure, dying to our rightness, to our wrongness, dying every moment and living into the Deep Now? It's a radical practice. Psychedelics, meditation, breath work, sexuality, martial arts, and extreme sports—all can become death practices. So practice resurrection. Die to all of it. And see who we are on the other side.

X.   **ABOVE ALL, BE KIND.** This one comes from Aldous Huxley, on his deathbed, on 200 micrograms of LSD. He held his wife Laura's hand and delivered four words: "Above all, be kind." None of it matters if we forget this part. It's worth returning to again and again.

Sacraments

The Ten Suggestions can be helpful as ethical guidelines, ways to steer through our own personal explorations. They don't provide clear direction for regulating our use of sacraments, though—the central experiences that are fueling everything else. And that's an issue: How do we strike the balance between liberation and structure in our relationship to the central experience of the Ineffable?

At their best, sacraments take us out of the day-to-day and give us a glimpse, however brief, of the sacred—of the world and of ourselves at our best. If you strip out the cultural specifics, most ritualized sacraments serve three functions—they work as metronomes, tuning forks, and training wheels. If we can make the most of that function-

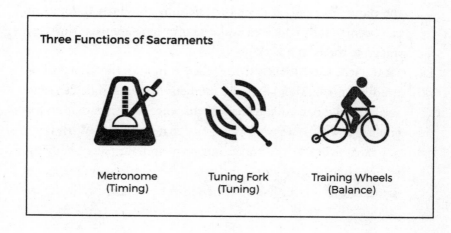

Three Functions of Sacraments

Metronome (Timing)   Tuning Fork (Tuning)   Training Wheels (Balance)

ality, we have a way to build sacramental rituals that serve us, rather than our serving them.

In the grind of life, we never know for sure if we are keeping the beat. If we're stressed or anxious we may play too fast, forcing the feel, instead of feeling the Force. If we're tired or depressed we might start to lag, perpetually late to the unfolding moment. But when we experience the global reset of a peak experience, our nervous system recalibrates, and we begin again on the One—the sunrise, the sunset, the seasons, our heartbeats. The metronome lets us know whether we are fast or slow and brings us back to the steady pulse of life.

In addition to our timing, we also need to calibrate our tuning. Life hurts. We get hit, knocked out of whack, and beaten out of tune. But functional sacraments give us the chance to hear the perfect pitch of the tuning fork again. They help us recognize whether we're sharp or flat. It can be hard to notice that slight shift in tone ourselves. It could be a loss of physical health, or inattention to key relationships, or a drop in professional drive. It might have happened imperceptibly over time, but now, faced with perfect pitch, the gap is obvious. The heightened perception of a peak state lets us hear that discrepancy clearly and recalibrate the instrument of ourselves.

Sacraments also serve as training wheels. They return us to center and prop up our balance when we wobble. They let us practice steering without the full consequences of falling over and getting hurt. This is the mechanism of action in MDMA with PTSD psychotherapy. The MDMA allows the traumatized person to feel supersaturated in love, safety, and security. That somatic anchor in their bodies, minds, and hearts is often strong enough that patients can practice living from that perspective. Thanks to the training wheels, it's possible to regain the feeling of living from a place of love. It doesn't last forever, but over time it lets someone practice turning that state into a new normal.

These three functions help us balance the heights of peak experience with the healing we all need to do. But they also offer a simple insight on how we should relate to them. They are tools to repair us from and prepare us for a life fully lived. Nothing more or less.

After all, musicians don't spend all of their time fiddling with metronomes and tuning forks. Aspiring cyclists don't keep their training wheels on any longer than they need them to find their balance. Musicians, as soon as they are on time and in tune, go out to find other musicians to play with. Cyclists, once they can pedal in a straight line, go out and explore the world. Sacraments offer us something simple: an experience of being on time, in tune, and in balance. The place we all started. A place we can return to. A place from which we can begin again.

Scriptures

For anyone who's already a part of an existing wisdom tradition, this one's straightforward. Sacred texts are in easy reach. Even if you have strayed from your family's beliefs, the scriptures that inspired your ancestors are probably all around you—showing up on holidays, on bookshelves, or in hand-me-down stories. They're there, waiting to be dusted off and rediscovered. If we return to them after having glimpsed the Sublime ourselves, many of them read entirely differently than what we might remember from childhood. "And every one of them words rang true, and glowed like burning coal," Bob Dylan once sang, "pouring off of every page like it was written in my soul." Embedded in the world's sacred texts is the wisdom of thousands of years of human history, insights, and reflection; we'd do well to remember.

But there is an inevitable amount of confusion and exclusion on those pages too. Many people today have drifted away from the faith of their grandmothers and grandfathers because they cannot locate their own experience in those stories. That has played a large part of the rise of the "spiritual but not religious" Nones. Others, not raised within a spiritual tradition, struggle to find their way back into scriptures written in fundamentally different times and places.

The question we need to ask: Are there scriptures that offer us both salvation and inclusion? Are there stories that can speak to us all? Because it would be a mistake to neglect the positive role that scripture can play beyond enforcing outdated doctrines. Our sacred stories bond us together, inspire us to do better, and heal us when we need it most.

Psychologists at Princeton's Social Neuroscience Lab, for example, have found that people who read narratives develop stronger social cognition than those who don't. When scanned, the brains of bookworms show more Default Mode Network activity in the area devoted to empathy. We're kinder and wiser when we can imagine the lives of others.

We're also stronger. Marshall Duke, a psychologist at Emory University, found that children who learned their family story across generations had a higher sense of self-esteem and self-control. They even had more resilience in the face of trauma.

And we inherit the most resilience when these intergenerational stories oscillate, mirroring the ups and downs of our own lives. "Our family is the best" turns out to be less helpful than "we've had a share of triumphs and disasters, and we're still here." Just like Kurt Vonnegut's Cinderella Story.

Interestingly, Vonnegut noted one other famous tale that shares that Down, Up, Really Down, Really Up shape—the scriptures of the New Testament. In that instance, it's the Down of Original Sin, followed by the hopeful Up of the nativity at Bethlehem, undone by the tragic Really Down of Good Friday, only to be redeemed by the Really Up of Easter Sunday. It seems we've always been suckers for a seat-of-the-pants yarn that works out in the end.

It might be time to dust off that trusty framework and start spinning more tales that inspire hope, resilience, and empathy. Cognitive psychologist Keith Oatley calls stories "the mind's flight simulator." We get to learn and practice what might be unforgiving in real life. We can harness the power of our imaginations to prepare us for what the world will inevitably throw at us. This is true of all narrative, but it is especially true of those that speak directly to our deepest yearnings. Who are we? Where did we come from? Where are we going? That's what scriptures do.

It's not only our ancient tales that can inform. Living scriptures are all around us, in poetry and prose. These sources include an even broader representation of voices and perspectives than traditional texts ever did. As we discussed in Chapter 7 on music, we have an amazing selection in the Arcana Americana—the book of redemption songs forged in the American experience. Gospel, blues, jazz, country, folk, and hip-hop speak to suffering and renewal as powerfully as any tradition ever has. We have tales of woe, of heartache and loss, and of triumphant renewal and revival. That testimony belongs to the world now. The answers were always in our texts. Some of the best just happen to be set to music.

Deities

So far, in exploring our tool kit for ethical culture we've steered clear of the most obvious bone of contention—the gods themselves.

It's one thing to introduce a provisional metaphysics, suggest some ethical guidelines, sketch out a cadence for sacraments, and present a case for scripture. All together, they outline a framework for Meaning 3.0 that blends both of the versions that came before it. Whether you call it a transcendental humanism or a rational mysticism, it leaves that "god-shaped hole in our hearts" safely vacant.

But we've come this far. We should follow our query to its inevitable conclusion.

On the one hand, for true believers, suggesting that we have any say in our relationship to the Divine smacks of presumption. "Man proposes," Thomas à Kempis observed, "and God disposes." On the other hand, for committed skeptics, trying to rehabilitate gods that have justified so much superstition and suffering might seem like backsliding. Progress, for these folks, leads away from, not back to belief.

If media theorist Marshall McLuhan was right and "we become what we behold," we should pay attention to what we behold. Everybody worships, after all. The only question is what.

That notion of becoming and beholding predates McLuhan by thousands of years. Tibetan monks and nuns have advanced practices where they contemplate wrathful and benevolent deities. At first they meditate to understand the complex nature of consciousness and all of the subtle contours and variations of the Buddhist mindscape. Over time, these contemplatives try to take on the qualities of the deities themselves. Rather than worshipping these archetypes at an arm's-length third-person I-It remove, they pursue the intimate communion of the second-person I-Thou and even attain the singular first-person I-I realization. The deities just provide a road map.

This approach isn't confined to "exotic" mountain kingdoms of the East. The medieval Christian practice of veneration of the saints shares a similar structure. The devout would approach the altar of a patron saint, light votive candles, kneel, and pray. Over time, contemplating the story of this sainted self would allow an aspirant to take on more of those qualities themselves.

While Church fathers did their level best to discourage what they feared could descend into idolatry, they never stamped it out entirely. Local pagan gods went underground as the Church exerted its authority, only to bubble back up as patron saints for every occasion. The Black Madonna of Chartres is one example. The Virgin of Guadalupe in Mexico is another. Kali and the Corn Mother, dressed up in different garb.

Veneration, beholding, and becoming are essential spiritual tools that we're always reinventing and repurposing. This kind of syncretic mashup of culture—mixing, adding, and morphing over time—is how religion has always been done. It's created rich and varied ecologies of the divine—catalogs that have allowed seekers to find their own challenges and aspirations in the pantheon of their faith.

Despite the smuggling of pagan gods back into the Christian catalog, there's a unique bug in the code of Western monotheism that remains. It's responsible for much of our current fixation with rapture ideologies and why we find them so familiar and irresistible. If we're serious about updating our relationship to deities, we're going to have to fix it.

* * *

Not long ago, I was watching *American Gods,* an adaptation of Neil Gaiman's book about a clash between the Old Gods and the New Ones in the United States. In a flashback, a colonial-era Irishwoman is visited by a leprechaun, and she thanks him for all the good things the faerie folk had bestowed over her life. He replies, "Oh, good and ill, we're like the wind, we blow both ways."

And that got me thinking about something Princeton religious scholar Elaine Pagels wrote about the origins of evil in the Western world. Pagels is one of the world's leading scholars on the Judeo-Christian tradition, and was part of the team at Oxford that translated the Gnostic Gospels of the Nag Hammadi scrolls. But she also unearthed some deep cuts from the Old Testament and found something fascinating in the book of Job.

The famous story of Job is the one in which God and Satan make a bet about the allegiance of this unlucky man, and then Satan kicks the living shit out of him to prove he's only faithful when things go his way. Job shakes his fist at God. Yahweh bows up on him. Satan laughs.

Except that's not actually how it happened—and how it did happen has set the stage for most of Western metaphysics and our current Intertwingularity. Like many classic constructions, the story of Job was started at one point by an original author and then added to and modified over time. What we take as Job's seamless narrative was actually cobbled together over the centuries.

It turns out that in the original formulation, it was only Yahweh and Job, and no Satan to be found. (And before we got Dante and the Romantics merging Lucifer with Satan, Beelzebub, and all things big-time baddy, *S'tan* meant the Adversary, or the One Who Opposes. Think of him more as a plot device than as evil incarnate—Satan doesn't appear anywhere in the Hebrew Bible in the way we think of him today.)

So the story of Job Author #1 had a plot problem—if the God of Abraham was simultaneously all-powerful and all-good, then why on earth would He do all these horrible things to poor old Jobey? It didn't pencil out. God was either all-powerful but kind of a dick, or He was all-good, and could never be so vengeful. In the twentieth century, this became known as "the Auschwitz problem"—namely, how could an omnipotent and omni-benevolent deity stand by and allow for the horrors of the gas chambers or Hiroshima?

Story of Job Author #2 felt the same, so in order to resolve this impossible plot tension, he invented a new character—*Satan*—and inserted an existential rant from Job in the middle of the tale that would have made Camus proud. It was an innocent fix to an obvious problem. Now God got to keep on keeping on in the all-powerful/all-good category, while the dirtiest deeds got outsourced to a villain. Problem solved.

Except, really, all it did was kick the can down the road a few thousand years and leave us with a massive theological hangover. Everyone from Saint Paul to Saint Augustine to Immanuel Kant and David Hume wrestled with it. They had to do backflips to explain the inexplicable.

It's really important to note here that this isn't usually how the gods roll. The Judeo-Christian monotheistic all-powerful/all-good setup was a radical mutation of the Pantheon. That's the bug in the code we need to fix if we're going to reboot Olympus.

If you think back to your Greek myths, Zeus, Hera, Hermes, Aphrodite, and the gang could help or harm humans, pretty much on their whim. The gods were petty, jealous, vengeful, prideful, powerful, creative, courageous, honorable, mischievous, and petulant. In other words, a whole lot like the humans who worshiped them. "Greeks who worshipped such gods had no need for Satan *since their prophets never claimed that their gods were unequivocally good*," Pagels explains [emphasis added].

Same with Odin and the Norse gods, same with the faerie folk of the Celts. Never can tell which way the Divine is gonna break—for or against you. "Like the wind, we blow both ways," quoth the leprechaun.

Same in indigenous traditions—Trickster gods abound. From Anansi and Iktomi to Coyote and Brer Rabbit, to their cartoon descendant Bugs Bunny, the Trickster is there to help us when we need it most, but to punk us silly when we need the reality check. Or sometimes, just because they feel like it.

"For if we believe that an all-powerful God created a 'very good' world, what happened to it?" Pagels wondered after she lost both her son and her husband to tragic deaths in the span of a year. "While the Buddha declared as his first noble truth that 'all life is suffering,' *Jewish and Christian theologians speak of 'the problem of suffering' as if suffering and death were not intrinsic elements of nature but alien intruders on an originally perfect creation*" [emphasis added].

In the weird way that philosophical legacies work, that simple move—cleaving good and evil neatly into two separate camps—gave us the seeds of late nineteenth-century mystical New Thought, which begat Norman Vincent Peale and the Power of Positive Thinking, which begat the New Age, which kind of brings us to our present Conspirituality moment, where growing numbers of us are stitching together outlandish mythologies in place of meaningful responses to a world going off the rails.

In these formulations, we refuse to accept that sometimes life is random, that sometimes good things happen to shitty people and sometimes shitty things happen to good people (karma be damned). If we refuse to acknowledge the Trickster element in life, then we have to go to almost insane, and occasionally pathological, lengths to prop up our Just So Stories where *everything happens for a reason*.

That's why rapture ideologies prove so tempting—they offer, in one seductive move, a resolution to all that impossible plot tension, where we look around a world that's making less and less sense every day, but somehow, naively, still insist that it's supposed to. Or that it ever did.

"There is no way to suppress change . . . not even in heaven," Lewis Hyde wrote in his book *Trickster Makes This World*. "Those who panic and bind the Trickster choose the [path of control and cataclysm]. It would be better to learn to play with him, better especially to develop skills (cultural, spiritual, artistic) that allow some commerce with accident, and some acceptance of the changes that contingency will always engender."

So instead of insisting that our gods are all-powerful and all-good, while shunting the unavoidable suffering of life onto shadowy forces of evil, can we heed the leprechaun's warning: Sometimes the Divine goes our way, sometimes it doesn't. And figuring out the Why behind that is beyond the ken of mortal folk. Instead, can we keep on doing our best to take radical responsibility for our lives and our part in the bigger scheme, but also hold it all loosely, and be as wary of false certainty as any other false idol?

* * *

So while many in the Spiritual But Not Religious camp may feel that they've outgrown belief in gods, there is a functional psychotechnology worth returning to. Much in the same way the flyover effect changed astronauts' perspective of life on this planet, contemplating deities can change our experience of life as we live it.

"We shape our tools," Marshall McLuhan went on to say, "and our tools shape us." In this instance, he wasn't thinking big enough. Our gods may have shaped us, but we also shape our gods. We may be in their image, but invariably they are also in ours. And if we forget to imbue our gods with a Trickster's sense of humor, to remind us that life is equal parts tragic, magic, and comic, the joke will inevitably be on us.

CHAPTER 14

Team Omega

All that crying won't do you no good (come on up to the House)
Get down off the cross, we could use the wood (come on up to the House)

—Tom Waits

The Jesus Meme

When I was a young and broke graduate student in Boulder, Colorado, my best cheap entertainment was to go to the local bookstore. I'd buy a bottomless cup of coffee and browse the aisles for random finds. One night, a local professor, Rabbi Zalman Schacter, was giving a free talk upstairs, so I dropped by.

Schacter was recounting his story as a young Hasidic rabbi in Manitoba, Canada. After discovering what he called "the sacramental value of lysergic acid" in 1962, he left his tradition to explore Buddhism, Sufism, and all things countercultural. Those were the days for that sort of thing and Schacter had jumped in willingly.

But then, on a trip to the Wailing Wall in Old Jerusalem, he found himself in a crisis of faith. He prayed for Divine guidance about whether he should pursue the teachings of the Buddha or commit to his practice as a Sufi mystic. Every time he asked, the voice in his head kept saying, "But, Zalman, you're a Jew!" He'd dodge, putting up an argument why Buddha or Allah had more relevance, or how communal hippie living was closer to true communion. The voice would return: "But, Zalman, you're a Jew!"

Eventually, he relented, returned to the United States, and started the Jewish Renewal movement. It brought updated Hasidic and kabbalistic elements back into the liturgy along with song, dance, mysticism, and meditation from other world traditions. In his own small way, his interfaith explorations had allowed him to return to his own lineage with fresh eyes and to reinvigorate it for himself and thousands of others.

He was funny, engaging, and full of beans. I identified with his rejection of his own tradition and his yearning for beliefs that felt more interesting, less corrupted, and more true than what he'd inherited. I went home, grabbed a beer, put on some music, and sat on the ratty futon that passed as our couch. Out of nowhere, staring at my own Wailing Wall, tears began to stream down my face.

I realized that despite my relentless study of everything non-European—Taoism, Buddhism, Sufism, and Native American culture, I was irrevocably steeped in the Judeo-Christian tradition. My mother was an Easter and Christmas Anglican, my father a reluctant atheist who tagged along to church when he had to. After leaving England as a kid, I'd been dumped in Catholic school, so I'd spent ten years observing their strange customs too—from First Communion, to Confession, to the macabre Stations of the Cross.

No matter how low a regard I held it in, all of my experiences, all of the coming-of-age stories I loved, from *One Flew Over the Cuckoo's Nest* to *Cool Hand Luke* to *Stranger in a Strange Land*, were steeped in the idiom of the tragic, sacrificial hero. It was the dominant motif of Western scripture, art, and music for two thousand years of history.

I couldn't escape it if I'd wanted to. If we're honest, none of us can. Believers or not.

That's what I wept for that night. The futility of pretending I even had a choice.

I realized that the Buddha was too transcendent to ever fully grab me. Effortless, graceful, inscrutable, he was like the Roger Federer of enlightenment. Siddhartha was a trust-fund prince who'd thrown it all away to seek enlightenment and found it. Then he beamed up to the mother ship while sitting under a massive fig tree. His *ethos*—his philosophical insight—was awesome, but his *pathos*—his painful lived experience—was, for me, a little lacking. I could not locate my own doubts, alienation, and confusion in his flawless performance.

Lao-tzu, the mythical Taoist sage, seemed like a dim legend. He arrived in those tales fully formed—a laughing mystic, with no particular details on how he got to where he was. Like the Dude in the Coen brothers' film *The Big Lebowski*, Lao-tzu just abides. Timeless. Steeped in the Way. Any suffering in this world is merely a lack of alignment to the Tao. All grace comes from surrender to It. As much as I still find Taoism indispensable while chasing flow in the mountains and oceans, I found it less helpful as a guide through the nitty-gritty of my own confused life on the flats.

If Buddha and Lao-tzu felt too transcendent and ahistorical for me, Muhammad felt too immanent and historical. He was a warlord, a general, and a brilliant strategist, after all. Like Sherman on his Civil War march to the sea, Muhammad's armies decimated their opponents. His laws were medieval and sparingly updated. I found the ecstatic writings of Hafez and Jalāl ad-Dīn Rūmī predictably inspired, but I did not especially resonate with the dictates of their broader faith.

That said, I had even less time for the bureaucratic platitudes and starchy observances of mainline Christianity. Even a brief reading of history revealed centuries of ruthless control and corruption, cloaked in the name of God. And in my own life experience, the church ladies on Sunday, the pervy priests fondling the altar boys, the lying and cheating schoolkids banking on Wednesday's confession to absolve them—none of it felt like home either.

Then I read Princeton professor Elaine Pagels's National Book Award–winning title *The Gnostic Gospels*. As one of the original translators of the Nag Hammadi scrolls at Oxford, she'd had a ringside seat in uncovering the forgotten gospels of Thomas, Magdalene, and others. And while New Age fabulists and pulp fiction like *The Da Vinci Code* have run wild speculating about esoteric Christianity, Pagels offered something else: a meticulous, scholarly examination of original texts and their implications for the first-century Church.

In case after case, Pagels showed how the pillars of the faith—ranging from the primacy of the pope and the bishops, to the miracle of transubstantiation, to the Virgin Birth—all stemmed from fierce battles for the power and direction of the organization. What I'd assumed was theological actually turned out to be political. That crack in the foundations gave me an opening to reconsider my experience.

Because what Pagels showed was that there really wasn't a singular and definitive historical Jesus. Our understandings of him and what he represented were irreducibly mediated through human interest and historical context.

Was he the divine Son of God, sent to earth to free us of our Original Sin? Was he a mortal man who became enlightened? Or a regular dude who didn't? Was he a fictional construct—a convenient grab bag of Middle Eastern solar gods and mystery cults? Or was he a cipher, an allegory cloaking a mystic's initiatory instructions? Was he really ever here at all?

So much blood and ink have been spilled trying to litigate these questions—typically with far more certainty and less curiosity than is helpful. But what if we've all been fundamentally missing the point in our striving for certainty, pro or con?

Because what is beyond doubt is that the *idea* of Jesus, the Jesus Meme, which includes all versions—god, man, and myth—has shaped the last two thousand years of human history more than almost any other human who has ever lived. That in itself, in all of its ambiguity, is worth a real reckoning.

Sure, there are flukes of history that changed the course of events. Emperor Constantine's conversion threw the weight of the Holy Roman Empire behind what might have fizzled as one more Jewish sect. The unlikely dominance of European colonialism spread those ideas around the world at the point of the sword. Without those simple twists of fate, maybe we wouldn't remember the fellow at all. But they did happen, and we do remember.

That was the other thing I learned from reading Pagels—the prospect that buried underneath two millennia of all-too-human bureaucracy, dogma, and politics lay a hidden tradition of personal illumination. And it represents one of the more significant chapters in the timeless struggle between the Priests and the Prometheans. Only in this case, the Priests were represented by Paul and the early Church fathers, and the Prometheans were the original initiates of Christ consciousness—the Gnostics. Stealing fire from the gods, and getting nailed for their troubles.

The Gnostics, alight with passion and I-I, and I-Thou experience of the divine, ran a somewhat unconventional growth strategy. They believed in the maxim "by their fruits ye shall know them" and membership was self-selecting by the light in someone's words and deeds. Women were often leaders and preachers. Art, music, and even sacred sexuality were common. They were mystic seekers, not institution builders.

But Paul and the orthodox Church fathers had a different approach. They cannily realized that if you only admitted those touched by the Holy Spirit, you'd never get anywhere. Instead, their growth strategy was closer to the dime-store motto "stack 'em deep, sell 'em cheap." Let everyone in, Jew and Gentile, regardless of spiritual attainment, and be sure to pass the collection plate. ABC. *Glengarry Glen Ross* style. Always Be Collecting. Heaven can wait.

That was the fork in the road they never told us about in Sunday school. We ended up with organized Christianity while the Christed

Ones got left by the wayside. That's not to say that two thousand years of organized religion is bankrupt or that it never produced genuine believers or served as powerful social glue. It did and it does.

But it is to say that way back in its earliest days, Christianity faced a schism between doctrinal authority and experiential liberation that has gone on to shape history and belief ever since. And maybe it's time to backtrack and consider that road less traveled.

* * *

Because let's face it—Christianity has some god-awful branding problems. For the faithful, there's still some meat on that bone. But for the unchurched, twice shy, or followers of different faiths? It's slim pickings trying to gin up enthusiasm for a Christian revival. It would be a mistake to even try.

But it would be an even bigger mistake to scrap it entirely. The Jesus Meme has been virally replicating for two thousand years. It's created a tremendous amount of momentum, resonance, and shared reference points recognized around the world.

What sticks with me most about the story of the Nazarene has little to do with canonical scripture at all. I've ended up reading most of the Bible, but in snippets from Shakespeare to Dante to Dylan. Samson and Delilah. Lot's wife. Cain whacking Abel. Abraham and Isaac down on Highway 61. Palm Sundays. Last Suppers.

Often, when you trace those allusions back to the original scripture there's only a couple of obscure lines of text. None of the drama, side characters, or color we remember. Do that often enough and you realize something—the text has been a leaping-off point for centuries, into art, song, and story—and that part of the Judeo-Christian tradition isn't constrained to the faithful—it's everyone's legacy. It truly belongs to the world now.

So, if the bad news is, we're almost out of time in a world devoid of Meaning. The Good News is that some of the answers have been right in front of us all along.

We'd be crazy not to make the most of that fact.

All Those at the Banquet

That problem of Christianity's lousy branding haunted me ever since that night with the rabbi. I kept finding myself drawn to the archetype of the Nazarene, and at the same time, repelled by much of what the organization founded in his name had to offer. I felt trapped, a confused and closeted mystic christic.

The idea that a flesh-and-blood mortal could feel a burning truth inside them, and seek to share it with the world, despite the betrayal and ridicule of those they were trying to help, while having to face personal doubt, despair, and uncertainty alone? That sounded more like the human experience we all have to live through than any of the more transcendent tales I'd found elsewhere.

Even stranger, the metaphors for "living a Christed life" that resonated with me most strongly—the ones that touched my heart when I was broken and gave me some encouragement to go on—weren't even Christian at all. But they seemed to embody the essence of those teachings better than anything I'd heard in parochial school.

Pema Chodron, the Tibetan Buddhist nun, writes in *When Things Fall Apart*, "To be fully alive, fully human, and completely awake is to be continually thrown out of the nest. . . . *To live is to be willing to die over and over again.*" Now that, I could wrap my head around. It established uncertainty and annihilation as a baseline, a sign that all was right, rather than that something was wrong.

Leonard Cohen, a Zen Jew, writes in his song "Anthem," "Ring the bells that still can ring / Forget your perfect offering / There is a crack, *a crack in everything / That's how the light gets in.*" Those lyrics gave me goose bumps. Instead of waging war on the broken parts of myself, Cohen offered permission to celebrate the woundings.

This whole Grace and Grit riff, testifying to the enduring human spirit, isn't just a Western concept. The Japanese have two related terms that speak to this sense of redemption within imperfection—*Wabi Sabi*, "flawed beauty," and *Kintsugi*, the art of repairing broken pottery with golden glue. Wabi Sabi is a philosophy of the imperfection and impermanence of all things, and how life is made even more exquisite by that realization.

Kintsugi takes that abstract philosophy and grounds it in the material, highlighting the uniqueness of each vessel's brokenness. It renders Cohen's "light getting in through the cracks" visible and celebrates it. Halle-fuckin'-lujah.

The Chinese have a version of their own. They call it *Chongxi.* "Chong" means to rinse out, and "xi" is joy. So chongxi is literally "joy bathing"—the belief that you can wash away misfortune with joy. Connecting ecstatic redemption to cathartic suffering appears to be an essential part of cultural immune systems everywhere—a map to find our way home.

Alice Walker, a sometime Buddhist and unrepentant pagan, writes about how marginalized African American artists used to greet each other in Jim Crow Atlanta. "'All those at the banquet!' they'd say and shake hands or hug. Sometimes they said this laughing and sometimes they said it in tears, but that they were all at the Banquet of Life was always affirmed."

Nearly everywhere you look around the world, you hear echoes of this theme. Life is hard, but beautiful. It's tragic and magic at the same time. We get knocked down, as the song goes, but we get back up again. That doesn't belong to any singular tradition, but it's sustenance we could all do with more of. All those at the banquet. All those at the banquet of life.

Hurtling Toward the Omega Point

There's a starman waiting in the sky
He's told us not to blow it
'Cause he knows it's all worthwhile

—David Bowie

One of the most interesting examples of a truly global mythology comes from renegade Jesuit priest Teilhard de Chardin. He felt compelled to bridge the worlds of faith and science but so thoroughly upset the Church fathers that they exiled him from his native France to China.

Many of his most controversial writings were banned until after his death. There were "such ambiguities and indeed even serious errors, as to offend Catholic doctrine," one Church communiqué read. We must "protect the minds, particularly of the youth, against the dangers presented by the works of Father Teilhard de Chardin."

But he was also a paleontologist who loved to dig up the bones of the ancient past. He helped unearth the prehistoric Peking Man in China and helped excavate the Piltdown Man in England (later revealed to be a hoax). Although he earned the praise of evolutionary biologist Julian Huxley (Aldous's brother), Teilhard's grand theories regularly upset biologists and physicists. Some of his ideas overreached or didn't hold up to developments in science or theology. Many academics dismissed him as a poetic kook.

Despite being shunned by the very gatekeepers of Faith and Reason that he was trying to unite, Teilhard captured the imagination of generations of writers and artists.

Science fiction writer and accidental mystic Philip K. Dick references him, as do Annie Dillard, Arthur C. Clarke, Flannery O'Connor, and Don DeLillo. Surrealist painter Salvador Dalí created his giant masterpiece *The Ecumenical Council* inspired by Teilhard's redemptive vision for the end of history.

For over half a century, his attempt to situate human evolution in the context of a cosmic unfolding has resonated widely. Judeo-Christian doctrine had the "in the Beginning" Alpha point down cold. Things got fuzzier when it came to the "at the End" Omega Point. Sure, there were the unhinged ravings of John of Patmos in the book of Revelation, but they spoke of a brute interruption to human history rather than an elegant culmination. There were Seventh-day Adventists and others, waiting around for the Second Coming, but those hoped-for due dates came and went. Time after time.

That's not how Teilhard saw it. In addition to the biosphere of all living things, and the atmosphere wrapping our planet, he intuited another element—the *noosphere*—literally the realm of mind. Back in the early twentieth century, that sort of notion seemed abstract, even mystical to readers. Today, in the age of nearly limitless digital information, instant memes, and perpetually connected humanity, the notion of a "realm of shared mind" isn't hypothetical anymore. The noosphere—our globally connected always-on shared mind space—supports seven of the top ten most valuable companies on the planet. Fiber-optic cables and Wi-Fi are our shared neurons. Bits and bytes are the new alphabet of our digital logos.

Teilhard imagined that across the arc of evolution we were becoming increasingly aware of both our individuality and our connectedness. The noosphere was growing. Over time, he saw that growth culminating at the Omega Point—literally the end of history.

"If the cooperation of some thousands of millions of cells in our brain can produce our capacity for consciousness," he wrote, "the idea becomes vastly more plausible that some kind of cooperation of humanity as a whole or a fraction of it may determine what [philosopher Auguste] Comte called a Great Superhuman Being."

He called this process of us becoming a Great Superhuman Being "Christogenesis." Literally, us becoming the body of Christ, together. Crucially, for our modern sense of individualism, Teilhard did not see this as a merging with some impersonal Borg or group mind. In fact, he saw the exact opposite. He envisioned the Omega Point as a simultaneous celebration of our uniqueness and our connectedness.

"The concentration of a conscious universe would be unthinkable if it did not assemble in itself . . . *every consciousness . . . remaining conscious of itself at the end of the operation . . .*" Teilhard writes, "each one becoming more itself and therefore more distinct from the others the closer it comes to them in Omega."

If we're trying to articulate an open-source Meaning 3.0 that provides universal scaffolding to build from, while honoring the uniqueness of different cultures, customs, and communities, this feels like a helpful framework to consider. The more we connect, the more we can, and even must preserve our differences. Mystical pluralism. Transcendental humanism. Anything more decisive risks a decline into fascism over time.

The Vietnamese Buddhist teacher Thich Nhat Hanh echoed this idea when he wrote, "The next Buddha will be a Sangha," meaning that the next Great Awakening would not be led by an individual avatar (a Buddha or a Jesus). Instead it would take the form of a dedicated community—the Sangha. This version of our salvation is collective and inclusive.

What happens, after all, when we grow up and stop waiting for a Second Coming? What happens when we're able to usher in the *Umpteenth* Coming—where so many people heed the call that there's nothing exceptional about it anymore? In these versions, the body of Christ, at the End of Time, is the whole lot of us.

Rapturists often fantasize that this Omega moment will be an eleventh-hour redemption that saves us from our impossible fate. It's a temptingly tidy fix for a bunch of wicked problems. Teilhard wasn't so optimistic. Even if we could solve the monkey puzzle of existence before we blow ourselves up, he wasn't sure everyone would come along for the ride.

"Will there be refusal or acceptance of Omega?" he wondered. "A conflict may be generated . . . the noosphere would cleave into two zones attracted respectively towards two antagonistic poles of adoration. . . . Universal love ultimately vitalizing and detaching only a fraction of the noosphere to consummate it—the fraction which will have decided to 'take the step' out of itself into the Other."

This matches closely to what we explored in Part One of this book— about the split between those committed to the global-centric Infinite Game and the ethnocentric Finite Game. The Infinite Game—which recognizes everyone's right to play and seeks to extend the Game to more and more players—is a practical expression of what Teilhard calls "Universal Love." Those who refuse to take that step and remain separate will be advocates of the Finite Game, who seek to win while others lose, and keep the spoils of the game for themselves.

This notion of some people stepping up to the task, while others are unwilling or unable, fits neatly on top of psychologist Abraham Maslow's pyramid of development. His model begins with basic survival needs at the base, narrowing as it goes up through individuation,

belonging, and actualization, all the way to Self-Transcendence—
which reflects a return to simple service of others.

Teilhard's notion of Christogenesis can really be seen as the final
step of Self-Transcendent people coming together around a shared
desire to help. In that light, the notion of a mythopoetic Omega Point
is really just a final flourish on what are broadly accepted stages of human development. It only sounds magical because so few of us have
gotten there yet.

This notion of a small group, "a fraction of the noosphere," to effect transformational change is echoed in the political sciences. Erica
Chenoweth at Harvard's Kennedy School has famously posited that
historic civil rights movements have required 3.5 percent of a population to reach a tipping point of transformation. For current environmental and social justice movements that number has taken on
almost mythical significance.

Skeptics have suggested that the large-scale interconnected crises we are facing today may present an order-of-magnitude greater
challenge than the prior case studies that Chenoweth based her work
upon. It's one thing, after all, to firmly insist on your right to sit at the
front of a bus that has enough gas in the tank to make it to its destination on time. It's another to try to transform that same bus into a
helicopter just as it sails off a cliff.

But since we're nowhere near amassing even 3.5 percent of
Omegans—truly surrendered humans joyfully committed to expand-
ing the Infinite Game—it seems like a decent milestone to shoot for.
Let's get there as fast as possible and take stock once we make it.

As we hurtle toward the final reckoning of the Omega Point, Teilhard envisioned exactly how it would all go down—a race of three intersecting curves: the viability of the planet, those drawn to inclusion,
and those dedicated to separation.

"In this hypothesis which conforms more closely to the apocalyptic
traditions," Teilhard suggested, "three curves would perhaps continue
to arise around us simultaneously in the future: the inevitable reduction of the organic possibilities of earth, [and] the internal schism of

consciousness as it becomes increasingly more divided over two opposing ideals of evolutionary movement."

In some kind of Cosmic Crisscross Crash, we'd be on the edge of our seats right until the last minute, unsure precisely how it's all going to turn out. "The Earth would end at the triple point where . . . these three curves would meet and reach their maximum at exactly the same moment," he proposes. "The death of the planet, materially exhausted; the tearing apart of the noosphere, divided over what form its unity should take, and *simultaneously, giving the event its whole significance and value,* the freeing of that percentage of the universe which has succeeded in laboriously synthesizing itself across time, space and evil to the very end."

You've got to hand it to the old Jesuit. He wasn't wrong. Scan the headlines today, rife with updates of shrinking icecaps, raging fires and pandemics, bitter civil unrest and social media flame wars, and we sure seem to be right on time for the End of Time. And those three curves—of planetary stability, Infinite Gamers, and Finite Gamers—are getting down to the absolute wire. We're not slouching toward Bethlehem anymore, we're hurtling toward it.

For those of us raised on Mount Doom and Mordor, X-wings and Death Stars, Muggles and Death Eaters, that feels about right. We're hardwired for tales of rebel misfits, at the eleventh hour and against all odds, saving the galaxy from overwhelming evil. Anything less of a nail biter, and it would hardly qualify as a worthy ending to the Greatest Story Ever Told.

So we've got that going for us.

Practice Resurrection

If we accept Teilhard's proposition—that the End of Time *might* culminate in some profound recognition of our shared humanity—the question is where to find that Omega Point. Our GPS won't cut it. The Omega Point, if it exists at all, will almost certainly lie way beyond where the sidewalk ends. It will be closer to finding Neverland. As Peter Pan reminds Wendy, the only way to get there is to follow the directions, "second star to the right, and straight on 'til morning."

Our GPS may not be able to help, but our CPS—our Cosmic Positioning System—might. And once we upgrade our navigational software, we find that the Omega Point has very specific coordinates. The corner of Everywhen and Neverwas. The intersection of Kairos and Chronos.

The ancient Greeks defined two very different types of time. Chronos is linear, discrete clock time. Marching inexorably from past to present to future. A horizontal move through space. We're all overly acquainted with Chronos these days—never enough of it, life ripping by in the rearview mirror. Frantic and bored at the same time. And no matter how successful or regretful we feel, never able to get any of it back.

The ancients also expressed the notion of Kairos, or sacred time, the Deep Now. It includes all instantiations, pastpresentfuture bundled into one seamless and sanctified moment. Kairos is life back in the Garden—outside linear time and its relentless march toward entropy and decay. Kairos is the vertical "axis mundi"—the World Pole on which our chrono-logical crossbeam hangs.

Buried deep in the esoteric traditions is a little-known interpretation of that intersecting crossroads. It's held by Rosicrucians (literally, those of "the Rosy Cross"), Gnostics, and even other Abrahamic religions like Islam that hold the "cruci-fiction" not as a literal description of a death sentence but as an allegory for the excruciating act of becoming an Omegan.

Christogenesis, in this hidden tradition, is only attained by the willing decision to hold oneself open to the timelessness of Kairos while remaining anchored to the fleetingness of Chronos. And to do it with an aching, beating heart right there at the crossroads of both.

This distinguishes the Omegans from the rapturists we've already discussed. Rather than trying to escape this human condition, Omegans submit to it. But they do so not in grim resignation or in forgetting their true nature—they do it while holding both, willingly.

And in completing that impossible task, they are transfigured into twice-born humans, or as Yale's Harold Bloom calls them, *anthropos*.

That juxtaposition—of being in the world (Chronos) but not of it (Kairos), is both the best and worst thing about the human condition: the blinding light and joy of peak experience followed by the inevitable return to the constraints of our flawed existence. It's a never-ending oscillation. And getting pulled between those two poles is both agony and ecstasy. Catharsis and Ecstasis. It's the Hegelian Dialectic to end all dialectics. Call it the Blissfuck Crucifiction. Scandalous, but accurate.

But getting unstuck in Time isn't easy. We are welded to Chronos. Our egos, our identity, our suffering, our pride, all of our fallible seeking, striving, yearning, craving humanness binds us to the mortal coil. Like getting to Platform 9¾ to catch the Hogwarts Express, you've got to risk smashing into a brick wall to make it to the other side. Because the nonnegotiable ticket price to get to Kairos? Dying.

Physical death is the most obvious, clumsy, and irreversible option to sideslip the gravitational pull of Chronos. Those who are lucky enough to have had a near-death experience often report glimpsing life outside of regular clock time. Its impact is often profound. But risking dying to finally feel alive is a fool's errand. Not safe, repeatable, or scalable.

We mentioned before how Tibetans have tried another approach. They spend their entire lives meditating and contemplating that mortal threshold in the belief that if they can cross it without flinching, they will get to step off the wheel of incarnation and suffering for good. But that's a lot of up-front commitment for one at bat. What if, after forty years of devout practice, you slip on the proverbial banana peel or get hit by that ever-lethal bus? What then?

Cantankerous poet and farmer Wendell Berry has a different suggestion.

> Expect the end of the world . . . Be joyful
> though you have considered all the facts . . .
> *Practice* resurrection.

That verse is inscrutable and provocative. "Be joyful, though you have considered all the facts" speaks to the freedom that comes from grieving fully and coming out the other side. It's a paradox reconciled.

But if we took his advice literally, how can we *practice* resurrection?

*   *   *

In the most literal way, we have to learn to get over ourselves. "If we can forgive what's been done to us," *Fight Club* author Chuck Palahniuk writes, "if we can forgive what we've done to others . . . if we can leave our stories behind. Our being victims and villains. Only then can we maybe rescue the world."

It's only when we die to our stories, our hopes, our fears, our pleasure, our pain, that we can glimpse what lies beyond all of them. Over the course of our lives, we catalog our stories, rehash our grievances, nurse our wounds, and justify our separation.

But that's just pride talking. Not the obvious posturing of "too cool for school" pride—but another more insidious sort. The pride of our suffering, our uniquely and Especially Important Difference. "Proud people," Emily Brontë observed, "breed sad sorrows for themselves."

We've spent so long meticulously collecting the stories of our grief, and using them as a shield against showing up fully, that when it comes time to toss them on the fire, we often hesitate.

Like the wife of Lot fleeing Sodom, turned to salt because she looked behind her. Like Orpheus unable to resist a backward glance into hell as he rescued his love, Eurydice—we can't help but second-guess grace and fuck it up right on the brink of redemption.

Because here's the thing about Kairos: If we make it, even for a moment, we realize that we're back in the Garden again. To try to measure that in chronological units—whether moments, minutes, or months—is irrelevant, and the wrong yardstick entirely. If we've spent even a second in Eternity, it's as good as Forever. There's no splitting Infinity.

Case in point: A decade ago my mother turned seventy. We had the whole family together on a lake in the Blue Ridge Mountains of Virginia, where we'd been going for decades to camp, fish, and water-ski. For a family of military brats and orphans whose lives had been stretched across three continents, this was as close to the Old Homeplace as we were ever going to get.

On that celebration night, we pulled out all the stops, erecting a giant dome tent, stringing it with lanterns and banners; music, smoked salmon, champagne—the whole bit. The matriarch of our clan was turning a milestone birthday and it felt appropriate to honor her with an epic bash.

Then as the sun was going down, my mother did something unexpected. Perhaps a little tipsy, or just officially out of birthday fucks, she went down to the dock, dropped off all her clothing, and jumped in the lake.

She'd been known to skinny-dip in the past, but typically years ago and under the discreet cover of darkness. We filtered down to the dock, and without any conversation or debate, we all took off our clothes and jumped in with her. Three generations of our family, from toddlers to elders, all splashing around in the lake, naked as the day we were born. Nothing like this had ever happened before, or since. It was an utter one-off of uninhibited joyful expression for a family of stuffy Brits.

As the sun set, a crescent moon hung there, perfectly above the trees. We were all laughing so hard it was difficult to tread water and stay afloat. The air felt liquid and full. The stars sparkled. After forty-five minutes of playing, splashing, and joking, we got out, hugged each other, and made our way to bed.

The next day, driving my brother to the airport, we looked back on it. "What happened last night?" I asked him. "I don't know," he said, "but that seemed like a state of family Grace for sure."

A month later my parents traveled back to England. A year later, almost to the day, my mother was dead of a cancer that had been secretly riddling her body for years. That skinny-dip birthday party was the last time we were all together, and it was the best time we'd ever had.

While it was tempting to wring our hands and lament our loss, the shining perfection of that evening didn't dwindle. It left us in awe, that if even for one moonlit swim, we had been together, in love with each other and with life. That's Kairos. To second-guess it, or to want more of it once you've tasted it, borders on ungrateful.

*   *   *

When Saint Paul said, "Love keeps no record of wrong," he wasn't talking about maternal forgiveness or romantic second chances. He was talking about Kairos. He was pointing the way toward the Omega Point.

If we are lucky enough to find or fumble our way to Kairos, the only thing to do is to drop to our knees and weep with gratitude. There's no second-guessing redemption. And that means there's no second-guessing the rocky road that got us there *either*. Our deepest wounds, our darkest nights, our hardest trials are all redeemed in that unfolding.

Like the old hymn goes, "Through all the tumult and the strife, I hear that music ringing. It sounds an echo through my life, how can I keep from singing?"

Chapter 15

Pondering the Yonder

*He who does not know the secret "die and become" will
remain forever a stranger on this earth.*

—Goethe

Reverse-Engineering Revelation

For most of human history, when mystics had a revelation, they came
back out of the wilderness and told everyone all about it. From those
original lightning-bolt insights grew up customs, rituals, and taboos—
calcifying that initial experience until it was barely recognizable—
crushed under the weight of cultural baggage. When these experiences
were rare, poorly understood, and nearly impossible to replicate, it
made sense to cherish and even fetishize the few glimpses we did get.

But that's exactly backward from how we should be doing it
now. Rather than doubling down again and again trying to explain
the Sublime from here, why not give everyone a ticket to ride? Let
them go and see for themselves? It's an experimental and experiential

approach—essential if we're trying to create an open-source methodology that works for different people around the world.

If we're sincere about trying to architect a flexible and inclusive replacement for doctrinal religion, this reversal is a key step. Rather than telling people what to believe, based on a distant and non-repeatable founder's revelation, we can share the methods that prompt belief. And let everyone make up their own minds and hearts. That's what the Alchemist Cookbook can offer—a chance to turn thousands of years of religiosity on its head and replace it with self-authenticating techniques of ecstasy.

* * *

If we take a minute to go back to our earlier inquiry, which was "How might we redesign Meaning 3.0 so it was open-source, experiential, and experimental?" then there's a bold step we need to take for Omeganism to become a viable mythology.

And that's how to find the Omega Point reliably. We may have dropped a pin in the map at the intersection of Kairos and Chronos, but we still haven't figured out how to get us all there in one piece.

"There are a thousand ways to kneel and kiss the ground," Rūmī reminds us, "there are a thousand ways to go home again."

He's right. But we've only got one nervous system. And that's our royal road to redemption.

In our survey of the Big Five techniques—respiration, embodiment, sexuality, substances, and music—there's a deceptively simple recipe that comes up time and again.

Maximize endocannabinoids, endorphins, dopamine, nitric oxide, oxytocin, and serotonin.

Increase vagal nerve tone and heart rate variability.

Shift your brain into baseline alpha and theta activity, with dips into gamma or delta waves.

Trigger a global reset of your brain stem with compounds such as nitrous oxide or ketamine or cranial-nerve stimulation (all these correlate with delta wave EEG induction).

Load your nervous system with pulses of energy in the form of electrical current, magnetism, light, sound, pain, or orgasm.

Align your spine, and engage your pelvis, limbs, and fascia for flexible movement and integration.

Alter the ratios of oxygen, carbon dioxide, and nitrogen in your bloodstream through deliberate organic or gas-assisted breathwork.

Play high-fidelity polyrhythmic music that entrains you out of your default mode network and serves as a carrier wave of your subjective experience.

Experience anamnesis—remember what it is that you forgot.

Stay awake. Build stuff. Help out.

With these simple tools we can reliably engineer an ecstatic death practice. You can call it the Blissfuck Crucifiction if you're feeling poetic. Or the Sexual Yoga of Becoming if you're more practical. Or Erotocomatose Lucidity if you're old-fashioned. But what we call it is ultimately far less important than what it does. It offers a global systemic reboot of our nervous system, and with it, our psychology and notion of ourselves.

And while death/rebirth rituals are as old as humanity, from the shamanic initiations of indigenous peoples to the Eleusinian Mysteries of ancient Greece, up until now they've been largely metaphysical and metaphorical. Thanks to advances in neuroscience and psychology, we have a much deeper understanding of how to prompt an experience that has been shrouded in mystery and misunderstanding. What used to be metaphysical or metaphorical is now simply physiological.

That changes everything. If we hope to democratize Nirvana, we can't rely on hand-me-down descriptions; we have to be able to go and see for ourselves. Reading inspirational quotes or gazing longingly at images from the Hubble telescope isn't going to cut it. We need the launch codes for actual liftoff.

Crucially, that experience of gnostic death/rebirth initiation is content neutral. What you glimpse or understand in that rarefied state is yours and yours alone. The psychological narrative that you choose to run could be agnostic as you mull the infinite wonders of consciousness. It could be theistic, as you commune with the gods and angels of your pantheon. It could be aesthetic as you marvel at the fractal symmetries of your mind's eye. There's room for all of it on Team Omega.

Believe what you want to believe. Just never lose the Faith.

(And don't die wondering.)

In that instant of living, embodied truth, "faith" doesn't mean blindly following someone else's dogma or doctrine. It doesn't mean superstitious obedience to priests or sky gods. Instead, it's something closer to what the Quaker theologian and Stanford chaplain Elton Trueblood described: "Faith is not belief without proof, but *trust without reservation.*"

We come to that unreserved trust—in ourselves, in each other, and in the universe—somatically. We feel it in our hearts and bones, or not at all. That's the gift and power of a fully transformative ecstatic, cathartic experience. We get to not only say but truly mean: "This I remember, and today I begin again."

*   *   *

Because here's the thing about getting a glimpse of Kairos. Not only is it autotelic, it's *autodidactic.* Autotelic just means it has its own reason or motivation for doing. Like dolphins surfing waves, or kids rolling down hills—we do it for the sheer love of it. But that autodidactic part? That means it's self-teaching or self-disclosing.

The information in Kairos has an uncanny ability to feel utterly unique, incredibly timely, and often packing a wicked sense of humor. Why that might be, no one's really figured out. But that it is so, appears to be beyond doubt.

Too often, we can't resist personifying this intelligence, anthropomorphizing it, deifying it, reifying it. We're storytelling monkeys who cannot, will not, let the Mystery stay the Mystery. The moment someone collapses all of that potential into the false certainty of an explanation, we distort what it was, what it is, what it could be. Most times, it's better just to let the Burning Bush burn.

Information Theory

We are a way for the universe to know itself. Some part of our being knows this is where we came from. . . . We're made of star stuff.

—Carl Sagan

We should at least *ponder* the yonder, though. If we're considering entrusting our lives and our futures to its self-disclosing insights, we need to have a provisional understanding of where the information in Kairos comes from.

Without engaging in metaphysical guesswork, we can explore several explanations of the Information Layer that don't require leaps of faith. They represent reasonable inferences from established science. That's not to say any of these will turn out to be true. Advances in theory, measurement, and exploration will certainly replace them with more accurate models over time.

But it is to say that it's high time we move from the reductionist materialism of the New Atheists and their blanket dismissal of truths that don't submit to microscopes or telescopes. We'll also need to steer clear of the other extreme. If we succumb to untethered magical thinking, we'll only end up swapping out dusty old fundamentalism with newer, shinier versions of the same.

It's possible to update both of those stances with a rational mysticism—call it the New Platonism. It still values reason, evidence, and logic but also leaves room for what lies beyond our ken. When navigating through terrain with no familiar landmarks, we need to be more precise with our compass bearings, not less. After all, it's much easier to stay found than it is to get un-lost.

What follows are four explanations for where the information in peak states comes from, starting from the most empirical to the more conjectural . . .

EXPLANATION ONE: *The Umwelt Effect*

At all times, the raw data of reality is blowing past us at millions of bits per second. Most of that time, our regular waking consciousness, tuned and calibrated to the "overworked primate" setting, ignores nearly all of it. That's what Henri Bergson and Aldous Huxley called the "reducing valve of consciousness." Our conscious mind, for example, processes information at about 120 bits per second. Our retina processes up to 11 million bits. In a non-ordinary state, we expand that reducing valve and our *umwelt*—or the portion of reality that we can perceive expands with it. Hopped-up neurochemistry, hyperconnected neuroanatomy, and optimized neuroelectricity let us pick up on more of what's swirling past us every second anyway. It may seem supernatural, but really it's just more data. For a strict materialist, this is the leanest, most Occam's razor–ish explanation. "The universe is full of magic things," Eden Phillpotts wrote, "patiently waiting for our senses to grow sharper!" All peak states do, then, is sharpen our senses enough to perceive a little more of that magic.

EXPLANATION TWO: *The Ancestor Effect*

In the past decade, a slew of studies have traced markers of physical and mental health getting passed down from generation to generation.

From remote arctic villages in Sweden to the descendants of Confederate POWs, survivors of the Holocaust, and long-suffering lab mice, we have suggestive evidence that there's some form of legacy memory—both biological and psychological—that we inherit from our families.

The field of epigenetics is very much in its infancy, and researchers debate findings and methods with every newly published paper, but there's a lot we are already learning from it. For example, methylation, i.e., the ability of genes to turn on or off depending on real-world conditions, RNA, a single-strand nucleic acid that signals to DNA, and histones, the proteins that DNA is scaffolded onto, are possible mechanisms by which we "remember" past generations' experience. If, in non-ordinary states of consciousness, our *umwelt* expands, we might somehow access that accumulated experience more consciously.

That kind of ghostly intuition would seem magical and definitely beyond our own personal knowing—like using a Lifeline Call in the game show *Who Wants to Be a Millionaire?*, but to our dearly departed instead of friends back home. As far out as that sounds, it's very much in keeping with indigenous and traditional cultures, from Native Americans to the Greeks and the Japanese. They each have "ancestor cults" where they seek guidance from those who have come before. Extend that back through multiple generations, and there's a distinct possibility that we hold within us, however dimly, some form of ancestral knowing that goes beyond culture and stories, and into the core of our biology. The latest science provides a plausible explanation for how that might be happening.

EXPLANATION THREE: *The Starstuff*

We share about 97 percent of the crucial building blocks of life—carbon, hydrogen, nitrogen, oxygen, phosphorus, and sulfur—with the rest of the galaxy. As Joni Mitchell sang, "We are stardust." The raw materials of our bones, blood, and brains, the complex chemistry that fires our synapses and pumps our hearts, all come from the detritus of the Big Bang. We are that big, and that old.

In *Living with the Stars: How the Human Body Is Connected to the Life Cycles of the Earth, the Planets, and the Stars*, Stanford University professor Iris Schrijver concludes, "Everything we are and everything in the universe and on Earth originated from stardust, and it continually floats through us even today. It directly connects us to the universe, *rebuilding our bodies over and again over our lifetimes.*"

It's right there, in our DNA. Since Watson and Crick's initial discovery, we've understood that our DNA contained the basic coding of all living things. More recently, we've begun to understand precisely how well those double helixes hold and store incredible amounts of information—up to five million times more efficient than current methods.

Yaniv Erlich, at Columbia's Center for Computational Biology and Bioinformatics, says, "DNA has several big advantages . . . [it's] been around for 3 billion years and humanity is unlikely to lose its ability to read these molecules." One group at the University of Texas recently encoded *The Wizard of Oz* in the universal language Esperanto onto a DNA strand. George Church at Harvard has managed to encode the 1902 silent film *A Trip to the Moon* onto a double helix. These examples concretely demonstrate the two-way street that connects data stored on DNA to our own lives and stories. We've moved from the realm of thought experiment to physical experiment.

If we follow these threads, they lead to a potentially startling implication. We are made of starstuff and share the chemical makeup of the galaxy. That much is known. DNA, responsible for the programming of all life, can be both encoded and decoded. It not only tells a cell to grow into a heart or a leg or a tree, it can hold a movie or the collected works of Shakespeare. And much, much more than that. It is one of the most efficient and resilient storage systems possible, across time and space.

In heightened states of consciousness, where our nervous systems are primed to perceive patterns and access information that isn't normally accessible through waking awareness, is it possible that we can somehow "read" the information in our genetic DNA? And if we can, however clumsily or intuitively, decode that data, what story would it have to tell us?

In the beginning, I Am. Before the moon and the stars, I Am. Before Abraham (or Instagram), I AM.

Only in this thought experiment, the grand "I Am" is *us*. Encoded in our bodies, decoded by our brains, we find that we are literally the Alpha and Omega—we've been here all along. The raw materials of carbon, hydrogen, nitrogen, oxygen, phosphorus, and sulfur, the phosphates and sugars of the DNA strand make up all of life, and all of us. And the anamnesis—the forgetting of the forgetting that so often accompanies glimpses of Kairos—could be a remembering of that simple fact.

As Iris Schrijver acknowledges, "Very little of our physical bodies lasts for more than a few years. Of course, that's at odds with how we perceive ourselves. . . . But we're not fixed at all. We're more like a pattern or a process. . . . This transience of the body and the flow of energy and matter led us to explore our interconnectedness with the universe." In that stunning recognition, each of us can see ourselves as Omegans. But we'll have to die to the illusion of our individual separation to glimpse it.

EXPLANATION FOUR: *The Information Layer*

The first three explanations for where the information comes from have been, however hypothetical, still material. *Umwelts* and expanded data processing. Epigenetic signals passed down from parents. Our own DNA serving as a hard drive for the periodic table of the universe. All still taking place within our physical bodies and brains.

This final explanation goes beyond that and considers the notion of a non-local source of all that inspiration.

For as long as philosophers have thought about it, they've supposed that there is a realm of reality beyond what our *umwelt* or five senses can perceive. That realm, they'd insist, is more true, more complete than anything we live in our day-to-day. Plato called it the Realm of Ideal Forms. There, everything that we could ever experience exists first, in abstract, idealized perfection. An apple or a chair on this plane, according to Plato, is merely a partial representation of the original that lives in pristine suspended animation Out There.

Plato and later Western scholars also entertained the notion of the Aether—a kind of invisible background substance of the universe. The Aether was literally considered the substrate of all physical existence, serving as the carrier for everything from light to sound. But after centuries of consideration, Victorian physicists Michelson and Morley disproved this notion. Their refutation set the stage for Einstein's theories of relativity and much of contemporary physics that came after.

But thinkers kept reaching for some metaphor to describe their glimpses of the Information Layer. Buckminster Fuller called it the Design Realm and credited his prodigious output in the fields of architecture, sustainability, and futurism to his access to that domain. He was merely transcribing what already was, he humbly maintained, not inventing new things from whole cloth.

In the twenty-first century, Hungarian physicist Ervin László called this hypothetical realm the A-field, or Akashic field, after the Sanskrit term for space. For him, the quantum vacuum stretches across time and space and carries information with it. If and when we access that field, we gain entry to a world of incredibly dense, non-local data. Think of accessing the A-field as closer to surfing the internet instead of picking the *Encyclopaedia Britannica* off the shelf.

For most of the modern era, pondering the Information Layer—whether the aether, or the noosphere, or something with "quantum" in the front of its name—was a dodgy career prospect. Scientists risked almost certain ridicule and marginalization for even considering that there was a There there, beyond thin air. After Michelson and Morley, those kinds of musings were decidedly *non grata*.

But they've never entirely disappeared, either. Lately, we may be coming full circle on the whole "where does the information come from?" inquiry.

The notion that the information doesn't come from anywhere, but that it is present everywhere, is one of the more intriguing hypotheses in contemporary physics. While most scientists hold that the universe is made up of combinations of energy and matter, or even timespace, others hold that at its simplest expression, the universe *is information*.

Nineteenth-century mathematician Charles Babbage, polymath and inventor of the "Babbage Engine" proto-computer, was one of the first to assert that information was central and elemental. But it wasn't until the 1980s that physicist John Wheeler, member of the Manhattan Project, collaborator on Einstein's unified theory of physics, and coiner of the terms "black hole" and "wormhole," brought that idea up to date.

In the spring of 1989, at the Santa Fe Institute, Wheeler presented a paper introducing his concept of "Its from Bits." "It from Bit," Wheeler wrote, "symbolizes the idea that every item of the physical world has at bottom—at a very deep bottom, in most instances—an immaterial source and explanation; that what we call reality arises in the last analysis from the posing of yes-no questions . . . ; in short, that all things physical are information-theoretic in origin *and this is a participatory universe*."

Wheeler's participatory universe echoes Teilhard's Omega Point. In both frameworks, consciousness and existence culminate into a self-aware singularity. "Physics gives rise to observer-participancy," Wheeler says, "observer-participancy gives rise to information; and information gives rise to physics." Round and round we go.

All of existence is encoded as information in the Either/Or of polar opposites, and according to Wheeler, we both observe that fact and participate in it. From the Up or Down of electrons spinning across the universe, connected in their polarities no matter how far apart—to the ones and zeros of computer coding, everything is a binary. Life or death. Fight or flight. Black and white. Friend or foe.

Male or female. Heaven or hell. Alpha and Omega. From the simplest building blocks of reality, to the survival mechanisms of single-celled organisms, to the vicissitudes of the human condition, we are hard-wired for contrast.

To explain how we might access the nearly infinite amount of information that makes up the universe, Oxford mathematician Roger Penrose has floated a theory that human brains, under certain specific conditions, are capable of quantum computing via microtubules in our neurons. This idea would provide a structural explanation for seemingly impossible acts of cognition or intuition. While Penrose earned universal admiration (a Nobel and a knighthood) for his work in mathematics, his theories of quantum consciousness have not been received as warmly. Max Tegmark at MIT did the math and concluded that Penrose was off by at least ten orders of magnitude in his calculations of our mental capacities. "It's reasonably unlikely," Tegmark stated in a paper, "that the brain evolved quantum behavior."

Stanford neuroscientist David Eagleman has cautiously resurrected an alternate explanation—what is known as the dualist argument of consciousness. The materialist argument insists that "mind" is only the by-product of activity in the brain. The dualist argument suggests that there is the hardware—the brain, and then there's signal that the hardware picks up—the universe of information that Wheeler was talking about. Eagleman writes in his book *Incognito*: "I'm not asserting that the brain is like a radio, but I am pointing out that it could be true. There is nothing in our current science that rules this out."

Jeffrey Kripal, professor of religion at Rice University and dedicated explorer of the weird and sublime, puts Eagleman's theory in broader historical context. "William James, Henri Bergson, and Aldous Huxley all argued the same long before Eagleman. Bergson even used the same radio analogy. This is where the historian of religions—this one, anyway—steps in. There are, after all, countless other clues in the history of religions that rule in the radio theory and that suggest, though hardly prove, that *the human brain may function as a super-evolved neurological radio or television and, in rare but revealing moments when the channel suddenly 'switches,' as an imperfect receiver of some transhuman signal* that simply does not play by the rules as we know them."

Einstein once said that "every true theorist is a kind of tamed metaphysicist." It was true of his friend and colleague John Archibald Wheeler. It was true of paleontologist and theologian Teilhard de Chardin. It could be true for us as well. With the advent of repeatable practices that deliver us into the Information Layer, we get to explore the vastness of inspiration that is available.

"Can we ever expect to understand existence?" Wheeler wondered. "Surely someday, we can believe, we will grasp the central idea of it all as so simple, so beautiful, so compelling that we will all say to each other, 'Oh, how could it have been otherwise! How could we all have been so blind so long!'"

Amazing space, how sweet the sound, we were blind, but now we see.

Becoming a HomeGrown Human

We've covered a fair bit of terrain so far. Starting with the collapse in meaning in Part One, and our need to harness evolutionary drivers in Part Two. In Part Three, we've dipped our toes into the field of culture architecture, and how to make the most of these powerful tools without making the same mistakes as past efforts to organize around peak states and healing.

But it does seem important to bring it all back home and show how this process of self-initiation can work, over time, in relationship with those we love most. Think of this as the final section in the field guide to becoming an Omegan.

What follows is a visual description of that process, which, if we follow courageously and consistently enough, can deliver us to maturity. Drawn in this way, it looks like an *Ichthys*, or what is often called the "Jesus Fish." Two arcing curves crossing over on one side to make a tail. It was popular in the early centuries of Christianity as a secret symbol among believers. Since the 1970s it's seen a revival and now adorns the bumpers of minivans everywhere.

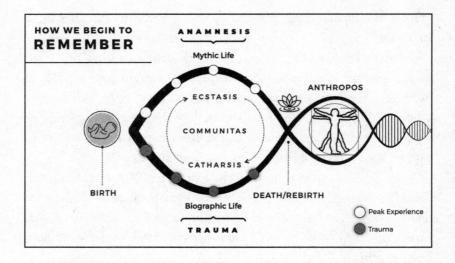

This isn't that. It just looks kind of like it. If there's a precursor to this version, it's probably science fiction writer Philip K. Dick's 1974 epiphany, when a mesmerizing delivery girl came to his door wearing a golden *Ichthys* necklace. As he recounts it, a burst of pink starlight shot out of her Jesus fish, knocked him flat on his ass, and prompted him to come unstuck in time. He spent the rest of his life trying to make sense of that encounter. So think of this version as less minivan bumper sticker and more PKD galactivation.

For now, let's keep it simple. We can call it the DNA Jesus Fish. This model is an approximate road map for the process of self-initiation into Anthropos. Of finding and living into life as a twice-born human. Of sourcing from the Information Layer, the Noosphere, or whatever we want to call it.

It starts, where all of us started, with our physical births. It ends, as all of us end, at our physical deaths. But in between, there's a lot of variation in how these brief lives of ours unfold. That's the bottom curve on the image. Along that arc of our biographical lives, bad things often happen. Tragedies, traumas, setbacks. Those are the dark dots. Adverse childhood events (ACEs). Adverse adult events. Sickness, divorces, betrayals, abuse, violence, despair. The wages of sin few are lucky enough to escape. Birth to death with a bunch of hits in between.

But if we're dedicated, talented, or just plain lucky, we might get a glimpse of something "More"—a taste of Kairos—that's the upper arc on the image, and it represents our mythic lives. It could have been a moment of awe in nature where time stood still—a gorgeous sunset or a shooting star on a campout. It might have been a concert with our favorite band with everyone belting out the chorus together, or a transcendent night with a true love where it seemed our heart would burst.

No matter how it happened, we cherish it, looking back on it as one of the few moments in life where everything made sense, where it all seemed worth it. But since it was only one point in time, there's no larger pattern to discern.

Unless it happens again.

And another time after that.

It takes three points to spot a trend, math nerds love to remind us. Once we've had a few of these breakthrough experiences (the dots on the upper arc), the next time we return to Kairos, the next time we experience anamnesis, and remember what's more deeply true, we also remember we've been here before. "The funny thing is that, despite all the newness, there's something about all of it that feels—well, the only way I can put it is that it's like coming home," Ann Shulgin, therapist, and partner to noted psychedelic chemist Sasha Shulgin, noticed. "As if there's some part of me that already knows—knows this territory—and it's saying Oh yes, of course! Almost a kind of remembering!"

Once we connect the dots backward and forward in time, we start to see the beginnings of a trend. The faintest outline of the top arc reveals itself to be the plot of our mythic lives. The mirror image of our biographic life. The best of what's in us to be.

Here, we're not living lives of quiet desperation. We're thriving. Inspired. Powerful. Purposeful. It feels like redemption for all the lumps and bumps, chaos and confusion, meanness and monotony of our day-to-day. It feels invigorating to get to lay our burdens down. We begin to remember who we truly are. Or at least, who we could be.

But we also see the traumas, woundings, blind spots, and workarounds of our lives with clearer eyes, and maybe even some compassion. If anamnesis reminds us of who we are at our core, it also gives us a laundry list of loose ends, dead ends, and amends. Things we haven't done but need to, things that aren't taking us where we need to go and we should stop, and apologies we need to make.

When, inevitably, the moment of grace recedes, and Kairos slips away and we return to regular life in Chronos, we have a choice: We can take that glimpse above the clouds, and all of the information and inspiration it offered, and use it to heal. We can take those peaks and use them to backfill our valleys. Or, we can succumb to spiritual bypassing.

When that happens, we pop up into a peak experience, look around, feel our turbocharged selves, and rather than looking back down at our day-to-day with renewed compassion and commitment, say, "Fuck it! I'm never going back to that!" The dirty dishes and smelly laundry, the mind-numbing job, the dysfunctional friends and family—all of it turns to ash in our mouths. The pain of seeing the light only to have to slink back into the basement feels too much. We dissociate and try to cling to our newly established mythic life.

We might go hog wild for a new ecstatic practice and community— whether breath work or tantra, or brain stimulation. We might start indulging in psychedelic "medicine work" that turns out to be a thinly veiled excuse for hedonism and sensation seeking. In extreme cases, we might even change our name to reflect our new identity, and start dressing in flowing linens, sandals, and mala beads. (For reasons linguists haven't yet pinned down, no one seems to change their name from Sally to Becky, or from Bob to George. Sally becomes Satchananda, or Devi. Bob becomes Vanguard, or Achilles.)

Whatever the coping strategy, if we get swept up in spiritual bypassing and refuse to come down from our highs, it just means there's that much farther to fall. These days there's no shortage of playmates in this high-altitude Land of the Lost.

*　*　*

There's another known issue navigating the path to HomeGrown Human that's worth mentioning: muddling our tenses. While most of modern psychology assumes that I am "me" and you are "you" and when we sit down together our clocks are synchronized, that's rarely the case. In fact, we're almost never truly sharing the present together. Our meatsuits might be co-located in space but not in time. We are lost in a sea of stories—painful pasts and fearful futures we want to avoid at all costs, or perfect pasts and fantastic futures we're desperately hoping to have more of. Rarely do we meet in the Deep Now together.

When we start cultivating our mythic lives, shuttling between Kairos and Chronos, things get even weirder. Typically, it happens something like this. We're fortunate enough to have some breakthrough—some glimpse of Kairos where we feel ourselves at full strength and remember the hidden thread of our deepest purpose. It's amazing, and we can't wait to get back home and deliver the Good News to the people we love.

We get back, heart blown open with literal en*theo*siasm—filled with Spirit. But then something totally unexpected happens. Our loved ones are just not picking up what we're laying down. We assume it must be because we haven't communicated how powerful and utterly life changing our experience was. SO WE SHIFT TO ALL CAPS. That will really let them know, we think, and hey, we're still riding the afterglow so we've got love to spare.

But that only makes it worse. The more we blast them, the farther back they stand. We start out certain we can win them over with our conviction, but it rarely works out that way. And it's largely because we came unstuck in time and aren't synchronized with our partners anymore.

When we have a breakthrough experience of our truest/highest/ bestest self, we conveniently forget our bad debts. "Sure, that Saul guy was a tax collector and a real sonofabitch, I'll admit, but hey baby, that's not me, *I'm Paul now*, can't you see?"

Our *leading* edge in Kairos gets precisely matched up with their *bleeding* edge in Chronos. Those closest to us aren't willing or able to trust the New Me, until we've acknowledged and atoned for the Old Me that might have hurt them in the past.

They're not wrong. We probably were selfish, hurtful, weak, or distracted back then. No matter how compellingly different we seem right now, they'd be a fool to just let down their guard and trust us outright. It's not until we are willing to come down off our high horse and shovel some shit that they can feel safe enough to work through the trauma that we may have had a hand in creating.

The temptation here, and it ruins marriages and destroys friendships, is to get sucked into a bypass. Frustrated by our partner's hesitance, or outright refusal to recognize our newest level of attainment, we can grow peevish. We might withdraw. Maybe into more "spiritual" books, or online forums, or our new friends who "get us" and speak our language.

Faced with weeks or months of tension we might even conclude, "You know, I'm just not sure we're on the same journey anymore. I think I might be more committed to growth/spirituality/healing than you are." And we might be. We really might be. Not every high school buddy or long-term spouse is drawn to the same things at the same pace. People absolutely do grow apart. Especially if we matched someone in an earlier phase of life we've now left behind, cracks can become gaps that become chasms.

But that's not always how it works. As often as not, the people who love us most are the ones gamely holding the bag when it comes to our disowned blind spots. And they can't trust us enough to let go of their own wounding to risk coming along for the ride of *our* lives. If we're unwilling to take responsibility for what we have done, and for what we have left undone, their decision to hold back is likely the right one.

Our own "personal journey," if unchecked, can lead to dangerous ego inflation and distortion. Any experience or insight that pulls us "up and away" from our relationships is probably half-baked. An experience that brings us "down and among" toward the least of our brothers (and sisters) is likely a more stable and trustworthy revelation.

That's where lineage teachers used to come in so handy, to ground us and remind us of the fundamentals we still need to work on. But these days, we've mostly ditched the traditions. We may be on our own, but we do still have each other. That's where communitas becomes the vital third leg of the stool. It provides balance, and accountability for our explorations in ecstasis and catharsis. It keeps us humble. It keeps us human.

No Place Like Home

If you submit to the process and don't succumb to the pitfalls, you come to realize that the shuttling between our biographic and mythic lives picks up momentum. One informs the other. Ecstasis inspires us, but also gives us the blueprint to heal. Catharsis mends us, and leaves us better able to integrate the insights we receive. Communitas connects us to each other in celebration and support.

Those three points become a flywheel, spinning faster and faster and propelling us through life. There's no cutting corners, there's no skipping steps. If we fixate on one element at the expense of the others, we fall out of balance. If we deny the sacred, the mundane will crush us. If we deny the mundane, the sacred will burn us. But once we accept both, we die to our lives of separation.

This is what we mean when we talk of this initiatory process as the Blissfuck Crucifiction. It really is the Agony and the Ecstasy. Both. Forever. We are off the hook of our neurotic searching for something more. But we're on the cross of bearing witness to the Full Catastrophe of the human condition. "Ain't no saint without a past," Dolly Parton reminds us, "or no sinner without a future." We're never fully fixed. We're never totally broken.

And the moment we stop trying to wriggle off that commitment, something beautiful happens. The arc of our biographic life in Chronos starts to lift up, inspired by our dedicated work of healing and integrating. Our mythic life in Kairos starts to bend down as well— grounded by our commitment to bring it all back with us. We begin to braid the two together.

When they finally intersect, at the crossroad of our lives, that's when we complete the alchemy. Like Dorothy in *The Wizard of Oz*, tired of her flat-ass and dusty life in Kansas, we have to run away to find what we're looking for. We seek magic, only to realize that there truly isn't any place like Home. The mythic characters of the Cowardly Lion, the Tin Man, and the Scarecrow reveal themselves to be the three farmhands back at the ranch. "Always *and already*," Indian philosopher Nisargadatta observes, "the Other World is this world, rightly seen."

We are reborn as Anthropos. We get to live as HomeGrown Humans. Rather than yearning for transcendence and escape, we come to appreciate the preciousness of these brief mortal lives. Isn't that why the gods and angels have always been jealous of us anyway? Humans are the existential mayflies of the universe. With life spans so brief that every moment matters to us, in a way that the immortals can never taste. We have prefrontal cortexes and opposable thumbs, and for a fleeting few decades we're here to love and lose, to fight and fuck, to create and destroy, to yearn and grieve.

If Carl Sagan was right when he said, "We are a way for the universe to know itself. Some part of our being knows this is where we came from . . . we are made of starstuff," then direct experience is the only way we get to validate that truth. Once we've proven it to ourselves beyond a shadow of a doubt, we're given the gift of returning fully to these lives of ours.

* * *

In Zen, there's a famous series of ten paintings called the Oxherding parable. They symbolize the search for enlightenment. When I first read it in college I was humbled to discover that what I'd assumed was the final destination of Awakening showed up on panel number four. Panels five through nine proceeded to highlight distinctions that sailed over my head. But the tenth panel is the one that really stuck with me. It showed a picture of a smiling potbellied old man with a walking stick.

"His doors and windows are locked. Even the wisest sages and scholars cannot find him. He is down in the marketplace now, among the people, with helping hands."

Anthropos, twice born, Adam Kadmon, bodhisattva—they've gone by different names over the ages. East and West.

But today, it doesn't even need to be that fancy. HomeGrown Humans are all around us. Teachers, farmers, and firefighters. Doctors, nurses, and parents. Soldiers, singers, and carpenters. Leading us to the Omega Point where we can unlock the intelligence and creativity in our bones. HomeGrown humans, being human, doing human, grieving human. Down among the people, with helping hands.

The Four Horsemen Cometh

Pestilence, War, Famine, and Death. Those were the old school Riders of the Storm, the four horsemen of the Apocalypse. Not an especially fun crowd to run with and definitely not going to take us where we want to go. If we're going to bring about "the unveiling"—we've got to do it in a way that cherishes life rather than destroys it.

To make it to the Omega Point, we'll need to hitch our wagon to four very different horses: Danger Mouse, Tank Man, Soul Force, and Radical Hope.

Danger Mouse

A couple of years ago, Andrew Huberman, a rising star in the field of neuroscience and a professor at Stanford, published a curious study in the journal *Nature*.

It, like many research papers in the field, focused on mice. But Huberman and his colleagues were asking a question that no one had figured out before. "What happens in the brain when we see something that terrifies us?"

Everyone has heard of the "fight or flight" mechanism. But just because it rhymes doesn't mean it's right. In reality there are two distinct responses to mortal threat, one for fleeing and freezing and the other for standing and fighting.

The thalamus lives near the center of the brain and functions like a traffic roundabout—a hub relaying sensorimotor information to the cerebral cortex. There are two crucial hubs it talks to—the *xiphoid nucleus*, which triggers "salience reducing" (don't you look at me!) behaviors, and the *nucleus reuniens*, which prompts "salience enhancing" (you want a piece of me?) behaviors.

Not surprisingly, regular mice favor freezing and fleeing. When faced with the overhead shadow of a looming bird of prey, over 90 percent hightail it for cover. Only 2 percent engage in confrontational behavior like thumping their tails, and they're only brave enough to try that once safely under shelter.

But when Huberman stimulated mice's *nucleus reuniens*, something else happened. The mice got braver. Instead of running for the hills, they stood their ground. "Activation of the ventro-medial Thalamus (vMT)," Huberman writes, "consistently increased arousal and saliency-enhancing 'courageous' behaviours . . . in the direct presence of a perceived threat." When faced with the looming shadow of a bird of prey, they turn, face the danger, and beat their tails on the ground. It's the rodent equivalent of Bruce Lee's famous beckoning "bring it on" gesture.

Huberman wanted to know if he was manipulating these poor mice and sending them to their doom. But given the choice between seeking this stimulation, or getting left to their own devices, the mice actively sought it out. "Increases in arousal induced by vMT stimulation are rewarding," he wrote in the paper, "that is, they have positive valence."

It's not just mice that seem to crave courage. We do too. In a pair of earlier studies Huberman noted that "self-stimulation of the [comparable] human brain area . . . is strongly reinforcing, even more so than activation of areas associated with sexual arousal." We'd rather be brave than get laid. That's saying something.

That tiny little cluster of neurons called the *nucleus reuniens* that makes us braver, so we can face the danger instead of run from it? In Latin, it literally means "the seed of reunion." Sown in the fertile ground of Meaning 3.0, it's our courage that could bring us together.

Tank Man

When you think about it, we don't need to slice up the brains of rodents to prove how essential courage is in our lives. In all of our legends and myths the story is always the same. David and Goliath. Odysseus and the cyclops. Frodo and Sauron. Harry and Voldemort.

That little mouse against the looming hawk was never going to be a fair fight, and neither were those others. But somehow they work out. If we leave enough space for Grace.

We memorialize that moment of truth. It's King Leonidas giving his speech to the three hundred Spartans facing down a hundred thousand Persians. It's Thelma and Louise clasping hands as they drive off the edge of the Grand Canyon. It's the boys of *Dead Poets Society* standing up on their desks to recite "O Captain! My Captain!" to their doomed teacher.

It's "Tank Man" in Beijing's Tiananmen Square in 1989 calmly standing in front of a column of armored vehicles. It's the Greensboro Four sitting at the Woolworth's lunch counter in 1960, politely asking to be served. It's the string quartet on the *Titanic*, picking up their instruments and playing "Nearer My God to Thee" as the ship goes down.

It's every moment, some famous, most anonymous, where a person, with their back against it, chooses to sacrifice safety and security to do what must be done, with as much courage, grace, and dignity as they can muster.

*　　*　　*

If this was just a roll call of fictional and historic moments of heroism it would only be worth so much. Cheap sentimentality won't get us where we need to go. We have to mine this vein for practical insight.

Those stories are so arresting because we love to imagine ourselves as those heroes. We like to believe that when the hawk looms, when the battle cry goes out, we'll heed the call.

Except most of us wouldn't. "We don't ever rise to the occasion," the Greek poet Archilochus observed, ". . . we sink to the level of our training." Or, as boxer Mike Tyson put it more succinctly, "Everybody's got a plan until they get hit."

That's why we need to raise the level of our training. And the only training that's up to the occasion is death practice. If we don't practice transcending our survival programming, at the crux, we'll flinch. Almost every time. The storied exceptions only prove the rule.

By practicing resurrection, we come back, again and again, to that singular point where we have the chance to move beyond a life of seeking pleasure and avoiding pain. Even, and especially, if our life depends on it. In that instant we are presented with the chance to step off the hamster wheel of Chronos and willingly step up to the cross of Kairos. Consequences be damned. Once we've died and been born a second time, dying again doesn't seem so hard.

For anyone who's grown despondent, overwhelmed by all of the graphs measuring all of the things in an unraveling world—we have to take refuge in this simple fact: We're wired for courage at the deepest levels of our being. While it's easy to fixate on dramatic examples of heroic sacrifice, there's even more power in the infinitesimal courage of the day-to-day. A sleep-deprived mother working three jobs to feed her children. A schoolkid protecting the bullied on the playground. A stranger offering the homeless some kindness or comfort. A tired, anonymous man, standing in front of a phalanx of tanks, saying enough is enough.

Our courage is always there, dormant but potent. When we act on it, it sends shock waves through time and space. That's the only exponential curve that bends in the right direction these days. It's our force multiplier. Our ace in a hole of heartache.

* * *

Nancy Koehn, historian at Harvard Business School, writes in her book *Forged in Crisis* about five leaders, Antarctic explorer Ernest

Shackleton, President Abraham Lincoln, the German pastor Dietrich Bonhoeffer, who tried to assassinate Hitler, environmentalist Rachel Carson, and abolitionist Frederick Douglass. While each is more or less famous for their historic roles, Koehn emphasizes something deeper. "Intentionally, sometimes bravely, and with the messy humanity that defines all of us when we're at our most vulnerable, these people made themselves into effective agents of worthy change." In their moments of crisis, they had *no idea* what they were doing. And they did it anyway.

Their stories, Koehn notes, "are as astounding as any from the great myths, adventure novels, and films that we remember and return to again and again."

"In the process [of becoming courageous leaders], each of the leaders and the people they inspire are made more resilient, a bit bolder, and, in some instances, even more luminous," she writes. "When this happens, impact expands, and the possibility grows for moving goodness forward in the world."

Soul Force

The "possibility grows for moving goodness forward in the world." There's a term for this contagion of courage. It's called Soul Force. Martin Luther King wove it into his "I Have a Dream" speech in Washington, D.C. "Again and again," he said, "we must rise to the majestic heights of meeting physical force with soul force."

But those weren't King's words or ideas. He'd borrowed them twice over. One of his spiritual mentors was Howard Thurman, who in 1935 traveled to India as the first African American interfaith ambassador. There he met with Mahatma Gandhi and became steeped in the peaceful resistance the Indian lawyer called *satyagraha*.

On Thurman's return to the United States, he translated the Sanskrit term into something more accessible—Soul Force—and began sharing its power with Black ministers and activists. Until Thurman, nonviolent protest was a tactic of the civil rights movement, more than a central philosophy. It was a calculated move to not provoke the Bull Connors of the world. After Thurman shared Gandhi's message and King embraced it, Soul Force became the foundational strategy of social justice movements everywhere.

But Thurman was more a mystic than an activist. In one of those grace notes of history, he also delivered the sermon at the famous 1962 Good Friday experiment at Harvard Divinity School. Most accounts of that service focus on the headlines—seminarians were given the psychedelic psilocybin and many of them had profound mystical experiences that day.

But virtually nowhere can you find accounts of what they were thinking about, sitting in Marsh Chapel, watching the sunlight stream through its rose-petaled, stained-glass windows.

Everyone is familiar with the musical cadence of the Baptist preacher tradition. Martin Luther King epitomized it. Barack Obama rode its rhythms into the White House. Thurman sounded nothing like that. His voice was a rumbling baritone. His cadence was irregular and marked with as much silence as sound. In the closing minutes of an hour-long Good Friday sermon in a chapel of tripping mystics, he told the story of hearing "an anguished voice crying out, 'Forgiveness.'

"I went out and searched and found a man in the throes of crucifixion. I said, 'I will take you down.' I tried to take the nails out of his feet, but he said, 'Let them be, for I cannot be taken down until every man and every woman and every child will come together to take me down.'

"I said, 'But I cannot stand to hear you cry. What can I do?' He said, 'Go about the world. Tell everyone you meet that there's a man on the cross, a man on the cross.' Tell everybody, everybody that you meet."

That man on the cross is *anthropos*. That cross lies at the intersection of Kairos and Chronos. A couple of thousand years ago, his realization was rare and remarkable. Today it's required of all of us. It's this recognition of our divinity and our mortality that delivers us to our full humanity. Every man, woman, and child. Every HomeGrown Human. Take out the nails, remove the thorns. Forgive ourselves and each other. Not to usher in the Second Coming, but to bring about the Umpteenth Coming. It's time to take him down. It's time for us to step up. Tell everyone.

Tell everyone you meet.

Radical Hope

We've got Danger Mouse confirming that courage is wired into us at the deepest levels of our brains. We've tipped our hat to Tank Man and all those who have done the impossible in the face of uncertainty and doubt. We've acknowledged the world-changing power of Soul Force. We need all of them, but we're not quite done.

The final horse we need to saddle up is Radical Hope. Regular old "whistling past the graveyard" hope won't be enough to save us from our demons or the darkness. We're going to need something stronger.

Because here's the thing: We might do everything we can and still not make it. "We live at a time of a heightened sense that civilizations are themselves vulnerable," University of Chicago philosopher Jonathan Lear writes in *Radical Hope: Ethics in the Face of Cultural Devastation*. "Events around the world—terrorist attacks, violent social upheavals, and even natural catastrophes—have left us with an uncanny sense of menace. We seem to be aware of a shared vulnerability that we cannot quite name."

Lear explores what it means when we have to give up hoping for a return to the old and familiar touchstones of our way of life. What can we do, how can we go on, if the world we grew up in ceases to exist? "The inability to conceive of its own devastation," Lear says, "will tend to be the blind spot of any culture."

In place of that quid pro quo bargaining kind of hope—where we put on happy faces and wait for the ship to right itself—Lear highlights a fundamentally different kind of hope, *radical* hope. "What makes this hope radical," he explains, "is that it is directed toward a future goodness that transcends our current ability to understand what it is."

That's something that comes through often enough in experiences of Kairos that it's worth underscoring here. Time and again, when entering the Deep Now, there is a persistent sense that somehow, in the end, it all works out. We make it to the Omega Point.

As we drift back down into our bodies, into our waking selves, and into our time-bound chronological existences, we realize we are blessed with the privilege of getting to live out these middle chapters of our own brief lives—not as isolated individuals, but as walk-on parts in a much longer and larger passion play.

Only now, we're freed from the burden of wondering if the impossible is possible. We can relax a bit, we can be kinder, more playful, more courageous—for ourselves and for each other, steeped in the knowing that somewhere, somewhen, somehow, *we have already one*.

And what's especially beautiful about that realization if it comes, is that it doesn't let us off the hook for showing up at full strength. Calvinist predestination doesn't work here. We can't just run out the clock, certain of the outcome. Because even if we've been blessed with a glimpse of the Happiest Ever After Ever, we also know it all comes down to a 51/49 nail-biter in triple overtime to win the Game. That means that every single calorie we burn, every breath we take, every stand we make, is essential to that final and triumphant tally.

Radical hope gives us perspective beyond the false certainties and certain vulnerabilities of our own lifetimes. We may not get to the Promised Land ourselves, but we keep on walking in the conviction that our children, or their children, might. The question's not having hope, as Cornel West reminds us, it's *being hope*. As we let go of our own personal references and preferences, we can reorient to the longer arc of humanity finding its way to the Omega Point. That really would be the greatest Cinderella Story of all time. Delivered from evil, at the stroke of midnight, or not at all.

"We are not expected to finish the work," the Talmud advises us, "nor are we excused from it." It's an impossible task, and we have to try anyway. We have everything we need to remake our world. We can affirm who we are and what we've forgotten. We can learn to weep rather than whimper. We can find our brothers and sisters who hear the truth in what we say.

"Only where love and need are one," Robert Frost writes, "and the work is play for mortal stakes, is the deed ever really done, for heaven and the future's sakes."

If we can do the work and recapture the Rapture, we might finally evolve from *Homo sapiens*, the ape who knows, to *Homo ludens*, the ape who plays. And what will we play at? The Infinite Game. Frost is right, the stakes are mortal. Our need may be great, but so is our love. Both heaven and the future are waiting to see what we do next.

This is the story of how we begin to remember. This is how we dance each other home.

If you're interested in learning more, ranging from references to research to tools to community, you can find it all at www.recapturetherapture.com.

Stay awake. Build stuff. Help out.

Acknowledgments

I'd love to thank all of the pioneers and brilliant minds who blazed this trail, HomeGrown Humans all. To Rick Tepel and Tony Dubler, my two best friends who knew me back when, how I wish you were still here. To my advisers: Lucille Clifton, who taught me poetry; Patricia Nelson Limerick, who taught me prose; and Vine Deloria Jr,. who taught me you could pray just fine with tobacco from a pack of Marlboro Reds. Wade Davis, for being a lyric poet, adventurer, and scholar all in one lifetime; Rick Doblin, for so fully embodying the twinkling message you bring to the world; Helen Fisher, for showing that sexy anthropology was actually a thing; Elon Musk, for moving more matter in the right direction than maybe anyone ever; Kimbal and Christiana Musk, for mighty good times in gorgeous places; Nicole Prause, for so bravely following your research wherever it's led; Andrew Huberman, for asking more questions I'm interested in (and then nailing the findings) than almost any scientist out there; David Eagleman, for being a masterful communicator as well as thinker; Adam Gazzaley, for sharing your Friday loft and your mind-bending inventiveness; David Deida, for poking out of your Cypress swamp long enough to remind me of the pointlessness of it all; Doug Rushkoff, for your integrity and insistence that it's all about Team Human; Erik Davis, for your techgnostic brilliance parsing the highest of weirdness; Roger Walsh, for sharing the notion of polyphasic consciousness, carbogen, and your higher wisdom. Jared Diamond and Yuval Harari, for stretching the box of what neuroanthropology could be; Tristan Harris, for your heart and your critiques of our digital lives; Jonathan Haidt, for being a voice of reason in unreasonable times; Michael Pollan, for being the writer I've quoted most often and widely; Bill McKibben, for taking a stand long before most of us got off our asses; Amy Cuddy, who I knew without asking was into the blues; Jason Silva, for ranting and riffing forever on. Jasen Trautwein and Grant Korgan for sharing the stoke at the Surf Ranch and the joy of perfect peeling barrels with me. To Kevin Conley, for keeping me company through the dog days of the summer of 2020, helping four hundred pages get written in five months flat. To my agent, Byrd Leavell, at United Talent Agency, who believed in a book about the end of the world, prior to it actually ending. To Karen Rinaldi, my fierce and fearless editor, who never flinched once, and only made this better. To Elaine Pagels, who modeled intelligent faith; Sue Phillips of the Sacred Design Lab, whose deep kindness renewed my faith in ministers; Pema Chodron and Alice Walker, for grandmother wisdom that soothes the soul. Curt Cronin, for trusting my heart and having my back. To Gary Snyder, my all-time hero, a mountain man, a family man, a poet and protector of Turtle Island. You are an axe, I am a handle, model and tool, craft of culture, how we go on . . .

Glossary

Adiam: A mystical name for Anthropos, or perfected Man. *Adi* is an honorific meaning "first" or "preeminent" in India and "jewel" in Hebrew. "I AM" is a statement of pure being first invoked by Yahweh. Adam is First Man. Ad-I-Am is Adam with the highest I at its center. A decent avatar for the future of humanity.

Agnosticism: The view that the existence of God, or the divine or supernatural, is unknown or unknowable. Robert Anton Wilson said that anyone who faces the burning bush of ultimate truth returns either insane or agnostic.

Alchemy: Commonly known as the effort to turn lead or other base metals into gold. In the esoteric traditions, sometimes thought to refer to the process of transforming human consciousness into higher forms of awareness.

Alpha: First. The beginning of time. Especially in Judeo-Christian eschatology. Also, in primate studies, the pack leader or dominant specimen in a group of animals.

Anamnesis: Literally, the opposite of amnesia. The "forgetting of the forgetting," a.k.a. deep remembering. It is the idea that humans possess innate knowledge (perhaps acquired before birth) and that learning consists of rediscovering that knowledge within us.

Apocalypse: The unveiling or revealing at the End of Time.

Arcana Americana: A neologism combining *arcana*—a secret scripture or esoteric text and *Americana*—the deeply American folk tradition. Distinguished by its syncretic combination of African, European, Jewish, and indigenous folkways and references to a consistent death/rebirth narrative combining suffering with redemption.

Armageddon: The ultimate showdown between Good and Evil before the final Days of Judgment.

Anthropos: The Greek word for "human." Mystical sense of perfected, integrated, balanced human. See also: Adiam, HomeGrown Humans, Vitruvian Man.

Big Five: Respiration, embodiment, sexuality, substances, and music—the strongest widely available evolutionary drivers to promote peak states, healing, and relational connect.

Blissfuck Crucifiction: The initiatory death/rebirth experience of becoming *anthropos* by deliberately harnessing deep pleasure and ecstatic consciousness to simultaneously hold the profound grief of the human experience. The convergence point between Kairos and Chronos. The spelling of cruci-*fiction* is deliberate—as an indicator of its metaphorical nature.

Catharsis: A deep sense of healing, usually with respect to trauma. Often energetically released.

Chronos: Clock time. Linear progression of past, present, and future.

Communitas: A deep sense of connection with others. Victor Turner's term for a profound gathering of people. See: Group Flow and the Quaker term "gathered meeting."

Culture Architecture: The discipline of bringing design thinking to solve social challenges—specifically by reinvigorating or innovating new forms of cultural practices based on anthropological understandings of human behavior. See also: Neuroanthropology.

Deep Now: See Kairos.

Ecstasis: Literally, "to step outside oneself." A deep sense of inspiration, or positive non-ordinary state/peak experience, often involving some form of ego death or dissolution.

Embodied cognition: The field of study based on the insight that bodies affect brains and brains affect bodies. Moving our physiology informs our neurology, and with it our psychology.

Epistemology: The study of the nature of knowledge, justification, and the rationality of belief.

Eschatology: The study of the Eschaton, or the End of Time.

Ethics: As opposed to morals, which are typically rendered in binary good and bad, thou shalt/shalt not terms. In ethics, it's not the act but one's relationship to the act that matters and determines its merit. Less common in traditional social structures, due to the requirement that an individual can practice personal discernment and accountability. Essential in higher levels of post-conventional explorations, where rigid categories give way to paradox, contradiction, and provisional certainty.

Finite games: Any form of social exchange with a one up/one down outcome, from commerce to military conflict to sexuality. See also: Infinite game.

Flow: An optimal state of consciousness resulting in peak mental and physical performance.

Garden (of Eden): A place of timeless perfection, outside of normal causation, not subject to sin, separation (or the Second Law of Thermodynamics). See also: Kairos, Deep Now.

Gnosis: A direct experience of the Suchness of Reality, or Source. Un-Englishable. Profound. Confounding (disambiguation: also a dissenting sect of early Christians who held a particular philosophy that this world is a prison of illusion created by a false god, the demiurge).

Gnosticism: Ancient religious ideas and systems that originated in the first century AD among early Christian and Jewish sects. These various groups, labeled "gnostics" by their opponents, emphasized personal spiritual knowledge (gnosis) over orthodox teachings, traditions, and ecclesiastical authority. Sometimes referring to a deeper worldview that holds this reality as false, and created by a false god (à la *The Matrix*).

Hedonic Calendaring: The practice of planning out the entire year around skillful access to peak states, ranging from supportive daily practices to weekly "sabbath" practices to monthly, seasonal, and annual events of increasing depth and duration. Intended to promote healthy alchemy and prevent addiction or insanity while avoiding the binge/purge dynamic common to most hedonistic exploration.

Hedonic Engineering: The practice of harnessing peak states in service of facilitating healing and integration, up to, and including, the reformatting of self-identity.

Hedonism: The pursuit of pleasure, often to excess.

Hierogamy: *Hieros gamos* (Greek). The sacred union between the archetypal man and the archetypal woman.

HomeGrown Humans: People who have completed their initiatory process and surrendered to their part. Fully alive. Deeply committed. Fearless. Joyful. Courageous. Kind. Steeped in the deep knowing of who they are and what is theirs to do. See also: *Anthropos*.

Homo Ludens: Johan Huizinga's term for "the playful ape." In this instance, people dedicated to playing the Infinite Game. See also: Anthropos, Home-grown Humans

Infinite game: James Carse's conceptualization of infinite games—where the point of the game is to keep on playing, as opposed to a finite game, where the point is to win. In the infinite game, one plays with the rules rather than playing within the rules.

Kairos: Sacred time. A location in time-space containing past, present, and future in one location. See also: Garden.

Liminal space: The "adjacent possible"—the transitional spaces between realms of reality. Tidal pools and edges of forests are liminal spaces, as are waking/dreaming states.

Logos: In the Western mystery traditions and mystical Christianity, it is "the word made flesh." A deep, mystical, and even invocatory truth. The most famous example kicks off the book of John, "In the beginning was the Word." Other examples are #truthbombs and the Rastafarian concept of Word Sound Power.

Magick: Distinct from rabbits in hats, magick is the art of bending reality to one's will. Practiced around the world, the Western tradition stems mostly from Greek, Egyptian, Persian, and Jewish lineages. Aleister Crowley added the "k" to distinguish it from lesser versions.

Meaning 1.0: Organized religion. Those who believed were saved. Those who didn't weren't.

Meaning 2.0: Global liberalism. The idea that markets, democracy, and civil rights would bring us into a world where everyone, not just the elect, were entitled to a fair shot at the good life.

Meaning 3.0: A combination of Meaning 1.0 and 2.0. Fulfilling the pro-social functions of traditional faith—inspiration, healing, and connection—

while fulfilling the inclusive promise of modernism—open source, scalable, and anti-fragile.

Metaphysics: The branch of philosophy that examines the fundamental nature of reality, including the relationship between mind and matter, between substance and attribute, and between potentiality and actuality.

Morals: Pre-defined "right" and "wrong" as established by a given authority. Thou shalt / Thou shalt not. See also: Ethics.

Mystery school: A community dedicated to direct experience of non-ordinary states and the truths contained therein. See also: Gnosticism, Platonism.

Neuroanthropology: An emergent discipline combining historical analysis with the findings of neuroscience and psychology to better understand human culture, ritual, and behavior, and to uncover the functional mechanisms of action underneath social forms.

Neuro-kinesthetic programming: Integrating the nervous system and physiology in service of overall heightened perception, cognition, and performance. See also: Embodied cognition.

Omega: The End. The final end point of history, as in "the Alpha and Omega." The End of Time. Teilhard de Chardin called the Omega Point the "body of Christ," where all awake humans would join together via the process of Christogenesis.

Ontology: The philosophical study of being. More broadly, it studies concepts that directly relate to being, in particular becoming, existence, reality, as well as the basic categories of being and their relations. Considering the base nature of reality.

Platonism: The philosophy of Plato that affirms the existence of abstract objects, which are asserted to exist in a third realm distinct from both the sensible external world and from the internal world of consciousness. Especially relevant for those experiencing the information richness of peak states.

Pythagoras: Ancient Greek philosopher who influenced Socrates and Plato. Founded a mystery school dedicated to embodied communal living. Articulated idealized theories of music and mathematics. Figured out some cool stuff about triangles, too.

Rapture: A story of impending cataclysm for the many, and the joyful redemption of the few. Or a sense of bliss or extreme, mind-eclipsing pleasure.

Rational mysticism: A worldview of philosophy that acknowledges non-ordinary states of consciousness and experience, but insists on bringing logic, evidence, and reason to their interpretation. See also: transcendental existentialism.

Redemption Songs: See also: Arcana Americana, and Bob Marley's tune of the same name.

Sexual Yoga of Becoming: One expression of Hedonic Engineering, combining erotic stimulation with breath work, soft-tissue massage, tremor release, trauma work, music, dance, psychodynamic work, music, and psychedelics. See also: Tantra.

Soul force: A form of courageous civil resistance coined by Howard Thurman and popularized by Martin Luther King Jr. (originally known as *satyagraha*, a concept of nonviolence first propounded by Mahatma Gandhi).

Spiritual bypassing: The pursuit of experiences encountered in non-ordinary states as a means to avoid the important work needed to be done in real life.

Tantra: The embrace of all that arises as source material for awakening and growth. Often associated with sexuality, but includes the dissolution of ego boundaries and working with all positive and negative aspects of intersubjective co-created reality.

Transcendental existentialism: The two-part notion that life is inherently unknowable, random, or meaningless (the existentialism) *and at the same time* filled with profound grace and beauty (the transcendentalism). See also: Agnosticism, Gnosticism, Rational mysticism.

Vitruvian Man: Leonardo's famous painting of a multi-limbed human inscribed with perfect proportion between squares, triangles, and circles. In our case, a visual representation of *Anthropos*—balancing head and heart, left and right, masculine and feminine, heaven and hell. See Amanda Sage's recent update of Vitruvian Human for a contemporary take on the classic.

Appendix

Sexual Yoga of Becoming Study

THE POWER OF STACKING

Combining practices like in this study provides two very specific advantages compared to stronger singular interventions—more responsive steering and shorter durations. If you use only one tool from the Hedonic Engineering tool kit—say, psychedelics or high-tech brain stimulation—then if things go sideways it can be much harder to correct. Your thrusters are set full throttle in one direction. Stacking methods together gives us the equivalent of trim tabs on a plane—we can add or subtract from our recipe, making micro-adjustments across several domains. It also makes it easier to reverse effects if someone runs into challenges.

Shorter durations also matter, for a bunch of reasons. For starters, not everyone has ten days to disappear for a silent Vipassana retreat, or twelve hours to invest in LSD therapy (which is a big part of the reason why psilocybin studies

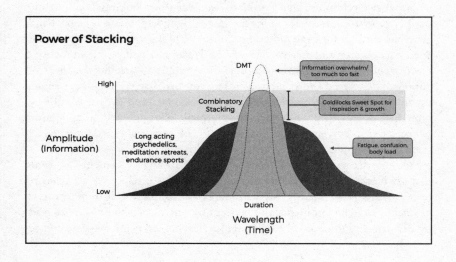

have taken precedence lately, their six-to-eight-hour duration fits better within working shifts at hospitals).

There's also the half-life factor to consider. If you're trying to get to the zone of peak inspiration on LSD or ayahuasca, for instance, you have to take a substantial dose that may grant you 60 to 120 minutes in that sweet spot of insight with hours managing the come up and come down on either side. If you're in a ten-day meditation retreat, you might have profound breakthroughs somewhere between days four and seven, with lots of sitting and suffering before and after. If, at mile seventy of an ultramarathon, you slide into the runner's high to end all runners' highs, it could make your year, but might take months to mend your beaten body.

That's not to say that kind of "earned wisdom" doesn't have a very real place in our efforts to mend and grow. It's just to say it requires large commitments of time and energy, leaves us exposed in the transitions between non-ordinary states and waking consciousness, and takes far longer to recover from and integrate.

Instead, by combining or stacking methods precisely, you can compress the duration while boosting the elevation. Not only does this fit more readily into busy lives and schedules, it also allows us to pay more attention to the insights we do receive and come back with fewer distortions, confusion, or fatigue. It's a game of amplitude over wavelength—height over time.

C³ Physicians

Subjects in the study who elected to pursue more intensive use of pharmaceutical compounds did so under the guidance of their own overseeing physicians who were able to make off-label prescriptions of the relevant substances. While we outlined the baseline protocols that subjects could follow, we left room for self-organizing experimentation within and across couples based on their own curiosity and creativity.

Sex-advice columnist Dan Savage advises that when looking for a romantic partner you want someone who fits the "3G's"—good, giving, and game. Kind, generous, and up for exploration. For anyone especially enthused by Chapter 8 on Sacraments, and Chapter 11 on the Hedonic Engineering study, we'd recommend you seek the care of a supervising physician who fits the "3C's"—curious, connected, and courageous. That means that (1) they are keeping up on contemporary research, MAPS trauma studies, and the use of off-label prescriptions; (2) they have access to informed colleagues and compounding pharmacies; and (3) they are willing to work with responsible patients and help them chart a course to fully dimensional health.

You may have noticed references to Schedule III and IV compounds—ones that are broadly available with a prescription. In this instance we are referring to cannabinoids (technically still Schedule I but legally available in most states), oxytocin (*not* to be confused with OxyContin), nitric oxide boosters (most readily ED drugs), intranasal or sublingual ketamine, therapeutic oxygen, and nitrous oxide. In order to access these you will almost certainly need a physical exam, a compelling and credible reason for use (the *DSM-5* has recently added "adjustment disorder" to its coded diagnoses, so if you are having difficulty "adjusting" to the state of the world globally, nationally, or personally, this could be a criterion to explore).

If any particular intervention or practice goes against personal, moral, legal, spiritual, ethical, or cultural norms that are important to you, simply skip that part. All you will need to do is increase the intensity or duration of the methods you do choose to compensate.

The breath work and PTSD study at Johns Hopkins is an example of how this can work. With Dr. Matt Johnson's leadership, we've designed a program that is specifically tailored to work in the Veteran's Administration, as well as in schools in South America, Africa, and India. We had to design a program that met the evidence-based requirements of large institutions such as the VA, while also being flexible enough and respectful of local cultures and belief systems not to threaten or undermine their values. Otherwise, a profoundly healing practice that unmoored people from their usual foundations could create controversy and blowback, ultimately making things worse, not better.

Because internal review boards have extensive restrictions on hands-on touch, we've substituted self-administered bodywork for therapeutic massage. Because non-ordinary states are usually interpreted via cultural norms and religious faith, we've backed off many of the frameworks that Stan Grof established in his holotropic breathwork (such as notions of past-life regression and re-birthing experiences) to something more neutral and open to interpretation by the subjects themselves. Because sexuality and substances are nowhere near ready for prime time, we omitted them entirely, while still seeking to replicate some of the same neurochemical and physiological shifts they prompt. So, of the Big Five, we only deployed three—respiration, embodiment, and music. And that should be more than enough to help sufferers of trauma heal and grow.

There's one additional sliding scale that's helpful for us to consider in the design phase: the range between high-tech/high-cost options and lower-tech/lower-cost options. With enough time, money, and cutting-edge equipment, you can pretty much get to wherever you want to go—but cost and access become real issues.

Three examples:

Adam Gazzaley, a polymath MD/PhD at UCSF, for example, has pioneered a multisensory immersion pod called the SensSync. It combines VR/AR with high-fidelity acoustics and biometrics that sense and respond to a user's physiology in real time. It's an utterly amazing experience, like inhabiting a video game that your body and brain are scripting in front of you. Next steps for the project include integrating this kind of immersion with psychedelic therapies for a maximally transformative experience.

But as of this writing, the only version lives at the Four Seasons Hotel spa in

Oahu, and retail units are expected to launch north of a hundred thousand dollars. It's a cutting-edge innovation, but it's not going to solve our scale issues any faster than buying everyone tickets to Mars.

Or if you are seeking to explore the kind of deep brain-stem resets we've been discussing involving the induction of the vagal nerve or transient hypofrontality (where the conscious executive functioning part of your brain goes offline for a moment), you could get access to the PoNS device we discussed in Chapter 6, some of the newest "vagal pacemaker" implants, or possibly even transcranial magnetic stimulation. But each of these involve expensive, regulated technology, accessible only with formal medical oversight, and typically not covered by insurance.

If you read Michael Pollan's *How to Change Your Mind* and are intrigued by the transformational promise of Schedule I psychedelics, you can submit your name to a research study and hope to be included at some point—but there are tons of exclusionary criteria and it can take a while. Even though the FDA is fast-tracking expanded access for MDMA-assisted psychotherapy, broad availability and affordability are still complex issues that need to be resolved. And repeat use beyond the one to three sessions typically addressed in studies is another issue: the FDA trials aren't even testing for neurotoxicity and other safety issues because, under their rubric, the drug therapy is considered a "single-use intervention." Off-label clandestine use, while prevalent, does not seem to be delivering the same sorts of consistent positive effects (see Age of Aquarius and Rave culture).

If we're sticking to our original IDEO design commitments, and wanting to make sure that solutions remain open-source, scalable, and anti-fragile, then we are drawn back, again and again, to leveraging our innate survival circuitry—respiration, embodiment, and sexuality (music and substances can be seen as effect amplifiers of the first three).

Participant Summary

We accepted twelve couples who'd expressed interest in this research and who had enough stability and focus to successfully complete a three-month longitudinal study. Length of relationship ranged from two to thirty years. While we attempted to represent a variety of experiences and backgrounds, our first criterion was relational and emotional stability. Gender, religion, relational format, and ethnicity are better represented in this cohort than economic background, which tended to skew toward the WEIRD (western, educated, industrial, rich, and democratic).

The Uribe-Sanchezes. Heterosexual, forty-something unmarried couple in San Antonio, Texas, in stable fifteen-year relationship with two grade-school daughters. Both Mexican American. Catholic background. He: architect. She: immigration lawyer.

The Waley-Divines. Gay couple, unmarried. Live-in committed relationship of six years. Mid-forties and early fifties, respectively. Entrepreneurs in Boulder, Colorado. Puerto Rican and Irish ethnicity. Secular Jewish and Catholic background, "spiritual but not religious" (SBNR).

The McNeelys. Lesbian thirty-something couple. Married. Three-year relationship. Split time between Boston and Los Angeles, California. One partner is an MD, the other a former pro soccer player. SBNR.

The Trables. Heterosexual couple. Thirty-year marriage in Annapolis, Maryland. One son, one daughter, high school age. Both Caucasian. Nonreligious. He: insurance business owner. She: charter school administrator.

The DeMerwes. Heterosexual couple. Ten-year marriage in Austin. South African and American. One son, one daughter, both elementary school age. Atheists. He: business owner. She: commercial real estate broker.

The Daubes. Heterosexual couple. Twelve-year relationship in San Francisco. Secular Jewish Americans. Two sons, grade school age. He: finance executive. She: interior designer.

The Duboises. Heterosexual couple. Twenty-five-year marriage in Washington, D.C. Asian American and Caucasian. One son, one daughter, both college age. "Christmas and Easter" Methodist background. He: aerospace engineer. She: lawyer.

The Davises. Heterosexual couple. Five-year open relationship in Los Angeles. African American and Armenian. No children. Baptist background, SBNR. He: banker and crypto currency specialist. She: event producer.

The Comforts. Heterosexual couple. Ten-year marriage in Bozeman, Montana. No children. Caucasian. SBNR. He: digital marketer. She: real estate.

The Lins. Two-year open relationship (not primary spouse) in Atherton, California. Asian American and Jewish background. No children. SBNR. He: private equity. She: gallery owner.

Objective Metrics

We wanted to track what we were doing. If this protocol wasn't helping people experience more peak states, healing, and connection—it probably wasn't worth the time or risks. So we identified a pair of objective metrics for each of those three categories. To better facilitate comparative analysis, we chose measurement tools that cross-reference to other studies in the field. This is no small point. If the nascent discipline of Hedonic Engineering stands a chance of addressing the Meaning crisis, we need objective, open-source research that can build on itself. Otherwise we'll remain stuck in the realm of unverifiable truth claims. Hopefully other academic and citizen scientists can use these initial baselines to advance their work.

We also included subjective self-reporting in the study, which while technically "anecdotal" would likely capture the experiences of the participants and provide context and color for the objective measure. (A selection of these responses is included in the findings below.)

Ecstasis Measures

Johns Hopkins Mystical Experience Questionnaire (MEQ30, weekly/episodic): This is the thirty-question instrument we mentioned earlier that measures sense of the mystical, positive mood, transcendence of time and space, and ineffability.

Flow State Scale (FSS, weekly): This is a nine-question assessment determining the level of mastery, engagement, and reward someone experiences in daily life.

Communitas Measures

IOS relational closeness scale (weekly): Inclusion of Other in the Self (IOS) scale is a simple instrument where raters score how close they feel to another based on a seven-point scale from completely separate, to partially overlapping, to totally merged.

PANAS positive affect scale (weekly): ten questions measuring positive emotions based on a five-point Likert scoring. The instrument also has ten questions measuring negative affect, which we omitted from this study.

Catharsis Measures

PCL 5 Trauma score (pre/post): The PCL-5 is a twenty-item self-report measure that assesses the *DSM-5* symptoms of PTSD. It does not take the place of the clinician-administered CAPS trauma assessment in dedicated trauma studies but can serve as a helpful initial benchmark.

Resting HRV (via Oura) (daily): Heart Rate Variability measured overnight by the Oura Ring, a biometric wearable device. Heart Rate Variability is a marker of how balanced our sympathetic (fight/flight) and parasympathetic (rest/digest) bodily responses are.

Cortisol Waking Response (weekly): Urine-based sampling upon waking to determine cortisol levels as an indicator of rest, recovery, and activation levels and as a measure of balance of the hypothalamic-pituitary-adrenal (HPA) axis.

The Protocol

We established a baseline-suggested commitment for the twelve weeks of the project.

Daily: Fifteen minutes clitoral stimulation of the female partner (or comparable genital stimulation for gay couple). This practice was intended to create a neurochemical baseline of priming and to serve as a comparison to the existing research on this practice.

Fifteen minutes of partner yoga, Thai massage, and myofascial release (with an emphasis on soft-tissue structural integration using basic tools like rollers, balls, percussive therapy guns, etc.).

Morning monitoring of sleep data and overnight resting Heart Rate Variability.

Journal entries.

Twice weekly: Sixty-minute sessions of Hedonic Yoga—fifteen-minute clitoral stimulation. Thirty minutes of exploratory sexuality and body work (using the Rule of 9s practice—which is a structured sequence of deep and shallow thrusting combined with breathing and eye contact. Nine shallow thrusts followed by eight shallow thrusts, one deep thrust. Seven shallow thrusts two deep thrusts . . . until nine deep thrusts, and then return to beginning with nine shallow thrusts. This is harder to pull off than it is to read about, and few couples successfully get in more than two or three sets before losing track). Fifteen minutes of breath work/closed-eye recumbent meditation to curated musical soundtrack.

Once weekly: One-hundred-and-twenty-minute fully integrated Hedonic Yoga practice. Fifteen minutes of clitoral stimulation, followed by mutual body work, including traction of joints and palpation of soft tissues, "edging" (bringing a partner up to but not past the point of climax), intensive hyperventilatory breath work followed by gas-assisted static apnea. The "52.1 Method"—fifty hyperventilations, followed by two deep breath holds with 100 percent oxygen, followed by one inhalation of nitroxygen and maximum-static apnea combined with pleasure/pain optimization. Fifteen minutes of closed-eye recumbent Savasana meditation to music. Documentation of insights.

Once monthly: Three-to-four-hour deeper dive with full exploration of all above practices plus potential addition of more intensive visionary elements—extended breath work, prolonged sexual and sensory stimulation, longer-acting compounds. Ideally timed to coincide with week of ovulation for female partner(s).

Partners were encouraged to explore and experiment within the Hedonic Engineering Matrix, selecting from Mild, Medium, and Spicy options, with an encouragement to "start low and go slow." They were then free to add additional intensity and complexity only after comfortably integrating prior practices. This approach is the opposite of a conventional study, which seeks to rigidly control for variables. By imposing minimal scaffolding, we were trying to support individual and collective exploration and innovation within boundaries.

The Findings

An unexpectedly interesting finding was the self-organizing innovation that arose within the study cohort. Instead of sharing specific instructions, we dumped out a bunch of LEGO blocks (in the form of the Hedonic Engineering Matrix and default practice schedule), showed how they can snap together in different configurations, and left a few potential recipes around to inspire creativity. That was the "liberating structure" of this experiment.

Over the course of those three months, couples continued to modify and innovate the beginnings of what can perhaps best be described as a Sexual Yoga of Becoming.

While we were able to gather some meaningful data from this study, not everything went as planned. First, the human factor. Four participants (two couples, not included in list above) pulled out of the program within the first six weeks, nullifying their results.

Mr. and Ms. N: "We said yes to this study because . . . we hoped that maybe it would help change things up for us. It really hasn't helped. If anything, it made things worse. We've got enough on our plates as it is, this isn't our hill to die on." For them, the focus and intensity of the training wasn't a good match with their relational status, despite initially hoping it could be.

The other couple who stepped out had dependent/caregiver issues and did not feel they had the ability to fully participate while balancing those demands. This is a common challenge for many families, especially those in "the sandwich years" with aging parents and growing children. It's a factor to consider in any broader applications of this approach.

Three additional couples had to manage similar issues (family commitments and relational challenges) but were able to complete at least three-quarters of the program and were included in the analysis.

Two couples completed the program but subsequently separated. This highlights the limitations of a twelve-week intervention to save or fix longer-standing issues in place of more established interventions.

On the measurement side of the study, we had to scrub the Waking Cortisol test, as sampling, collection, and testing weren't consistent enough across the cohort to remain valid. This breakdown illustrates the tension common to many study designs. Measure too little, and you risk missing the golden insight. Measure too much, or too often, and you end up with subject fatigue and a breakdown in compliance across data sets.

Additionally, we had no way to validate accuracy of self-reporting and had to take participants at their word. Like many dietary studies, where subjects over- or undercount calories consumed outside clinical settings, we had to accept their data at face value.

While the objective metrics offered some encouraging insights on the ability of Hedonic Engineering to prompt inspiration, healing, and connection, some of the most interesting data to come back from the Kitchen Sink Study were the subjective reports. We include a few representative examples here after the metrics for each section (lightly edited for clarity and consistency).

Communitas Results

Since this was a couples study, it makes sense to begin with the Communitas measures. After three months of dedicated focus, did partners feel closer and more connected to each other?

On the PANAS Scale initial baselines, the group averaged 2.1/5 for their identification with ten subjective happiness scores. By the completion of the program, that score had moved to 3.3—an increase of 24 percentage points.

(We do not know how persistent that effect was, as we did not conduct any long-term follow-up assessment.)

On the IOS Scale, which measured how close or separated partners felt from each other, the pretest average was 3.8/7 (indicating "some overlap" of intimacy). This moved to a 5.6/7 (indicating "strong overlap" of individuation and intimacy), an overall raw score increase of 26 percent.

In general, people felt happier over the course of this study, and more connected in their relationship with each other. This is not particularly surprising, as focusing on a relationship for three months is likely going to be more intentional than the default settings of most lives. But there were serious challenges as well—as evidenced by those who abandoned the program, or ended their relationship subsequently.

Even for those who completed the study, the practices often surfaced uncomfortable emotional and relational content that participants weren't always well equipped to face.

Ms. Dubois: "As soon as we felt we had this totally dialed . . . we hit a brick wall. Old stuff, from way back in our relationship where I had a brief affair, while Mr. D had been drinking and working too much. All of that came roaring back and I honestly didn't know if we'd make it as a couple—never mind sticking with this study."

Conversely, a man found that his commitment to his partner increased.

Mr. Waley: "I have to admit it—I've always had a high sex drive and a wandering eye, and the thing that always terrified me about 'settling down' was all the fun and adventure I'd be missing out on if I did. But now that we've been exploring this together? . . . It's expanding my life, not limiting it. . . . I feel like I can commit with no regrets."

A woman noticed the difference between roommate/teammate dynamics with her spouse and the increased polarization they experienced over the program.

Ms. Uribe: "When we first met we were constantly physical and romantic together, but over the past few years of my firm getting hectic and our kids, we'd just settled into teammate roles. But just doing the daily practice did something crazy to our attraction. It was like electro-magnets that build up charge from spinning. . . . I thought those feelings were in the rearview mirror! I feel like I've been learning sex through love, and Mr. U has been learning love through sex."

At least in theory, this heightened sense of positive connection (communitas) would serve as a supportive foundation for any potential healing and integration that participants might accomplish. To confirm that, we needed to assess the markers of physical and emotional stress (i.e., catharsis results) to see if healing was happening.

Catharsis Results

The resting HRV scale tracks physiological stress markers, measured by the millisecond variation in heartbeat rhythm. Seventy-five percent of normal healthy users have scores ranging from 46 to 72 milliseconds. A higher score is generally considered healthier. The group baseline was 60 milliseconds, and their post-study average was 66 milliseconds, indicating an overall increase in the health of their autonomic nervous systems. Women experienced greater improvement in this metric, experiencing a 9-millisecond increase, compared to the men, who only gained 3 milliseconds.

This loosely matched the results from the PCL5 Trauma Scale. The initial benchmark scored women at 42/120 points, meaning they had experienced more trauma, while men scored 34, for a blended average of 38 points. This placed the group on the lower end of the "Moderate Level of PTSD" band. Post-testing indicated a general reduction in those scores to the lower range of Moderate with 32 points. Women still scored in the Moderate range with 36, while the men dipped below into the Mild/Sub Threshold Level with an average of 28 points.

One woman had an unexpected regression into a traumatic incident from her past that she was able to meet with the support of her partner.

Ms. Trable: "This didn't really start happening until we were into the second month and got a little more comfortable with the extended sessions with lots of stimulation and more intense breathing—but when we were making love and holding eye contact I saw Mr. T's face start shape shifting. . . . At first I was really scared, because it reminded me of flashbacks of when I was molested growing up, but when I breathed through it and trusted him, it turned into something really powerful. . . . But without the love and trust I have for my man—there's NO WAY I would've felt safe enough to explore that. It still scares me, tbh."

A man reported a meaningful neurological/respiratory release from an improvised somatic healing session.

Mr. Daube: "We tried that Vagal Protocol we've been discussing on the chat [a modification involving the male partner wearing the Aneros prostate device, along with throat massage and abdominal palpation], and something broke open in me. When Ms. D started to push on my lower belly I felt all this shame and vulnerability rush through my body. . . . I never realized how much self-loathing and fear of weakness I was hiding in a rigid stomach. But she kept pushing deeper and deeper—almost like her hand was gonna press into my spine. Then I couldn't take it anymore and took a huge sucking breath. I cried in big giant spasms, and my whole body started trembling and shaking uncontrollably. Afterwards I felt calmer and more grounded than I can remember."

Another woman innovated an interesting variation on MDMA PTSD therapy, but instead of MDMA she used other state-shifting tools to put herself in a supersaturated state to revisit and rework a past traumatic memory.

Ms. McNeely: "We kind of stumbled into something—magical role play, I guess? . . . I found myself doing the breath-hold/gas and going down what we've come to call the Cosmic Fuck Tunnel, I found myself flashing back to a sketchy, deeply regrettable one-night stand I had during pledge week in college. But instead of being that nineteen-year-old girl, I was me—now. A fully empowered Turned On Woman. I got to relive that night and rewrite the script. Turned On me was there, showing that young boy exactly how to meet me. Calling the shots. Not putting up with any of his shit. Feeling my pleasure. It was super empowering. It's not that the old memory of what 'really happened' is gone. It's more like it's dimmer now, and the new version is fresher and in color."

The relatively low initial trauma scores of the cohort make sense considering that selection criteria for the study did not focus on previously diagnosed symptoms or adverse incidents. The range, or variation from highest to lowest scores, was greatest on the PCL5 of all six metrics we tracked, reflecting the asymmetric impact or absence of trauma in subjects' lives.

Additionally, women scored higher initially and remained above the "subthreshold" level in follow-up testing, but they did record the strongest improvement in resting HRV. This would indicate a positive neurophysiological reset of some kind, and a lessening of residual stress in their bodies. Since the PCL5 is self-administered, we would likely need to clinically administer the more robust CAPS test to separate out people's subjective self-reporting from a more accurate diagnosis.

Ecstasis Results

In assessing the category of peak experience, we wanted to try to capture both micro and macro non-ordinary state experiences. We wanted to see if there was an increase in easefulness and autotelic functioning (known as a flow state), along with any more significant experiences of mystical states.

The nine-question short version of the Flow State Scale measures overall, non-task-specific experience of autonomy, mastery, absorption, and purpose. The pretest measured a 3.4/5 score (68 percent). The posttest scored 4.2/5 (84 percent), for a 16 percent boost in overall raw score. There were no significant gender differences. The baseline scoring tracks closely to what our organization has assessed with thousands of subjects. The final result is higher than what we have observed after completion of a six-week digital training, which is to be expected given both the increased duration and the physical embodiment of this twelve-week program. There is ample selection bias in both these results though, as people interested in taking a course on peak performance (or an hedonic engineering study) may have a greater proclivity for attaining these states, a conscious awareness of them, or both. But in general, participants did report a significantly higher incidence of timelessness, effortlessness, and selflessness through their weeks in the study.

The final score to consider is the Johns Hopkins Mystical Experience Questionnaire (MEQ30). Initial benchmarking of prior life experiences placed the men at a 2.5/5 in the "Slight" mystical experience category, while the women scored a 3.1/5, breaking into the "Moderate" category. Final results saw an overall average of 3.95, with a men's score of 3.8 and a women's of 4.1, elevating them into the "Strong" category of mystical experience.

One woman found that combining the sonic driving of music with coordinated movement, breath, and stimulation meaningfully boosted access to non-ordinary states. (We would hypothesize that this type of "neurosomatic discombobulation" might knock out executive functioning and Default Mode Network activity, leading to a visionary state, but we were not able to test this during this study.)

Ms. DeMerwe: "Okay. Maybe we were slow figuring this out? . . . We do the 15 min stroking prep, then do some body work together on the bed. Then we'd take turns edging each other (orally) while one partner relaxed and did the breath work. With [cannabis] edibles and nitroxy onboard, we found ourselves naturally synching our movements, breathing and touching to the pulse of the music. I know that sounds corny—'Make love to the music!'—but when we would do it—especially to that playlist the group's been sharing—we would come unstuck in time! It was the dreamiest, easiest way to unlock really visionary spaces—it felt like horizontal dancing!"

A man reported an intense visionary experience, combining a full selection of options from the Hedonic Engineering Matrix, including prescription compounds.

Mr. Davis: "Week Ten we finally dialed in what we called the Whole Enchilada . . . breath work, blending pleasure/pain, working with cannabis and nitrous, and dialing our space and music. Then we added in oxytocin and ketamine nasal spray. WOW! We ended up doing spontaneous yoga on our backs—pushing and pulling on our bodies and joints, doing backbends and massaging each other's bellies—it felt like getting in a month of yoga in an hour. By the time we actually got around to lovemaking it was super intense—but we also got . . . insights into our life—where our daughter was suffering in school, and even why we have the circle of close friends we do—it was like looking at our life through a crystal ball."

A few of the couples coordinated with their functional medicine doctors to develop some substantial innovations (their report is the first full expression of the Vital Respiration Protocol we outlined in Chapter 5, "Respiration").

Mr. and Ms. Comfort: "Week Ten. We figured we'd really go for it. So we got our doc to prescribe us Meduna's mixture [carbogen, a 70 percent oxygen/30 percent carbon dioxide blend], the nitrogen [70 percent nitrous oxide/30 percent oxygen], and the [oxytocin-ketamine] nasal spray. We did our regular warm-up, body work, scene setting—even added in the Vagal nerve stack too [anal plugs plus throat massage/traction]. . . . We did the breath prep and the carbogen just as the dark music came on loud (I had a blindfold on too). It was awful! . . . But Ms. C. just kept her hand on my heart and belly . . . I was lost in the underworld and barely remembered I had a body. But then we switched to the nitroxygen blend right as the music went celestial. I lost all track of time and space. I was just floating. Peaceful. Extreme tension followed by total release . . . I was looking down on my whole life, this whole human experience from another dimension. It felt super familiar too—like I'd always known this? . . . It felt like we'd just hacked some kind of timeless death/rebirth ritual. It's been four days, and I'm still trying to figure it all out."

Both genders reported meaningful increases in their mystical states, with almost as large a variation in range as the PCL5 data. Some users had profound level 5 breakthroughs, while others could be classified as close to level 1 or 2 nonresponders. While there were no consistent gender differences in the incidences of flow state among the cohort, when it came to stronger, potentially mystical experiences women pulled ahead. This was consistent with the clitoral stimulation study, as well as Padmasambhava's ancient assertion of women's capacity in this domain. The rate of overall increase and the final scores indicated a higher incidence of strong mystical experiences than many current psychedelic studies.

* * *

If we were to really try to put proof to a key thesis of the book, that we need to move as rapidly as possible to global-centric consciousness, then we would hope that boosting inspiration, healing, and connection would accelerate development to those higher stages.

To do that, we would need to have pre- and post-tested participants' stages of consciousness. Two of the most rigorous metrics come from Harvard—the Maturity Assessment Profile first developed by Jane Loevinger and then augmented by Susanne Cook-Greuter, and the Lectica assessment developed by Zak Stein and Theo Dawson. If it could be reliably established that hedonic engineering practices not only reduce trauma, boost mystical states, and heighten connection but also expand perspective and problem-solving, then we'd really be into meaningful territory. This validation awaits further study as it was beyond the scope of this pilot.

Participant Journal Reports

The following are excerpts (with original anonymized naming) from the weekly journal entries that participants kept over the course of the three-month experiment. All members were on their own recognizance to be exploring with the oversight of their own C^3 physician/therapists/clergy and to ensure that they were observing all applicable legal, moral, ethical, professional, and medical guidelines. They were also free to "adapt rather than adopt" and explore their own unique innovations within the boundaries of the experiment. (Lightly edited for clarity and consistency, grouped under categories of experience type. Some of these entries were partially excerpted in the prior summary.)

Initial Experiences with the Protocols

Ms. V: "At first, it felt awkward and kinda forced to have to schedule our sessions. We've always thought of ourselves as spontaneous—especially when it comes to our love life. But once we got over that, we started valuing the 'sexual fitness' time, knowing that it was going to be there no matter what—and with kids in the house, we definitely found it easier to squeeze in these smaller chunks of time together than if we'd been holding out for a full romantic date night."

Ms. O: "I found it really uncomfortable to be on the receiving end of the 'fifteen-minutes' practice. I realized that all of my life I've been so conditioned to be a pleaser that to just lie back and receive sensation, and not even have to stress about climaxing (or satisfying my partner), was incredibly difficult for me."

Ms. Y: "Once I got used to the routine (and I made sure to set up our space nicely and put my favorite music on my headphones), I found that I could get into some pretty dreamy spaces during our [daily fifteen-minute] sessions. Only time I've felt something similar was during long mountain runs or ninety-minute intense yoga—but this was much faster to get to same place."

Mr. Z: "To be honest, I wasn't looking forward to the daily practice much at all. Figured it was gonna be kind of boring to just sit there and 'twiddle my thumbs.' It was way harder than I'd expected. Paying attention and really learning to go slow and soft was, for me, a good challenge and it forced me to really tune into Z's signals, which I thought I had dialed, but realize I kinda didn't! I'd never realized how much I was wired for harder, faster ever since learning to masturbate as a teenager. This felt like I had to reprogram my entire arousal routine."

Mr. S: "When I first looked at the calendar for this study, my heart sank. We've really fallen off the horse as far as romance goes, and the idea that we had to make time to have sex three times a week seemed pretty excessive. I mean, who has time in their life for that? But a month into this, it's almost the opposite. We can't wait until our next session."

First Exposure to Peak States

Ms. Q: "First time we tried the deeper-dive weekly session, there was too much going on to really relax and experience it. It was like going to a tango class and all I could think of was getting the steps right. But the second and third weeks? OMG! When we finally got the breathing and edging together, along with the music? I found myself on another planet. I came back laughing and crying, it was so beautiful."

Mr. U: "At first, we set it up so I was in the 'driver's seat' for our weekend sessions. Figured I'd rock my lady's world. But then, when it came to my turn [with the gas-assisted breath hold], I dissolved into this place where I heard a voice say, 'So, this is where you've been sending your lover without any idea where she was going?' I felt like a total fool—like I'd been given a dunce cap and had to sit in the corner!"

Ms. T: "I didn't have what I would call my aha moment until now [week 5]. It was my turn to do the edging/breath work process, and when I held my breath and Mr. T stimulated me, right as the song kicked into another gear, everything went still, I felt like I'd slipped outside of time. I saw perfectly how I'd been afraid of my big creative project at work and how it all traced back to a spelling bee I choked at in grade school! It sounds crazy—but it made total sense—I'm still thinking about it."

Mr. Q: "Our weekly 'Sabbath' practice has turned into something pretty indescribable. It makes me think of that 'vomit comet' airplane that does those big roller-coaster loops in the sky and leaves everyone weightless, like they're in space. Doing the protocol and the vital respiration breath hold, it feels like we're taking turns lobbing each other into zero G—but for our minds. When I'm there, I can think anything I want, about anything I can think of, with a 300 IQ for five to ten minutes. It's like jacking into the mainframe of a cosmic computer!"

Relational Experience of Sustained Practice

A note from one of the couples who dropped out of the study:

Mr. O: "Sorry to say, don't think this study is for us. We gave it an honest start, but then things got pretty uncomfortable. I know this was supposed to enhance our intimacy, and we did try that—but that meant getting more intimate with some pretty major problems in our relationship (mostly unresolved sexual history stuff). We're gonna bow out, maybe try some couples therapy, but, to be honest, I'm not that hopeful. Not the right time or approach for us."

A note from a woman in a couple who dropped out:

Ms. N: "I said yes to this study because Mr. P was so excited by it and I guess I thought/hoped that maybe it would help change things up for us. It really hasn't helped. If anything, it made things worse. We can't even agree on how to do the 'daily fifteen' together. I get mad at his controlling, he gets mad at my nagging. Pretty soon, the mood is done, and we don't even want to talk to each other. We've got enough on our plates as it is, this isn't our hill to die on."

Ms. R: "When we first met, we were constantly physical and romantic together, but over the past few years of my business getting hectic and our kids, I didn't realize how much we'd just settled into teammate roles. We still cared for each other, obviously, but the spark had kinda fizzled. But just doing the daily practice did something crazy to our attraction. It was like electro-magnets that build up charge from spinning. We couldn't wait for our Tuesday/Thursday sessions, and by Sunday I couldn't think of anything else. I thought those kinds of feelings were in the rearview mirror!"

Ms. Z: "Our 'romantic hookups' still happen, but adding sexual fitness—something we commit to ahead of time and just do—I didn't know that was an option. Now I treat it like flossing my teeth or going for a run—we do it because we know we feel better having done it."

Mr. N: "I have to admit it—I've always had a high sex drive and a wandering eye, and the thing that always terrified me about 'settling down' was all the fun and adventure I'd be missing out on if I did. But now that we've been exploring this Hedonic Engineering together? It's not even in the same ballpark! I feel like I'd trade all the flirting and novelty in a heartbeat to keep going down this road together. It's expanding my life, not limiting it. For the first time in my life, I feel like I can commit with no regrets."

Ms. V: "At first I was a little irritated and self-conscious about the daily stuff. Then I relaxed and basically surrendered to it. It felt good, and my days seemed a little lighter. It wasn't until [this couple took a two-week hiatus due to a family event] and we stopped that I actually realized how much of a positive difference it had made. I guess I was like a frog in a hot tub! But those two weeks I felt more stressed, was snapping at Mr. V, and had a harder time falling asleep. Wasn't until we got back home and started practicing again that I felt that tension go down again. I'm getting used to this 'new normal'! Can't believe we were trying to make it through the grind without it before."

Mr. Y: "Since college, I'd pretty much settled into a familiar evening routine where I'd have a couple of beers and maybe a joint. It's been how I decompress from work and turn my brain off. Since we've been doing this practice, I've found myself wanting that less, and even saving up our 'state shifting' to do together on our weekend sessions. I'm like a boy scout now—six days a week;)."

Intimacy and Trauma

Ms. M: "Actually, we've kind of run into an issue that's pretty scary for us. I'm concerned this is becoming an addiction? At first I was pretty skeptical that anything out of the ordinary was gonna happen. We both had our fun in college and in our twenties—I figured this would be pretty tame in comparison. But once we started doing the daily and weekly stuff, especially combining with substances, it became something we started doing all the time—like Sunday practice every day. I'd joke that I was like Charlotte in *Sex and the City* [where she gets a Rabbit vibrator and her friends have to stage an intervention]. But now I'm seriously having to question priorities and whether this is 'too much of a good thing'?"

Ms. W: "Once we got the hang of things and kind of settled into a rhythm that worked for us (about weeks three to six) we started consistently getting 'there.' We were literally high-fiving and laughing on the bed some days. But as soon as we felt we had this totally dialed and couldn't miss getting to what we started calling 'the Yum,' we hit a brick wall. Old stuff, from way back in our relationship where I had a brief affair, while Mr. W had been drinking and working too much. All of that came roaring back and I honestly didn't know if we'd make it as a couple—never mind sticking with this study."

Later related entry by Ms. W:

"It was confusing to go from such high highs to low lows. If we hadn't had the other couples going through this, I'm not sure what would've happened. But we stuck with it and kept going with our practices. Some days it felt awful. We literally hated each other's guts! But we did it anyway. (That was a complete change for me, as I used to withdraw and withhold sex when I was pissed at him.) Then, all of a sudden, we were back in the Yum again! It felt like psycho-archeology—just burning through all the layers of our relationship."

The Ws hit two more rough patches over the course of the study.

"The second one was just as hard and confusing. I actually ended up spending a couple of nights away at a girlfriend's house, it got so bad. But by the third time, we could kind of remember the pattern, so it didn't knock us so far off track. One night we wrote a Post-it note: 'Remember—we did this ON PURPOSE!' and stuck it on the fridge. That saved us more than once! Now when we get to those rough patches, we know they're coming, and keep practicing through them. It's weird—you don't actually have to talk about all your problems all the time. At the end of a session we often feel better, and half of the stuff we were fighting about just doesn't seem that important anymore. (that doesn't mean we're out of the woods, it just means we're slowly learning some new ways to deal when things get sh*tty)."

Ms. X: "This didn't really start happening until we were into the second month and got a little more comfortable with the extended sessions with lots of stimulation and more intense breathing—but when we were making love and holding eye contact, I saw Mr. X's face start shape shifting—he flickered between a madman, a Viking, even an almost demon-looking dude, before coming back to himself. At first I was really scared, because it reminded me of flashbacks of when I was molested growing up, but when I breathed through it and trusted him, it turned into something really powerful. It was almost as if we weren't just me and him anymore—we were every man and every woman ever—like we weren't just doing our work, we were doing 'the work.' But without the love and trust I have for my man—there's NO WAY I would've felt safe enough to explore that. It still scares me, tbh."

Mr. Z: "I'm a pretty type-A alpha kind of guy, but this week we tried that Vagal Protocol we've been discussing on the chat [a modification involving the male partner wearing the Aneros prostate device, along with throat massage and abdominal palpation], and something broke open in me. When Mrs. Z started to push on my lower belly, I felt all this shame and vulnerability rush through my body—I flashed to my Army dad making me stand up straight with shoulders back and my gut sucked in. Same in high school and college locker rooms. I still catch myself looking sideways in the bathroom mirror to make sure I've still got a six pack. That whole time, I never realized how much self-loathing and fear of weakness I was hiding in a rigid stomach. But she kept pushing deeper and deeper—almost like her hand was gonna press into my spine. Then I couldn't take it anymore and took a huge sucking breath. I cried in big, giant spasms, and my whole body started trembling and shaking uncontrollably. Afterward, I felt calmer and more grounded than for as long as I can remember—I can actually feel my center now as I'm writing this."

Mr. X: "This is kind of awkward to write about. I was raised by liberal parents in NYC, a feminist mom, progressive schools, etc, and I always considered myself super-respectful of women. When Ms. X first wanted to explore more intense sensation play and pleasure/pain I was really conflicted. It was so against everything I thought a 'good guy' did, and there's literally no models for how to do this outside of porn, which seems not okay and not safe. Then our second month special night, Ms. X started to playfully tease me into whipping her—but she called me out on how confused I was. 'You're whipping me like a little boy who doesn't know what he's doing,' she said, 'and that makes me not trust you. Whip me like a strong man!' she said. 'Whip me like a dangerous man,' she said. 'Whip me like a good man!' she said. 'Whip me like a loving man!' Each time I tried to do what she'd asked. It was powerful to have her lead me like that, and really interesting to explore all of those different flavors. Her trusting me let me trust myself. We both realized violence and disrespect have nothing to do with exploring more intensive sensations. You can want the latter without ever having to put up with the former."

Deepest Dives—Innovations with the Protocols

Mr. S: "Week Ten we finally figured out what we called the 'whole enchilada.' We were pretty comfortable by that point with the breath work, blending pleasure/pain, working with cannabis and nitrous, and we had our space and music pretty locked. Then we added in oxytocin and ketamine nasal spray. WOW! We ended up doing spontaneous yoga on our backs—pushing and pulling on our bodies and joints, doing back bends and massaging each other's bellies—it felt like getting in a month of yoga in an hour. By the time we actually got around to lovemaking it was super sensual—but I also got a ton of insights into our life—where our daughter was maybe suffering in school more than she'd told us, and even why we have the circle of close friends we do—it was almost like looking at our life through a crystal ball."

Ms. U: "Coming into this third month has been fun, fun, fun! Also heavy. Every week seems to bring up something we need to work through. Sixty days of daily stimulation have left me feeling much more open, more playful, and more relaxed. I like this version of me better. On our weekend sessions especially we've been getting to some pretty amazing places, and last weekend something happened where we kind of stumbled into something—magical role play, I guess? I've never been into the whole 'sexy nurse/French maid' thing—always seemed objectifying and cheesy. But when I found myself doing the breath hold/gas and going down what we've come to call the Cosmic Fuck Tunnel (not mine, my partner said that one), I found myself flashing back to a sketchy, deeply regrettable one-night stand I had during pledge week in college. But instead of being that nineteen-year-old girl, I was me—now. My fully empowered turned-on woman. And I got to relive that night and rewrite the script. Turned-on me was there, showing that young boy exactly how to meet me. Calling the shots. Not putting up with any of his shit. Feeling my pleasure. It was super-empowering (and crazy hot;). It's not that the old memory of what 'really happened' is gone. It's more like it's dimmer now, and the new version is fresher and in color. It's almost like I can time-bend and go back and reclaim my past from my present."

Ms. Z: "This one's a little embarrassing, but the more we got into this whole 'sexual fitness' space and really committed to it, the more I gave myself permission to explore my own edges and desires. And something I've always been curious about was having two lovers at the same time. But that's so risky for a woman to admit! What are the odds of having a boyfriend/husband and then finding another trustworthy guy to explore that—and if I did really let go or like it, or not like it, then what would happen? Would I get slut-shamed if it ever got out? Would my husband ever look at me the same? Seemed too risky. Then [Ms. Q] shared on the chat about some of the toys they've been experimenting with, and I finally plucked up the courage to try it. Not the extra lover part—but the experience of making love to two men with just my man actually present and toys standing in. Holy Smokes! We played fancy dress-up, arranged the bedroom mirrors so we could see and be in the scene at the same time. I felt alive, in charge, and fully stimulated. It was like I unlocked some ancient temple priestess in me. Even dealing with the kids and lunches this morning, it all felt more doable—less crushing. Like I had a little secret I could come back to that only I knew. It was like I 80/20'd a threesome—80 percent of the fun and learning, and only 20 percent of the risk!"

Mrs. W: "Okay. Maybe we were slow figuring this out? But OMG it seems so simple now that we have! We do the fifteen-minute stroking prep, then do some acro yoga together on the bed [partner-balancing yoga practice that is often taught in conjunction with traction-based massage techniques]. Then we'd take turns edging each other (orally) while one partner relaxed and did the breath work. With [cannabis] edibles and the N_2O on board, we found ourselves naturally synching our movements, breathing and touching to the pulse of the music. I know that sounds corny, or obvious 'make love to the music!'—but when we would do it (especially to that playlist the group's been sharing), we would come unstuck in time! It was the dreamiest, easiest way to unlock really visionary spaces—it felt like horizontal dancing!"

Mr. Y: "Week ten. We figured we'd really go for it. So we got our doc to give us access to Meduna's Mixture [carbogen, a 70 percent oxygen/30 percent carbon dioxide blend], the nitrogen [70 percent nitrous oxide/30 percent oxygen], and the [oxytocin-ketamine] nasal spray. We did our regular warm-up, body work, scene setting—even added in the Vagal nerve stack, too [anal plugs plus throat massage/traction]. And we mixed up our music playlist, so we had some darker, heavier stuff in there, followed by more angelic tracks. We did the breath prep and the carbogen just as the dark music came on loud (I had a blindfold on, too). It was awful! I felt like I was dying, like one of those horror movies where you're buried alive. But Ms. Y just kept her hand on my heart and belly. The music was frightening and emotional—I was lost in the underworld and barely remembered I had a body. But then we switched to the nitroxygen blend right as the music went celestial. I'm not sure what did it—but I lost all track of time and space. I was just floating. Peaceful. Extreme tension followed by total release. Truly heavenly. I was looking down on my whole life, this whole human experience from another dimension. It felt super familiar too—like I'd always known this? But somehow was just remembering it again. It's been four days, and I'm still trying to figure it all out. It felt like we'd just hacked some kind of timeless death/rebirth ritual."

Index

About the Author

Jamie Wheal is the author of *Stealing Fire: How Silicon Valley, Navy SEALs, and Maverick Scientists Are Revolutionizing the Way We Live and Work* and the founder of the Flow Genome Project, an international organization dedicated to the research and training of human performance.

His work and ideas have been covered in *The New York Times, Financial Times, Wired, Entrepreneur, Harvard Business Review, Forbes, Inc.*, and TED. He has spoken at Stanford University, MIT, the Harvard Club, Imperial College, Singularity University, the U.S. Naval War College and Special Operations Command, Sandhurst Royal Military Academy, the Bohemian Club, and the United Nations.

He lives high in the Rocky Mountains in an off-grid cabin with his partner, Julie; two children, Lucas and Emma; and their golden retrievers, Aslan and Calliope. When not writing, he can be found mountain biking, kitesurfing, and backcountry skiing.

www.recapturetherapture.com
www.flowgenomeproject.com

ALSO BY JAMIE WHEAL

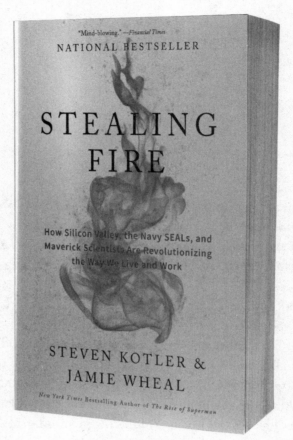

STEALING FIRE
HOW SILICON VALLEY, THE NAVY SEALS, AND MAVERICK SCIENTISTS
ARE REVOLUTIONIZING THE WAY WE LIVE AND WORK

National Bestseller • CNBC and Strategy + Business Best Business Book of the Year

Over the past decade, Silicon Valley executives like Eric Schmidt and Elon Musk, Special Operators like the Navy SEALs and the Green Berets, and maverick scientists like Sasha Shulgin and Amy Cuddy have turned everything we thought we knew about high performance upside down. Instead of grit, better habits, or 10,000 hours, these trailblazers are harnessing rare and controversial states of consciousness to solve critical challenges and outperform the competition. *Stealing Fire* is a provocative examination of what's actually possible; a guidebook for anyone who wants to radically upgrade their life.

ALSO AVAILABLE IN DIGITAL AUDIO